ISSUES & TRENDS IN
HEALTH

ISSUES & TRENDS IN
HEALTH

by
Rick J. Carlson, J.D.
and Brooke Newman

THE C. V. MOSBY COMPANY
ST. LOUIS • 1987

MOSBY

A TRADITION OF PUBLISHING EXCELLENCE

Design: Liz Fett

Editing and Production: Publication Services

For information contact The C. V. Mosby Company, 11830 Westline Industrial Drive, St. Louis, MO 63146.

Printed in the United States of America

Library of Congress Cataloging-in-Publication Date

Carlson, Rick. J.
  Issues & trends in health.

  Bibliography: p. 357
  1. Health.   2. Self-care, Health.   I. Newman, Brooke.   II. Title.   III. Title: Issues and trends in health.   [DNLM: 1. Health.   2. Health Promotion–– popular works.   WA 590 C284i]
RA776.C317   1987   613   87-26331
ISBN 0-8016-0958-5
PS/VH/VH   9   8   7   6   5   4   3   2   1   01/A/006

Rick J. Carlson, J.D.

Rick Carlson has worked as a consultant in the health policy, health futures, and health promotion fields since 1968. Currently, he is the President and Chief Executive Officer of the Primary Prevention Program and PHCard Systems, as well as president of The NewHealth Group, a consulting firm based in New York and Aspen, Colorado.

He has served as chairman of the California Governor's Council on Wellness and Physical Fitness, was the first director of the California Trend Report Project sponsored by the Naisbitt Group, and was invited to be a Visiting Fellow at the center for the Study of Democratic Institutions in Santa Barbara, California.

He also has organized, through the Rockefeller Foundation, the University of California Medical Schools, the Blue Cross Association of America and Institute of Medicine of the National Academy of Sciences, a series of major public policy conferences on issues related to medical care and the promotion of health. As a member of the Institute of Interdisciplinary Studies, he became one of the prime architects of the Health Maintenance Organization program, drafting legislations that initiated the HMO movement across the country.

Mr. Carlson has written several books on health and human services, including *The End of Medicine, The Dilemmas of Punishment, The Frontiers of Science and Medicine,* and *Medicine & Future Directions in Health Care*. He currently is writing a book entitled *New Health*.

Mr. Carlson received his Juris Doctor degree from the University of Minnesota in 1965.

Brooke Newman

Brooke Newman has worked as an editor, researcher, and freelance writer since 1966. She has written articles for magazines and newspapers, and has worked at Simon & Schuster and Time-Life Science Books. She was a contributing author of PLEASURES (by Lonnie Barbach) and worked with Leon Uris on JERUSALEM.

A 1966 graduate from Sarah Lawrence College, she went on to do graduate work in architecture at the School of Environmental Design, University of Colorado. Most importantly, however, she is the mother of four children and the wife of Rick J. Carlson. They live in Aspen, Colorado.

To Nikos, Samantha, Blue, and Joey, without whom this book would have been done a year earlier.

PREFACE

We are entering a new and interesting period in human evolution, especially in the more developed countries of the world, where we have become preoccupied not only with the control and treatment of disease, but also with the maintenance and enhancement of health. This was altogether to be expected from the success of measures for the control of disease, especially the infectious diseases and those resulting from poor nutrition, both types of which can be controlled by improvements in hygienic conditions and other basic requirements for health. The successes achieved by such means have been advanced further by the biomedical sciences and by greater attention to the avoidance of risk factors and to ways and means for avoiding the stress associated with the way of life that prevails in the twentieth century.

The growth in size of a population of older individuals and all that this implies, not to mention the liberation of youth and the possibility of making wider choices throughout life, creates a need for this guide for the perplexed which Brooke Newman and Rick Carlson have so ably put together. They and the contributors to this volume reflect a wide array of points of view and approaches for use by those who seek a source of information and guidance in their active, responsible participation in protecting, maintaining and enhancing their own health.

The day may come when it will be said that we are experiencing an epidemic of health to which this book has contributed.

by **JONAS SALK, M.D.**

CONTENTS

PART I   A FRAMEWORK FOR HEALTH

1 Rick J. Carlson, J.D.   The New Health Revolution, 2
2 Norman Cousins   A View of Health Promotion, 6

PART II   HEALTH EMPOWERMENT: YOURSELF

3 Tom Ferguson, M.D.   The Trend Toward Self-Responsibility, 10
4 Brendan O'Regan   Healing: Synergies of Mind, Body,
                                   and Spirit, 15
5 Steven E. Locke, M.D. and   The Healing Factor, 29
  Douglas Colligan
6 Daniel Goleman, Ph.D.   Meditation and Relaxation: An Overview
                                   of Their Applications, 38
7 Dennis T. Jaffe, Ph.D.   Biofeedback: Technology and
                                   Awareness, 41

PART III HEALTH EMPOWERMENT: YOUR ENVIRONMENT

8 S. Leonard Syme, Ph.D.   The Importance of the Social Environment
                                   for Health and Well-Being, 50
9 Leonard Duhl, M.D.   The Health of Cities, 58
10 Robert A. Aldrich, M.D.   Children and Youth in Cities: The Story
                                   of Seattle's Kidsplace, 63
11 Phillip Polakoff, M.D.   Occupational Diseases, 70
12 Lowell S. Levin, Ph.D.   Health Empowerment: An Approach to
                                   Community-Controlled Self-Care
                                   Development, 77

PART IV   STRESS AND STRESS MANAGEMENT

13 Ken Dychtwald, Ph.D.   Stress: What It Is and How It Affects You, 86
14 Dean Ornish, M.D.   Stress and Coronary Heart Disease–
                                   New Concepts, 93

15 Paul Rosch, M.D., F.A.C.P.   Stress and Organizations: Reducing
                                        the Stress of Community Life,   104
16 Dennis Jaffe, Ph.D. and   Burnout: Renewing the Spirit,   112
    Cynthia Scott, Ph.D.

PART V   NUTRITION AND DIET

17 Sheldon Margen, M.D.   What Is a Balanced Diet, Anyway?,   122
    and Michael Schwab
18 Kathryn Kolasa, Ph.D., R.D.   What Do You Need to Know About
                                        Some Dietary Supplements?,   135
19 Joan Dye Gussow, Ph.D.   Is Natural Better? And Other Questions
                                        About Health Foods,   152
20 James S. Turner, Esq.   Controlling the Chemical Feast: How
                                        To Survive the Expanding Crisis in Food
                                        Safety,   157
21 Anne M. Fletcher, M.S., R.D.   Diet, Nutrition, and Weight Control,   165

PART VI   EXERCISE

22 John W. Farquhar, M.D. and   The Relationship of Fitness To the Prevention
    Christine L. Farquhar, M.A.   of Disease and the Promotion
                                        of Health,   178
23 Ralph S. Paffenbarger, M.D.   Exercise and Reduced Risk of Coronary
    and Robert Hyde, M.A.   Heart Disease,   183
24 Joan Ullyot, M.D.   Which Sport Is for You?,   192

PART VII SPECIFIC HEALTH ISSUES

25 Edward M. Brecher   Caffeine, Cocaine, "Crack," Alcohol, Heroin,
                                        Marijuana, and Other Mind-Affecting
                                        Drugs,   200
26 Philip R. Lee, M.D. and   Patients and Pills: The Consumer's Role
    Helene Levens   in Assuring Safe and Effective Drug
    Lipton, Ph.D.   Use,   221
27 Clement Bezold, Ph.D.   The Future of Pharmaceuticals,   230
28 James F. Fries, M.D.   Can Health Promotion Enable People to Live
                                        Healthier Lives Into Later Life?,   236

29 Ralph Paffenbarger, M.D.   Exercise and the Aging Process,   242
and Robert Hyde, M.A.
30 Ruth G. Newman, Ph.D.   Some Myths and Realities About Aging,   254
31 Meredith Minkler, Ph.D.   Social Networks and Social Isolation
Among the Elderly,   259
32 Dale C. Garell, M.D.   Motivating the Adolescent: Special Needs
and Approaches,   266
33 James C. Gordon, M.D.   Crisis in Adolescence: An Unexpected
Opportunity for Growth,   276
34 Michael Lerner, Ph.D.   Varieties of Integral Cancer Therapies,   283
35 Tom Ferguson, M.D.   What You Should Know About
Smoking,   300

PART **VIII**   THE HOW-TO OF HEALTH CARE

36 American Hospital   Health Promotion: Your Hospital
Association (Elizabeth Lee)   and You,   308
37 Lori Andrews, J.D.   A Patient's Rights Primer,   316
38 David Sobel, M.D., M.P.H.   Medical Tests for Healthy People,   323
39 People's Medical   A Guide to Health Insurance,   330
Society (Charles Inlander)
40 Jonathan Fielding, M.D.   Health Risk Appraisals: A Consumer's
and Tracy Rodriquez   Guide,   347

PART **IX**   BIBLIOGRAPHY

41 Rochelle Perrine   Bibliography,   357
Schmalz, M.L.S. (Planetree)

PART I A FRAMEWORK FOR HEALTH

1 **The New Health Revolution**
Rick J. Carlson, J.D.

2 **A View of Health Promotion**
Norman Cousins

1 THE NEW HEALTH REVOLUTION

Rick J. Carlson, J.D. has worked as a consultant in the health policy, health futures, and health promotion fields since 1968. Currently, he is Special Adviser to the Primary Prevention Program and PHCard Systems, as well as president of The New Health Group, a consulting firm based in New York and Aspen, Colorado.

Mr. Carlson has written several books on health and human services, including *The End of Medicine, The Dilemmas of Punishment, The Frontiers of Science and Medicine, Medicine & Future Directions in Health Care* and, currently is writing a book entitled *New Health*.

Mr. Carlson received his Juris Doctor degree from the University of Minnesota in 1965.

This book has an uncompromising premise: the health field has changed so dramatically in the last 10 years that most of what we know about health and medicine today is obsolete and increasingly irrelevant.

A second premise is almost as crucial: much of what we are learning about health casts the individual as the central actor in the pursuit of health (though not so much as "holistic" medicine purists and "wellness" faddists might think). Hence, unlike more traditional times when everyone depended upon the family doctor for guidance, what the individual knows today is far more important and far more likely to lead to a healthy life.

Essentially the health field is undergoing a radical shift that will affect medical practice and research. Individuals will be profoundly affected in the ways they seek better health care, as will the health institutions. This shift will have far-reaching effects on the American economy, too, touching the individual, the neighborhood, the community, and larger institutions, including government. Finally, this shift will affect many of our social interactions as people live longer, treat disease more effectively, and respond to new health practices.

Remember back a dozen years ago. What kinds of questions were you asking about health? How important was your health? What kinds of health problems faced you, your family, and your friends? What were you doing about them?

What was your hospital like? What types of services and programs did it offer? Did you have health insurance? Was the cost of medical care an issue?

What problems did you solve on your own without a physician? Did you believe everything your family doctor told you? What about this "holistic health" stuff? Had you heard about health promotion and wellness? Had you heard the term *immune system*?

You probably didn't ask any of these questions in 1975. Few people really cared enough then to formulate such questions, much less to find the answers. But do you care now? If you do, what has happened in the last 12 years to make you care? Have any of the following occurrences since 1975 affected your personal health practices?

- The National Cancer Institute has published reports and sponsored conferences on the relationships between diet and nutrition both in preventing and treating cancer.
- The National Institute on Heart, Lung, and Blood Disease published new guidelines in 1984 for the treatment and prevention of hypertension which encourage nonpharmacological approaches, emphasizing physical fitness, nutrition, and stress control.
- The holistic health revolution emerged, flowered, then disappeared, as much from indifference as suppression, *because* it served its purpose in stating the obvious and in reminding many practitioners of truisms they were neglecting.
- The Institute for the Advancement of Health was founded in 1983 with a prestigious board and the mission to "further the scientific understanding of how mind-body interactions affect health and disease."

Since 1975, the health promotion movement has become a decided reality, with community programs emerging daily and with more employers developing or expanding employee programs at the worksite. "Wellness" programs abound, particularly in hospitals, and behavioral medicine programs flourish as mind-body links in health and disease are explored. New "prevention" centers have appeared, most prominently at the Pasteur Institute in Paris.

Consumers are changing longstanding habits in response to new health information (see the Gallup Poll results in *American Health*, March, 1985) and the self-help industry, which exceeded $17 billion in sales in 1983, is rapidly approaching the $30 billion mark. Health food restaurant franchises are opening throughout the United States, and the hottest new field in biomedical research is psychoneuroimmunology, which purportedly studies the relationship between emotional, psychological, and neurological states, and the body's immune system and capacity.

Investor-owned health care companies and HMOs are growing to the point where some have become prime candidates for corporate takeover. Hospitals have been merging, and offering new services, including birthing centers, women's health programs, sports medicine programs, "urgi-care" and "surgi-care" facilities, and health promotion and fitness programs. Holding companies are springing up to permit diverse corporate initiatives in the name of health.

These are fairly impressive events. I doubt that anyone could have forecast more than a few of these events in 1975. In fact, whenever I am asked, "What are the new ideas coming along in the health field?" I reply, "What more do you want?"

The growth rate in the health care industry over the last 12 years has been unprecedented and is largely due to a fundamental change in the way people think about their health. Bernie Tresnowski, president of the Blue Cross and Blue Shield Association in 1985, was asked by *The Wall Street Journal* why people were spending less time in hospitals. He replied "The movement [of consumers] out of hospitals and into new places and forms will continue. . . . The underlying reason it will happen is that this is what people want." (February 27, 1985)

In 1975 I wrote *The End of Medicine*, a book that launched a debate that continues today about the role of medical care. Ten years ago health was considered the consequence of good medical care. Today, as important as medicine can sometimes be, we know that health is far more than good medicine.

In *The End of Medicine*, I suggested that radical, even revolutionary, change would occur in the near future. The changes that are occurring today are the result (as are all truly profound changes) of shifts in the way we perceive things, of deep conceptual change. In 1975, some of these new ideas about health had just begun to crystallize. We had begun to think, if not necessarily to act, holistically about our health. We had begun to recognize (or more accurately, to remember) the critical role of the individual and of the capacities of the mind, attitude, and emotions. We began to see that medicine that treated only the physical symptoms of a patient whose illness resulted from stress, was medicine that in far too many cases could only palliate that illness. Only then did we begin to see that such medicine was a very costly enterprise, given the limited recovery it could produce.

Today we are in the midst of a revolution launched by changing ideas and articulated at the level of institutional change. The health care system is fiercely competitive. Hospitals are merging with national firms. Insurance companies are offering health care, and hospitals and clinics are offering insurance plans.

Changes in medical care are the result of changing attitudes and values—not mergers, acquisitions, and hot new marketing schemes. Most of what's happening at the organizational level in health care is the result of turf wars, "my organization is bigger than your organization," the adult male's equivalent of adolescent locker-room comparisons.

And yet, what are the consequences of these changing values and attitudes? What real difference will it make to the person interested in his or her health in 1995? If the "health seeker" in 1975 had known what was in store in the next decade, what an exciting set of opportunities could have been anticipated. Even on a more pragmatic lev-

el, what if the health-conscious investor in 1975 had had a few bucks to invest in a small company proposing to film Jane Fonda doing aerobic exercises?

The changes yet to come in the health field are much more dramatic than those occurring in the last 12 years, as truly revolutionary as those changes were. We have just barely begun to learn the new ways of health. As we continue our passage away from the highly mechanistic views that shaped our modern medical system, we will enter very new and different terrain.

Take Care was recently opened in Seattle by Group Health Cooperative of Puget Sound, one of the oldest and largest HMOs in the country. Group Health realized that with all the interest in self-care, a retail health store in a commercial shopping area might work—and it has. In the first 6 months of operation, Take Care revenues were way ahead of projections and might even be higher if the medical staff at Group Health allowed the store's management to sell vitamins and minerals, always a staple of consumer self-health wants. With the success of the first outlet, Group Health is already planning two more stores in Seattle, and has firm plans to franchise Take Care across the country.

As another example, theories about nutrition have changed dramatically in the 1980s. In the 1970s, any suggestion that nutrition had any connection with the onset or treatment of cancer would have been met with incredulity or, more likely, derision. But in June 1985, the American Cancer Society placed an ad in *American Health* magazine entitled "A Defense Against Cancer Can be Cooked up in Your Kitchen." The ad advised readers that a diet high in fiber, rich in vitamins A and C, and low in nitrites, salt-cured foods, and animal fats would help prevent cancer of the colon.

This book covers a spectrum of change. But there is one clear constant: In virtually every instance, the issues and topics addressed by contemporary commentators places the individual at the center of the health scene. Governments, communities, groups, health care providers, and (increasingly) employers do play very important roles. And undeniably, for some individuals, their responsibilities for their health are of less importance at given times—indeed, for the very poor and dependent, obtaining a decent livelihood is the central health issue, and any talk of personal responsibility for health is unrealistic at best and small and mean in any event.

Still, for the majority of us, the choices we make and the lives we choose to lead will determine our health. And this is the realization that is at the core of the New Health Revolution.

2 A VIEW OF HEALTH PROMOTION

Norman Cousins has written 16 books, including *Anatomy of an Illness, Human Options,* and *The Healing Heart.* For more than 25 years he was editor of *Saturday Review.* He is currently on the medical faculty of UCLA.

People are not machines. Neither are physicians mechanics. The interaction between patient and physician begins with confidence and respect—confidence by the patient in the physician and respect by the physician for the imponderables that can represent a vital fraction in any equation of treatment and recovery.

In his final piece for *The New England Journal of Medicine,* editor Franz Ingelfinger wrote: "If we assume that physicians do make patients feel better most of the time, it is chiefly because the physician can reassure the patient or give medication that is mildly palliative."

In a sense, every patient-physician relationship is a psychosocial venture. It is as erroneous to deny or disparage a role for attitudes in healing as it is to contend that they are an alternative to competent medical attention. Just learning about the fact of severe illness can sometimes create feelings of helplessness, hopelessness, anxiety, and panic, with well-known physiological penalties. The wise physician recognizes the need to provide emotional support for the environment of treatment. The physician cannot guarantee that his approaches will work, but what is of greatest concern to the patient is that everything possible is being done on his behalf.

It would be absurd to say that patients should not be given the best that medical science has to offer in view of the possibility that patients may feel angry or deceived if medical treatment hasn't worked. For the same reason, psychological bolstering should not be withheld out of fear that patients may react adversely if the downward course of the disease is not halted. In any case, medical science and psychological support go hand in hand. Guilt feelings are far more likely to occur when things that should have been done are not done. It is commonsensical to believe that most patients have a better attitude when they have a partnership with their physicians than when they feel sidelined and helpless.

Paying attention to a patient's emotional needs and to the quality of life; helping the patient to mobilize his inner resources when confronting a difficult challenge; creating an environment in which the physician can do his best; relieving feelings of panic and helplessness; being mindful of the needs of family and friends—all these come under the heading of psychosocial and psychological factors.

In the course of my assignment to lecture to students at the UCLA School of Medicine on the "medical humanities," the sessions producing the most intense discussions concerned patient-physician relationships. Resource materials for such discussions were far from skimpy and included such teachers and philosophers of medicine as Montaigne, Sir William Osler, Oliver Wendell Holmes, Francis W. Peabody, Lawrence J. Henderson, Walton Hamilton, Hans Zinsser, William Carlos Williams, Richard Selzer, and Walter Cannon. One thing in particular, however, troubled me about the exchanges as they progressed. The discussions were lively enough, but it became apparent that many of the students tended to regard the entire area of patient-physician relationships as soft. They seemed reluctant to attach appropriate importance to the physician's communication skills, to medical ethics, or to the circumstances of a patient's life. Certainly they were justified in regarding as primary the measurable information yielded by diagnostic technology or textbook approaches to treatment, but it was also important to consider the factors that affected patient cooperation and confidence. Even if we couldn't readily quantify compassion or communication skills, was it at least possible to gain increased respect for these aspects of medical practice? Why shouldn't a broad cultural background be regarded as essential in the practice of medicine?

I brooded over these questions, then I realized I needed additional evidence, if only of a suggestive nature. Accordingly, I undertook a mailbox survey in the Westwood, California, area on the general subject of patient-physician relationships. We distributed about 1000 questionnaires not far from the UCLA campus.

The questionnaire was accompanied by a letter stating its purpose—namely, to stimulate discussion among medical students about the way patients select and appraise their doctors. Participants were asked to give their answers or opinions to three questions: Had they changed their physicians in the past five years, or were they considering changing now? Why had they changed or why were they thinking of changing now? Did they have any suggestions to make about the education of medical students?

Altogether 563 responses were received—an unusually high figure, we were told by polling experts, considering that the questions called for written answers and the respondents had to supply their own postage and address their own envelopes.

We turned the responses over to the department at UCLA that, with the aid of computers, tabulated such materials. In due course, we received a survey report.

In presenting the report to the students, I was careful to emphasize the curbstone and informal nature of the survey, underlining the fact that it was in no way to be regarded as scientifically constructed or statistically significant. It was undertaken mostly for the purpose of supplying us with rough clues about patient's attitudes. Certainly, the base was much too confined for the survey to be considered remotely representative of patients as a whole. It was made clear to the students that the replies came from a single neighborhood that was up-scale in education, professional status, and income (a fact that seemed to impress some students who intended to go into practice).

The most striking fact emerging from the survey was that 85% of the respondents either had changed physicians in the past 5 years or were thinking of changing for reasons other than relocation, the physician's retirement or death, and so forth.

Only 25% of those who had changed physicians cited incompetence on the part of the physician as the reason for doing so. It was clear that competence was taken for granted. A medical diploma and an ability to meet other requirements appeared to offer adequate assurance of capability. Why, then, did they change physicians? The bulk of the respondents changed for a wide variety of reasons having to do with the style or personality of the physician, including poor communication skills, office atmosphere of clutter or disorganization, inability to reassure the patient,

and personal habits or characteristics (e.g., smoking, obesity, or lack of cleanliness).

In presenting the results of this survey to medical students, I reminded them that within the next decade the United States will have a surplus of 40,000 to 50,000 doctors. Laws of supply and demand will create an increasing respect for approaches and values now described as "soft." The net effect of the survey is that I now have little difficulty in gaining serious attention for the wide array of factors that go into a strategy of treatment. And, now that psychoneuroimmunology is attracting increased attention in academic circles, a far more auspicious environment exists than before for discussing the factors surrounding illness and medical practice. The question is not now—anymore than it has been—whether physicians should attach less importance to their scientific training than to their relationships with patients, but rather whether enough importance is being attached to all the factors involved in effective patient care.

PART II HEALTH EMPOWERMENT: YOURSELF

3 The Trend Toward Self-Responsibility
Tom Ferguson, M.D.

4 Healing: Synergies of Mind, Body, and Spirit
Brendan O'Regan

5 The Healing Factor
Steven Locke, M.D., and Douglas Colligan

6 Meditation and Relaxation: an Overview of Their Applications
Daniel Goleman, Ph.D.

7 Biofeedback: Technology and Awareness
Dennis T. Jaffe, Ph.D.

3 THE TREND TOWARD SELF-RESPONSIBILITY

Tom Ferguson, M.D. received his medical degree from the Yale University School of Medicine. While still a medical student he wrote a doctoral dissertation on the role of self-care in American medicine, taught a self-care class for first-graders, and founded the journal *Medical Self-Care*. *Medical Self-Care* has now grown from a student project to a respected and influential national bimonthly. The *Wilson Library Bulletin* recently named it the nation's outstanding health magazine. He is the medical editor of the *Whole Earth Catalog*, and is a contributing editor of *Prevention*. He is a regular contributor to *American Health*.

His books include *Medical Self-Care: Access to Health Tools, The People's Book of Medical Tests* (with David Sobel, M.D.), and *The Smoker's Book of Health*. He has received the National Educational Press Association's *Distinguished Achievement Award* and the *Lifetime Extension Award* for his writings "on the rapidly expanding area of self-help." His work has been cited by author John Naisbitt in his book *Megatrends* as representing "the essence of the shift from institutional help to self-help."

He lives in Austin, Texas with his wife and daughter, and writes and speaks widely on self-care and the future of health.

In the past decade we have become a health-conscious society. We are increasingly better informed about health issues, more capable of maintaining our own health, and more discriminating when choosing professional health care providers. Dr. Tom Ferguson outlines four key trends in our society that he sees as resulting from a health care revolution of major proportions: the shift from professional care to self-care; increased options in medications and treatment; decreased hospitalization in favor of home care; and increased availability of health information.∎

It's easy to forget that as recently as the mid-1970s people who exercised regularly, ate whole wheat bread, and preferred bottled water to mixed drinks were considered "health nuts."

There are a lot of health nuts around these days. The young and early-middle-aged adults among them are now called yuppies or baby boomers, but the new health consciousness is affecting people of every age.

It is now commonplace, in visiting a business office, to find a little clump of smokers huddled outside the door, furtively puffing away. One can put in an evening's serious party hopping and never be offered anything stronger than lite beer. It is possible, in some circles, to go for weeks without seeing a single chunk of red meat or a slice of white bread. Vitamin sales are at an all-time high.

This growing trend toward self-care is not limited to the healthy. Those with health problems are also taking a greater degree of responsibility. Health consumers in increasing numbers are requesting more second opinions, demanding clear explanations, and reserving final decisions about diagnosis and treatment for themselves. In many cases they are choosing to consult alternative practitioners or, with or without the support of their health professionals, they are developing their own methods of dealing with their problems.

Such changes have already begun to affect the use of professional health care. People who practice self-care use fewer professional services. A University of Chicago study found that self-caring persons spent 26% less on hospital bills and 19% less on physicians' services.

A HEALTH CARE REVOLUTION

Although these and similar changes have taken place gradually, it is not difficult, looking back, to see that we are roughly a decade into a health revolution of major proportions, a revolution that has already produced profound and lasting changes. This trend toward increasing self-responsibility in health shows every sign of continuing.

The self-care health market has become one of the fastest growing parts of our economy. Americans by the millions are investing in stationary bicycles, weight machines, and other exercise equipment. At the same time they are turning away from liquor, cigarettes, and high-fat foods. Firms that provide self-care goods and services are, on the whole, doing extremely well, while manufacturers who have fallen victim to the new health consciousness are being forced to take desperate measures. A recent Bacardi rum ad proudly expounds the fact that a rum and orange juice contains *less* alcohol than a glass of white wine. Hiram Walker recently introduced a line of low-alcohol Häagen-Dazs cream drinks. Seagram is testing a no-alcohol wine.

The tobacco industry has been hit hardest of all. Since the first Surgeon General's report on smoking in 1964, per capita smoking has plummeted 39%. The proportion of Americans who smoke is at its lowest point in decades—and is still falling. Even the president of the Reynolds Tobacco Company now admits that in the long run—it may take a century or two—the smoking custom will probably die out altogether.

We are buying more self-care books. Between 1977 and 1981, estimated sales of health-related books increased by over 1,100%. We are reading more health magazines: Between 1970 and 1980, sales of special interest health magazines more than doubled. We are buying more at-home diagnostic tests: Between 1984 and 1990 the sales of the top three at-home diagnostic tests are expected to grow by nearly 300%.

ESTIMATED SALES OF AT-HOME MEDICAL TESTS
(Figures are in millions of dollars)

Test	1984	1990
Blood sugar monitoring	$177	493
Blood sugar monitors	65	211
Colon cancer screening	40	130
Total	$282	$834

THE NEW HEALTH CARE SYSTEM

One could go on and on citing similar figures, but it might be more interesting to break off at this point and ask exactly what this all implies? Is there a pattern behind these many changes in the way we think and act about health? I believe that there is. When medical historians look back at the last quarter of the 20th century, I believe that they will see it as a period in which we moved from an *old* health care system built around the doctor, the hospital, and the clinic to a *new* health care system built around the individual, the family, and the home.

Structuring a health care system around the individual might seem a contradiction in terms. Isn't health care, after all, what doctors and nurses do? Under the old model, yes, but not under the new model. If health care is the process of keeping oneself—or someone else—as healthy as possible and managing health problems when they occur, then it is clear that the great majority of health care is now and always has been self-care.

I've found it useful to think of health care as a stool with four legs: tools, skills, information, and support. Let's suppose one has a sliver in one's foot. Many of us, provided with a good pair of tweezers, a good light, and a clean needle, could probably take it out. We might have trouble, however, if we lacked light, tweezers, or needles (tools), the required hand–eye coordination (skill), if we did not understand the proper way to go about it (information), or if we had been advised that one should not do such a thing (support).

THE OLD SYSTEM

In the old physician-centered health care system, the assumption was that the tools, skills, information, and support were to be placed at the disposal of the physician. Tools included such things as scalpels, operating suites, electrocardiographs, penicillin tablets, and cortisone injections. Skills included things like taking a throat culture, performing a physical exam, or doing brain surgery. Information was to be found in medical journals and textbooks and at medical meetings. Support services were provided by hospitals, laboratories, nurses, and the doctors' office staff.

But if we employ the assumptions of the new health care system centered around self-care, we see things a little differently. Tools will include devices to promote wellness—running shoes, exercise bikes, relaxation tapes, workout

videotapes, etc.—and devices used to detect, manage, and treat disease—blood pressure cuffs, otoscopes, prescription and over-the-counter drugs, and a growing number of at-home laboratory tests to detect such things as pregnancy, blood in the stool, or time of ovulation.

Medical skills now passing into the lay domain include taking a throat culture, taking of blood pressure, and prescribing the best over-the-counter drug for oneself.

Information includes knowledge of preventive measures (nutrition, exercise, stress reduction), disease management (arthritis, cancer, high blood pressure), and medical consumerism (making decisions about surgery, drugs, and medical tests, and checking up on your own medical care).

Support consists of educational programs, self-help groups, medical consumer organizations, and health workers who encourage and support self-care. In the case of home health care, support also includes respite and services for those caring for a family member with a chronic illness.

A number of current historical trends—many of them identified by John Naisbitt in his book *Megatrends*—underlie the sweeping change toward self-responsibility in health. The four trends described below are among the most important.

TREND ONE: THE SHIFT FROM PROFESSIONAL CARE TO SELF-CARE

In medicine as in other economic areas, laypeople are now doing an end run around professionals, using new institutions, new technologies, and new methods of communication to deal with problems directly rather than relying on professionals. This shift is occurring in all economic sectors.

Ten years ago, if you had a sum of money to invest, you probably put it in the bank. The bank would invest your money, pay you a fixed rate of interest, and pocket the difference. Today we are much more likely to invest that money ourselves in a money market account, a mutual fund, a certificate of deposit, or elsewhere. We have realized that bankers do not have a monopoly on investing.

In the same way, we have realized that doctors do not have a monopoly on health. Under the old system, consumers were encouraged to believe that doctors could "fix" virtually any health problem. Under the new system, we know that there is frequently little the doctor can do, but that if we take reasonably good care of ourselves, we will rarely need a doctor. It is an irony of medical history that as a result of the current medical malpractice crisis, the American Medical Association is now waging a public relations campaign to convince consumers not to expect too much of physicians.

TREND TWO: FROM "ONE ILL, ONE PILL" TO MULTIPLE OPTION

Forty years ago, most things were done in a pretty standard way. When there *was* a choice, it was usually of the either/or variety: Dad went to work. Mom stayed at home and had 2.4 kids. You either got married or you didn't. You drove a Ford or a Chevy. When you ordered ice cream you could have either vanilla or chocolate. All bathtubs were white. All telephones were black. That was the way it was.

It was much the same in health care. You went to the doctor, gave a history, and described your symptoms. The doctor would ask some questions, thump you a time or two, perhaps order a few lab tests. Then out came the little white pad and you received a prescription.

That's not the way it works any more. Consumers can now choose from multiple options—Naisbitt calls this today's "Baskin-Robbins society," where everything comes in at least 31 flavors. Today the new car buyer may choose from among more than 750 different models. There's a store in New York that sells 2,500 different types of light bulbs. There are currently 207 different brands of cigarettes.

There are more choices in health care as well. Most conditions can be treated in a variety of ways. If a pill is required, there frequently are a number of choices among different drugs in different dosages. Consumers now expect to be able to consider several alternatives and to choose the one that seems best to them. This may mean choosing between several possible drugs or taking no drug at all. It may mean visiting another doc-

tor, seeking a second opinion, or asking advice from any one of a growing number of alternative practitioners. Or it may mean using exercise, nutrition, relaxation, visualization, psychological approaches, or other nonspecific pro-health measures to help deal with the problem.

TREND THREE: THE HOME AS HEALTH CENTER

According to home health care industry sources, roughly 25% to 30% of patients now in hospitals don't really need to be there. They could be cared for just as safely and much more economically at home. Millions of patients have already avoided needless hospitalization, making home health care the most rapidly growing part of the health care system.

The rapid growth of home care is partly the result of new at-home versions of tools previously available only in the hospital (e.g., the equipment needed to perform kidney dialysis, parenteral feeding, and cancer chemotherapy), the explosive growth of at-home medical testing (e.g., blood pressure, blood sugar, portable EKG monitors) and the emergence of home health professionals who work principally in patients' homes (e.g., nurses, pharmacists, physical therapists, and rehabilitation therapists).

The home has always been the center of wellness activities. New at-home devices (e.g., exercise machines, exercise videos, relaxation tapes, pulse meters, home whirlpool baths, stationary swimming devices, and computer-based nutrition support systems) now make it possible for the health-active individual to do things at home that formerly could be accomplished only at a well-equipped health club.

TREND FOUR: HEALTH CARE AS INFORMATION FLOW

In some ways, the health information explosion has been the most dramatic of all. In 1977, self-care books accounted for only 3% of total nonfiction bestseller hardcover sales. Only four years later this figure had increased to 23%—a 1200% increase in total sales.

Health coverage in periodicals has experienced a similar growth. Circulations of special interest health magazines more than doubled between 1970 and 1980. There has been an explosion of health information in general publications as well. Three of the nation's most widely read weekly publications—*Time, Newsweek,* and the Sunday *New York Times*—have recently instituted special health sections or editions. The future offers electronic access to elaborate new health databanks accessible by home computer.

SELF-CARE AND THE FUTURE OF HEALTH

But a continuing trend toward self-responsibility will not in itself be enough to ensure the full flowering of a health care system built around the individual and the family. If the four legs of health care are indeed *tools, skills, information,* and *support,* and if the tools and the information available to future generations will outstrip the imagination of even the most wild-eyed self-care advocate, then the remaining potential bottlenecks to the development of self-care will be the lack of individual health skills and the lack of professional support for self-care.

Thus we are left with two pressing issues of public policy:

- **Health literacy** The health education currently offered in our schools does little to equip our children to deal with today's health realities—let alone those of the future. I believe it will take a commitment to health literacy comparable to this nation's earlier commitment to literacy in English to prepare our children to use these new medical devices and to understand the broad range of health information that will be available to them.

- **Professional support for self-care** Students aspiring to the health professions should be selected for their aptitude to encourage self-responsibility and to support responsible self-care. All clinicians should be competent in the skills of communications, negotiation, and interpersonal relations. Clinicians in practice should be evaluated regularly by the consumers they serve, and these evaluations should be given considerable weight in determining salary and advancement.

4 HEALING: SYNERGIES OF MIND, BODY, AND SPIRIT

Brendan O'Regan is Vice-President for Research for the Institute of Noetic Sciences.

Brendan O'Regan has always had the imagination to catch the significance of new ideas that most people would have a hard time classifying, much less understanding. And it is usually the case that whatever new theory Brendan decides to explore eventually will become an accepted topic of research in the health field. Brendan was interested in synergies of mind and body long before anyone else could see even a tangential relationship to human health. And although much of what Brendan addresses in this article is now being explored in legitimate research circles, some of it is still best viewed as a glimpse into the future.▪

In the past 5 to 10 years, some dramatic shifts have occurred in the cultural understanding of the mind/body relationship— although the pendulum may be about to swing back toward a "new conservatism." On the one hand, mainstream popular publications like *Time, Fortune, The New York Times*, and *The Wall Street Journal* have reported favorably on developments in the field of so-called holistic or alternative practices. For example, a cover story in *Time* in 1983 discussed the work of Carl and Stephanie Simonton, whose early work using imagery and psychotherapy techniques with cancer patients was described as follows:

"Bizarre as it seems, the technique has helped significant numbers of terminally ill patients survive beyond all expectations," says psychiatrist Sanford Cohen of Boston University. "How they do it, we do not know."

Statements like this reflect the fact that many practitioners have observed firsthand the positive impact that techniques such as guided imagery, relaxation, and meditation can have on the quality of life of seriously ill patients. Curiously, it also reminds us that proponents of the prevailing view in science and medicine find it easy to accept negative, "psychosomatic," or stressful linkages between mind and body, and hard to accept positive, healing, or disease-altering linkages between psychological and physiological processes. What seems to be the root of this problem is the fact that until recently we have had no sense of what the mediating pathways linking mental and physiological events might be. The worlds of psychology and neurology are only beginning to link up regarding the complex phenomena of higher order cognitive function, human emotions, and personal beliefs. It is one thing to note that these all obviously affect behavior, but it is seemingly quite another to suggest that they might alter the internal molecular environment in ways that can affect how we heal. Further, until recently there has been an even larger distance practically and conceptually between the worlds of the neurologist and the immunologist. Most studies of the immune system were conducted in animal sys-

tems and/or in vitro, and so the immune system seemed essentially autonomous from the nervous system. Now with the recent emergence of the new field of psychoneuroimmunology—which studies the links between the mind, the brain, and the immune system—we are at the beginning of time when it will not seem so strange that strong psychological support may positively affect host resistance and potentially alter response to disease. So the problem has been the great distance between the experiential claims of the practitioners of alternative techniques and the experimental world of medical research.

However, even the world view of the so-called alternative practitioner is finding a small modicum of acceptance in selected areas of current medical practice. For example, there is now evidence showing that even people undergoing standard radiation therapy can tolerate its highly unpleasant and toxic side effects better if they are simultaneously practicing some of these techniques or undergoing psychotherapy. Ironically, it seems to be this evidence that is convincing the normally skeptical establishment to use these techniques. When hypnosis, guided imagery, and meditation function effectively as aids in the use of conventional chemotherapy and radiation techniques by modifying the behavior of patients, the questions that are usually raised about their usefulness seem to be asked less frequently.

THE NEW MIND/BODY SKEPTICISM

On the other hand, the popular acclaim in the culture at large for the positive view of the mind/body relationship is also beginning to be assailed by others in the medical professions. During the past 10 years, practitioners of the so-called alternative techniques have often had to endure charges of charlatanism, the accusation that they were unethical in their handling of cancer patients or others with terminal illnesses, and the suggestion that to claim that psychological processes can be effective in altering the course of disease was "not science." The most conspicuous assault in recent times was launched last year by *The New England Journal of Medicine* when it published its editorial suggesting that all links between positive mental attitude and survival should be regarded as merely "folklore." The excuse for that diatribe against the entire field of alternative practices was a paper that studied, by unproven methods, a collection of cancer patients, many in advanced stages of disease, who could not be helped by any known therapy, physical or otherwise. Then generalizations were made from the conclusions of this study that were then extrapolated upon by one of *The New England Journal's* editors, Marcia Angell, to a degree that won criticism from a host of professional researchers all over the U.S. Ironically, a paper had appeared a few weeks before in *The Lancet*, England's older equivalent of *The New England Journal*, which showed that in a 10-year follow-up study, the only factor found in common among these unusually long-term survivors was what the British researchers called "fighting spirit." *The New England Journal of Medicine* staff obviously wrote their editorial while unaware of the work of their British colleagues.

Perhaps the major reason for this negative reaction in the medical establishment is that some practitioners of alternative techniques argue that their use not only enhances quality of life but also extends the actual length of life or survival time. And it is certainly true that exaggerated claims are not hard to find. A whole host of people have published claims that they can cure all manner of illnesses by the power of the mind alone. An even more controversial proposition is that remission may sometimes be facilitated by the use of alternative therapies. There is, as yet, no data base of any substantial kind regarding the frequency of remission, and so there is no way to solidly support such claims directly (see below). These claims have raised great concern in those who argue that the proof is not yet in and that we should not offer false hope to patients. This is, in general, exactly the proper kind of concern, if it is expressed as a concern and not a conclusion. The public should be protected against false claims and false hope. Strangely enough, little concern is voiced about the ethics of the opposite possibility, i.e., what Dr. Naomi Remen has termed "false despair." The offering by the physician of unduly negative expectations that can ultimately add up

to false despair is not a casual matter. Just as a placebo can bring about positive changes, a "nocebo" or negative placebo is associated with negative changes and side effects.

PLACEBOS: HIDDEN PATHS BETWEEN MIND AND BODY

We worry about false hope, yet pay little or no attention to the consequences for the patient of false despair. What might lead one to believe that psychological factors such as hope and expectation *can* lead to physiological change? As Dr. Joel Elkes of the University of Louisville has observed: "I have never understood why so powerful an instrument of healing as the placebo could have been dismissed in arrogant disdain by our profession rather than viewed as a precious resource deserving the most careful and thorough scrutiny."

There are many reasons for this situation. In the introduction to their impressive volume, *Placebo—Theory, Research, Mechanisms* (The Guilford Press, 1985), Drs. Leonard White, Bernard Tursky, and Gary Schwartz write: "The dominant view of placebo is that its use is mandatory in clinical trials, but unethical in clinical practice." This volume stands alone today as *the* single most comprehensive treatment of placebo research ever compiled.

Another possible explanation for distrust of the placebo revolves around the skittishness that its use must inevitably produce for the medical professions, since it challenges the basis on which they believe their knowledge and techniques to function. As Dr. Adolf Grunbaum has pointed out:

Surgery for angina pectoris performed in the United States during the 1950's turned out to be a mere placebo. Unbeknownst to the physicians who practised before the present century, most of the medications they dispensed were at best pharmacologically ineffective, if not outright physiologically harmful or even dangerous. Thus, during all that time, doctors were largely engaged in the unwitting dispensation of placebos on a massive scale. Nay, even after the development of contemporary scientific medicine some 80 years ago, the placebo effect flourished as the norm of medical treatment.

The revelation that surgical procedures for

angina pectoris did not objectively benefit patients suggests that similarly careful evaluation should be conducted today in other areas, such as the burgeoning coronary bypass industry. Some studies indicate that bypasses are often fully occluded 6 months after this expensive and traumatic procedure, and yet the patients continue to report positive health outcomes. One can only wonder if 10 years from now we will look back on bypass surgery as yet another placebo effect in which the well-being of the patient resulted from the triggering of the innate self-repair system.

When one realizes that variables responsive to placebos include reaction time, grip strength, pulse rate, blood pressure, pain, short-term rote memory, cough, mood changes, angina pectoris, headache, seasickness, anxiety, hypertension, gastric motility, dermatitis, pain symptoms from a variety of sources, and self-perceptions of relaxation and activation, it seems clear that the range of bodily systems that can become involved is quite varied. Therefore, deciding just where to begin and/or how to limit the variables in any investigation seems a daunting task. As Adolf Grunbaum has pointed out: "The medical and psychiatric literature on placebos and their effects is conceptually bewildering, to the point of being a veritable Tower of Babel."

However, that is usually the feeling at almost any time when science first approaches a complex problem. The first stages of rigorous investigation always involve the recognition of just how complex the problem is. Next comes the effort to systematize the data and search for patterns within it. We may just be about to enter this phase of placebo research at the present time. Many of the crucial pieces of initial data have been with us for some time, but it seems that it is only now that a systems perspective is being applied in an attempt to integrate the information across disciplines. Indeed just such an approach is advocated by White, Tursky, and Schwartz in the concluding chapter of their book.

It also seems clear that just as the placebo system is powerful, it also has its limits. The fact that the time curves of response to drugs *and* placebos parallel each other suggests that place-bos at least partially involve the pharmacological processing of chemical substances released by the action of the placebo—although in this case they are the product of the "doctor within," as Norman Cousins has called it.

However, just as the surgeon's scalpel can be used to heal or to kill, the placebo may have both positive and negative effects. A recent paper in the *World Journal of Surgery* described tests of a new chemotherapeutic agent which was being tested routinely against a control group given a placebo in the usual double-blind manner. The placebo turned out to have side effects which made 30% of the control group lose all their hair! One can only assume that since most people know that chemotherapy can have such a side effect, the negative expectation of hair loss somehow brought it about. (This use of the term "side effect" can often seem bothersome. Given the poor results of so many forms of chemotherapy, one can't help but wonder if some day we will realize that what we thought of as "side effects" may really be their main and only effect of any importance.) False despair, therefore, can adversely affect a patient. To create it, even with the intent of being ethical, flies in the face of every piece of evidence we have about the power of the placebo effect (see *Investigations*, vol. 2, No. 1, 1985). Somehow, false hope is unethical and false despair is not.

WHO RESPONDS TO SUGAR PILLS?

A part of the problem here is that what can be hope to one person will not seem anything like hope to another, and styles of healing can differ widely between one person and another. So what can we say about the kinds of people who respond to placebos?

A study done by Dr. Charles Moertel and others at Carnegie Mellon University in Pittsburgh in 1976 asked: Who responds to sugar pills? Is one particular personality type more prone to the placebo response? The importance of this question was neatly explained by Moertel:

The ubiquitous presence of the placebo responder renders completely unreliable any uncontrolled trials of drugs for symptomatical palliation. Lasagna and associates have pointed out that even in the controlled clinical trial, the influence of the placebo responder may produce serious distortion of results. He may change the slope of the dose response curve and consequently the sensitivity of the experiment; he may cause the optimal dosage of a drug to be seriously underestimated; and if he has a strong representation in an experimental group, he may so dilute the data that an effective drug may be discarded.

In view of the dominant role the placebo responder plays in our clinical practice, it is disconcerting that we know so little about him.

The preliminary answer from this study was that yes, certain types of people respond more to the placebo effect than others. Specifically, of the 288 cancer patients in the study, 112 (39%) claimed 50% or greater pain relief from dummy medications. Who were the responders? In this study, Moertel and his associates found that:

Patient groups showing an increased placebo response included those with a high level of education, farmers, those with a professional occupation, women working outside the home, and patients who were widowed, separated or divorced. . . . Particularly vulnerable to placebo effect is the very self-sufficient individual with heavy responsibilities who is thrust into the unaccustomed dependency of disabling illness.

In commenting on these results, Moertel and his colleagues noted that the patient who had a traumatic interruption of a marriage through death, separation, or divorce was strikingly more vulnerable to placebo effect than either the currently married patient or the patient who had never married. However, the study's finding that a high level of education correlated with high placebo response is not supported by other studies; for example, one study by Lasagna showed the very opposite correlation, i.e., there was a higher level of education in the *nonresponder*. Strong correlations were found, however, between strong placebo response and occupation. The placebo response got stronger and stronger as

one moved from unskilled workers to skilled nonnonprofessionals to professionals. Farmers clearly led all the groups in having the highest response.

Who did not respond? According to Moertel and his colleagues, those patients significantly immune to the effects of placebo included the married woman without children, the patient with a low educational level, the housewife, and the unskilled worker. One of the clearest correlations here involved the childless married woman: "Among the 14 childless women who were currently married, there was not a single placebo responder."

However there is no clear consensus today on just how reliable the differences identified by Moertel and his colleagues actually are or whether they hold for any given individual in all circumstances. Other studies that have attempted to identify a "placebo-prone personality" have yielded conflicting results. It seems that an individual can be a high responder in one setting and a low responder in another, so the overall concept of a "high responder" does not generalize as easily as it was once hoped it would.

PLACEBOS AND MIND/BODY PLASTICITY

A natural extension of this kind of thinking is to ask the question: are there conditions of mind and/or body that actually facilitate the plasticity of the overall system in ways that make the kind of natural self-repair induced by placebos more likely? In turn, we must ask: do these kinds of states, if they exist, involve significant components of the unconscious mind? The evidence seems to weigh in with an overall yes, although it has to be said in the same breath that the evidence is uneven and hopefully it will become clearer. Specifically, there do indeed seem to be states of mind that facilitate plasticity of the mind/body relationship. Data from medical anthropology has shown that various dissociative states, trance, prayer, and other spiritual practices, such as meditation and the forms of concentration intensified by Yoga, Zen and Buddhist practices, can enhance healing. We in the West have found ways of accelerating some of the results through technological forms of feedback, but the fact remains that the realization that these things are possible came to us initially from these Eastern practices. Today, another important source of such extraordinary natural plasticity is coming from the field of multiple personality research where it is possible to observe dramatic shifts in physical conditions seemingly as a result of shifts in personality alone.

These phenomena of relaxation, meditation, and dissociation all seem to involve, at one level or another, a shift in the relationship between conscious and unconscious levels of awareness. They also involve aspects of the mechanism of attention and expectancy. In turn, they are mind-states that include elements of unconscious processes, whether by virtue of association in the psychotherapeutic sense or by virtue of symbolic recall. They are indeed those states of mind most often directly associated with the symbolic aspect of mental processes, imagery, reverie, and the like. And after all, the idea of the pill or medical procedure as symbol seems to be the core of the placebo effect itself. If one of the basic languages of the brain is the world of image and symbol, then surely we should look carefully at that area of the mind/brain that we know to be most closely involved with processing this aspect of our mental lives. In the end we may have to understand that the functional states of mind, like hope, expectancy, and positive or negative feelings about self that appear to affect the placebo response, will have to be broken down into their subcomponents involving shifts in attention, dissociation, and imagery. The psychophysiological expression of these states is presumably the path to the triggers of placebo.

This symbolic aspect of the placebo, though it is perhaps its most obvious property, is also the most difficult one around which to build a science. It is interesting to note two different lines of thinking that have emerged concerning this aspect of the placebo—one from Dr. Howard Brody of Michigan State University, and the other from Dr. David Bohm, a physicist at Birkbeck College in London. Some years ago, Brody proposed the adoption of "a meaning model" for the placebo effect:

This theory asserts that a positive placebo response will be most likely to occur when three factors are optimally present: the meaning of the illness experience for the patient is altered in a positive manner, given the patient's preexisting belief system and world view; the patient is supported by a caring group; and the patient's sense of mastery and control over the illness is restored or enhanced.

This theory attempts to refine the notion of "expectation" so as to yield more easily falsifiable predictions, and also highlights the cultural dimensions of the phenomena, so that the pertinence of cross-cultural studies in medical anthropology to placebo research can be shown more clearly.

One of the main points here is the fact that symbolic processes *have* been shown to elicit a variety of emotional and behavioral changes, as in hypnosis research, autogenic training, and aversive conditioning procedures, and so we should not be surprised that the symbolic process of the placebo does this, too. The symbolic process of the placebo involves the creation of an *expectancy* that some kind of healing will result. There are many kinds of expectancy, and the ones most relevant here appear to involve the expectancy that one can predict and/or control what is happening to one (note Brody's third factor above). Dr. Mark Laudenslager and others at the University of Colorado have shown that uncontrollable, unpleasant events affect the immune system and seem to facilitate the growth of cancerous tumors, whereas the same events, when controllable, do not have the same negative immunological consequences. So our sense of expectancy is linked closely to our feelings about the need for control, and the lack of control can have a high cost.

The cognitive approach to placebo research is to examine how expectancy affects behavior directly. According to Dr. Richard Bootzin of Northwestern University, if a person has the expectation of being able to cope with a problem, he or she will be better able to do so. This can directly affect the physician/client situation and, as Bootzin suggests:

We have already seen that it is possible to induce changes in anxiety and mood through verbal and imagery techniques. The person receiving a supposedly effective therapy may reduce the number of self-defeating thoughts and images in which he or she engages and may increase the frequency of coping self-statements and positive images.

It appears, therefore, that it may be through the avenue of cognitive science that a sensitivity to the mental process aspects of the placebo will emerge.

Working from a very different line of argument, Dr. David Bohm has been writing recently on the notion of *meaning* as the link between mind and matter. In a series of recent lectures, Bohm pointed out that the relationship between physical and mental has usually been considered in terms of the "psychosomatic": *psyche* comes from the Greek word for mind and *soma* means the body. The term "psychosomatic" therefore embodies the notion of a split between mind and matter. However, Bohm argues that:

In my view, such a notion introduces a split or fragmentation between the physical and the mental that does not properly correspond to the actual state of affairs. Instead I wish to suggest the introduction of a new term, "soma-significance," to emphasize the unity of soma with significance and, ultimately, with "meaning" in all its implications and possibilities.

Bohm's argument is elaborate and complex and involves a detailed consideration of the feedback loops that exist between soma (the physical) and significance (the world of meaning). It may be that in the near future we will see a synthesis between this model of reality coming to us from physics and the phenomena of the placebo effect.

Admittedly this is not simple territory to try to analyze. But is it really enough to leave things as they now stand with the balance more often weighted toward the negative end of spectrum? However, what all this also highlights is the fact that so much about healing is informational and communicative in nature. If all levels of the patient, both conscious and unconscious, are listening to the physician for clues and interpretations of his or her condition, one can only imagine that modern medical training should begin to pay very careful attention to training the communication skills of physicians. There must surely be a middle ground here that allows a person's psychological resources the benefit of support and

encouragement, even in the face of negative odds. A willing spirit can indeed make weak flesh walk, sometimes even in the face of overwhelming odds to the contrary.

SPIRITUAL HEALING: MYTHS OR MIRACLES?

However, if one feels that exaggerated claims are made by those practicing various alternative methods, they pale in comparison with the claims made by many in the realm of spiritual healing. Although some are doubting that the relatively slow processes involved in remission exist, there are others in the realm of spiritual healing reporting dramatic changes occurring with a suddenness and rapidity that is nothing less than astonishing.

But, one may ask, is there really any evidence that the spiritual does play a measurable role in healing? Or are spiritual factors at such a highly diffused end of the spectrum of influences that their role is always likely to remain intangible? Spiritual healings so often seem to strike like lightning that one is left with the feeling that to study it scientifically would be like trying to grasp a thunderbolt. A simple way to consider spiritual healing in scientific terms is to ask whether or not these nonphysical aspects of the human being can ever act as significant activators of the healing system. Most mainstream cancer researchers seem to believe that the impact of the nonphysical systems can never be as powerful as drugs or surgery. Yet some of the claims in data on miraculous healing suggest otherwise.

The most accessible examples of well-documented spiritual healings are those kept by the International Medical Commission at Lourdes in France. These cases are examined by an international medical team that applies quite stringent criteria to the cases. In fact, of the 6000 or so claims that have been submitted since 1858, a total of 64 have been accepted as "miraculous" by the Catholic Church. The list of conditions that were healed makes interesting reading, with quite a wide range of diseases involved. They include cases of various kinds of cancer—including some where sarcomas of the bone "filled in" within a matter of hours. They also include cases of multiple sclerosis and Parkinson's Disease. In the late 1800s there were many cases of remission from tuberculosis, which of course are no longer seen today since it can now be cured with drugs. It is interesting that the medical commission's first question about any claim is whether or not it can be explained as a remission. If so, it is dismissed from further consideration as a "miraculous healing" since remissions are considered natural, not supernatural!

Of course, Lourdes is not unique in this regard. There are now similar, less well-documented claims being made concerning an apparition of the Virgin Mary that has been appearing in the little village of Medjugorje in Yugoslavia since June 24, 1981. Millions of people from all over Europe have visited this tiny place, and some 250 cases of extraordinary healing have been reported. Again, the variety of conditions affected is impressive, though there seems to be a bias toward conditions with psychosomatic components, according to the Franciscan monks observing the situation. Even so, conditions involving tumors and various kinds of cancer are amongst the current records. What is perhaps most interesting is that this is continuing to happen on a daily basis at the time of this writing. To date, two teams of doctors and scientists from France and Italy have visited the village and made a variety of measurements on the boys and girls who claim to witness the apparition—during the time of their experience of it.

Some people of a deeply religious persuasion are, of course, convinced that the conditions of healing are always spiritual and outside of science. Others continue on a more scientific course in the belief that ultimately both scientifically measurable and spiritually important factors will be found to be involved. A highly intriguing example of this proposed hybrid between the scientific and religious realms has emerged recently in the form of the study done by Dr. Randy Byrd, a cardiologist and former assistant professor of medicine at the University of California, San Francisco. Byrd did a double-blind, randomized study of 393 coronary care unit patients at San Francisco General Hospital. A computer chose 192 patients to be prayed for by prayer groups. The other 201 patients were not prayed for and none of the patients knew whether they were being prayed for or not. *The Medical Tribune* reported the results of the study as follows:

The subjects of prayer suffered fewer complications in three areas:

PATIENTS PRAYED FOR	PATIENTS NOT PRAYED FOR
Three required antibiotics	Sixteen required antibiotics
Six suffered pulmonary edema.	Eighteen suffered pulmonary edema.
None required intubation.	Twelve required intubation

Interestingly, Byrd recruited Protestants, Catholics, and Jews throughout the country to pray for specific patients in the designated group. As Byrd described it:

Each person prayed for many different patients. But each patient [in the prayed-for group] had between five and seven people praying for him or her. As part of the study, the people praying were given the name of the patient, the diagnosis, and the condition. They were asked to pray each day, but no specific amount or way of doing it was specified.

It remains to be seen what science will think, given that the typical methods of a double-blind scientific study have yielded positive results like this. What is especially interesting here is that the patients did not know that they were being prayed for, and yet one group did better than the other. The number of patients involved certainly seems large enough for the study to be statistically significant. It will be important to repeat this study with more refined experimental designs.

Anyone willing to look carefully at this evidence comes away with the sense that there are not only many factors in healing still unknown to us, but that certain kinds of spiritual conditions do indeed seem to be associated with dramatic kinds of healing.

NEUROTRANSMITTER PLASTICITY: THE NEW APPROACH TO SELF-REPAIR

Those with rigorous scientific training who have recently become sympathetic to the role of the mind and spirit in healing have unfortunately been left by holistic practitioners without much of the kind of hard evidence needed to back up many of their claims. Hence we face a series of dilemmas in our search for a scientific understanding of the healing process and whether it is affected by mental and spiritual factors. The fact is that we know very little about how such interventions work when they do succeed and nothing at all about why they don't work for certain people.

However, this situation may be about to change if the right kind of research progresses in the next few years. Dr. Jonas Salk observed during an interview on the mind-body issues: "The holistic approach is really what it is, and we're now positive that the mind, in addition to medicine, has powers to turn the immune system around to defend itself against disease or illness."

Some might regard this statement as going a little beyond the evidence to date. But the slow but steady emergence of data from fields like psychoneuroimmunology, positive emotions research, remission research, and biomagnetism suggests that Salk will prove right in the long run. However, the notion that there might be an unknown, more generalized self-repair or healing system has received little attention from researchers in any formal way. It seems that one of the first contemporary writers to identify the concept of a healing system per se was Norman Cousins in his book *Human Options* [1981], where he pointed out:

Over the years, medical science has identified the primary systems of the human body—the circulatory system, digestive system, endocrine system, autonomic nervous system, parasympathetic nervous system, and the immune system. But two other systems that are central to the proper functioning of a human being need to be emphasized: the healing system and the belief system. The two work together. The healing system is the way the body mobilizes all its resources to combat disease. The belief system is often the activator of the healing system. (p. 205)

Given the wide range of evidence for the existence of unusual or extraordinary healing, it seems clear that there must indeed be some unknown set of conditions and/or systems that can be switched on to bring it about. As we mentioned earlier, many new developments are leading to a new view of the whole process of healing and self-repair. As we slowly begin to fill in the picture of mind modulation of the immune system, the endocrine system, and the neuropeptide system, the links between the spiritual, the mental, and the physical may become clearer.

In considering the feedback loops that exist between psyche and soma, one recently discovered property of the nervous system may be especially useful conceptually. This is the property of molecular and neurotransmitter plasticity in the brain. Neurotransmitters are the chemical agents of communication between the neurons of the brain. It was originally thought that the brain used only two neurotransmitters: acetylcholine and another one resembling epinephrine. Now we know that there are more than 50 different molecules that can act in the role of neurotransmitters. Indeed, these molecules are to be found not just in the brain but in other parts of the body as well. The growth in our knowledge about these "communicator molecules" (carriers of meaning in Bohm's language) has coincided with the emergence of another major concept in our understanding of the nervous system, i.e., its plasticity and its ability to use more than one neurotransmitter to communicate between neurons. Previously it was thought that the relations between neurons were more or less "hard-wired" and that once they were linked up within the developing organism, they were basically locked in to that wiring—in part by their presumed use of a specific neurotransmitter for transmission of their messages.

It is now known that any given neuron seems to have the ability to switch from using one type of neurotransmitter to another and thereby alter the messages it sends *and* the region of the brain to which it sends signals. As Dr. Ira Black from Cornell University recently wrote:

It is becoming increasingly apparent that the transmitter status of a neuron represents a dynamic, changing process, influenced by multiple extracellular factors, including afferent and efferent innervation, proximate nonneuronal cells, and hormones. Consequently, neurons may respond to environmental information by altering transmitter phenotypic expression and, presumably, the signals sent to other neurons.

It is now believed by some that this is a property of neurons in the adult brain and not just in the developing organism. Since placebos clearly seem to require that a basic change in the modus operandi of the brain/mind take place, it is tempting to speculate that such neurotransmitter plasticity of neurons may be a logical route for the brain to choose in mediating the placebo response. Such plasticity may prove to be the molecular key to placebo effects, allowing as it would the actual physico-chemical modes of transmission from the same site to change from one type of signal to another.

It is also known that neurons can effectively involve themselves with more than one neurotransmitter or neuropeptide at the same time. This kind of work is underway, involving the ratios of substance P to acetylcholine at the synapse. It could well be that the subtle shifts of mind involved in hope and expectancy on the molecular level could involve just such shifts in neuron to neurotransmitter relationships. One of the important sources of new thinking in this field is Candace Pert and her colleagues at the National Institute of Mental Health. Writing in the Journal of Immunology in 1985, Pert and her colleagues state:

A major conceptual shift in neuroscience has been wrought by the realization that brain function is modulated by numerous chemicals in addition to classical neurotransmitters. Many of these informational substances are neuropeptides, originally studied in other contexts as hormones, "gut peptides," or growth factors. Their number presently exceeds 50 and most, if not all, alter behavior and mood states, although only endogenous analogs of psychoactive drugs like morphine, valium, and phenocyclidine have been well appreciated in this context. We now realize that their signal specificity resides in receptors (distinct classes of recognition molecules) rather than the close juxtaposition occurring at classical synapses. Rather precise brain distribution patterns for many neuropeptide receptors have been determined. A number of brain loci, many within emotion-mediating brain areas, are enriched with many types of neuropeptide receptors, suggesting a convergence of information at these "nodes." Additionally, neuropeptide receptors occur on mobile cells of the immune system; monocytes can chemotax to numerous neuropeptides via processes shown by structure-activity analysis to be mediated by distinct receptors indistinguishable from those found in the brain. Neuropeptides and their receptors thus join the brain, glands, and immune system in a network of communication between brain and body, probably representing the biochemical substrate of emotion.

This new informational systems view of the healing process seems likely to deeply transform our overall view of what happens in healing processes and promises to "make sense" of many previously inexplicable claims. In his recent book, *The Psychobiology of Mind-Body Healing*, Dr. Ernest Rossi observed:

Neuropeptides, then, are a previously unrecognized form of information transduction between mind and body that may be the basis of many hypnotherapeutic, psychosocial, and placebo responses. From a broader perspective, the neuropeptide system also may be the psychobiological basis of the folk, shamanistic, and spiritual forms of healing (that share many of the characteristics of hypnotic healing) currently returning to vogue under the banner of "holistic medicine."

It seems therefore that a basic logic is unfolding here; the many complex linkages between mind, brain, body, and cell are beginning to emerge at long last. The net result may make sense of some things we have dismissed from medicine and may make us dismiss from medical practice some attitudes and behaviors towards patients we have allowed out of ignorance of the impact they can have on people's lives and the course of their disease.

REMISSION: THE PEAK OF SELF-REPAIR?

It seems most likely at this point in time that the most powerful scientific evidence for the idea of an unknown self-repair system will emerge from the study of the phenomenon of spontaneous remission. There are thousands of references in refereed medical journals to this most dramatic form of self-repair. The largest study ever done of the world medical literature on remission has recently been completed by the Institute of Noetic Sciences in California. An initial search of the medical data bases yielded a total of 9000 references to the subject, i.e., there were 9000 cases where the topic was mentioned somewhere in a paper. A closer analysis led to a smaller number of papers that were either totally about the subject or had a major portion of the paper devoted to some aspect of the topic. To date we have assembled more than 2500 such papers from over 830 different medical journals in hard copy and also stored all the titles and abstracts of these in an electronic data base. It does not take long to realize after reading that many papers on the subject that surely something is going on here! It is no longer intellectually respectable or medically informed to shrug and say that it is all an artifact of misdiagnosis, as so many have done. The data base is as interesting in showing which diseases do not exhibit any tendency toward remission as it is for those that do seem to remit more often. Certain kinds of cancer, such as melanoma, seem "remission prone" while others, such as lung cancer, rarely seem to remit.

But one may well ask: Is remission researchable? Does it occur without treatment? And, if so, why and in whom does it occur? There are many cases of remission that occur even though the person has never received any medical treatment. There are literally hundreds of cases like this reported in the world's medical journals. So the phenomenon is there, but the detailed studies of it are not. Until the biological and psychological markers of spontaneous remission are mapped, we can only guess whether the necessary preconditions for remission are physical and/or psychological in nature. Indeed, there seems to be some progress along the lines of purely biological markers.

If the work of Dr. Jorge Yunis of the University of Minnesota is made public and verified by other scientists, a significant step forward in understanding the genetic basis of remission may be made. Yunis' work builds on the 1955 discovery that each human cell typically contains 46 chromosomes. Each chromosome contains hereditary information in the form of long strings of DNA, which in turn instruct the pancreas to produce insulin, brain cells to make neurotransmitters, and so on. He has tried to identify which genes are associated with various diseases, birth defects, and the like. But our ability to do this is limited by our ability to see the chromosomes themselves. The early staining techniques that made them visible allowed us to see only about 640 bands on each chromosome. Yunis claims to have devised techniques that allow him to see up to 10,000 bands per chromosome! This high-resolution chromosomal analysis allows a much finer analysis than ever before, and Yunis now claims to be able to tell more precisely than anyone else just how genetic defects are associated with everything from the major diseases to the shape of your face and when your hair will turn grey. An interview in *Omni* in March 1986 quotes Yunis as saying:

For example, if a patient's cancerous cells have an upside-down segment on the sixteenth-largest chromosome, chances of survival are excellent: the patient is likely to go into complete remission. Patients with an extra copy of the eighth-largest chromosome have a fair prognosis: average survival is ten months. Multiple chromosomal defects foretell the bleakest outlook: the patient is likely to die within ten weeks.

The problem with this claim is that Yunis has so far refused to publish the details of his technique of examining chromosomes on the grounds that it will cause all kinds of ethical problems. Specifically, he wonders what would happen to someone's chances for either employment or health insurance if a genetic screening technique that could reliably predict that the person will come down with cancer at the age of 35 were used on a drop of their blood at birth. This position may be justified, but if history is any indicator, it is only postponing a problem, not solving it. Discoveries in science seem to know no national or institutional boundaries, so the chances are that whatever Yunis has discovered will sooner or later be rediscovered by others. If this kind of work is verified by other scientists, then we can expect to see dramatic advances in our understanding of when to expect remission in certain kinds of people and perhaps how to facilitate it in those who lack the genetic predisposition toward it.

Other work on the molecular biology of remission-related issues is proceeding apace. The pioneering work of Coley in the early part of this century, using bacterial infections to stimulate the immune response in cancer patients, has led to the discovery and isolation of the factors produced by these methods. So today Dr. Lloyd Old and his colleagues at Sloan Kettering are testing something called Tumor Necrosis Factor, which was isolated as a result of studying Coley's early work. Thanks to the new genetic engineering techniques, the powerful biological factors can be cloned and produced in large quantities by companies like Genentech and Cetus. Other new pharmaceutical companies such as Ribi Immunochem in Montana and Cell Technology Inc., in Colorado are also testing what they claim are less toxic variants of this approach with, they say, startling results. These approaches involve the stimulation of the patient's own immune system to produce its own interferon, its own colony stimulating factor, and other important components of the immune system. The results of tests on animals with these substances have been impressive enough to allow these companies to begin human clinical trials recently.

Of course, we now know that psychological processes also affect immune function—a fact not known before 1977. And although there is no really systematic evidence to suggest that "healing is all in the mind," a survey of the existing literature on remission only makes one wonder all the more about these possibilities, since frequently one finds the only clue in a given report to be the fact that the patient experienced some profound change in outlook—psychologically or spiritually—and then began to recover. This information is certainly too "soft" to warrant going any further at this time, but one's curiosity is left somewhat piqued by these anecdotal reports.

THE ELECTROMAGNETIC FACTOR

Just as there is an important effort afoot to understand the role of the mind and the brain in healing, there is yet another fledgling science trying to establish itself which also has an important contribution to add to the healing puzzle. This is the slowly growing area of biomagnetism or electromagnetic biology. Nobel Laureate Albert Szent-Gyorgy pointed out many years ago that the charge on the surface of a cancer cell is opposite to the charge on the surface of a healthy cell, and he suggested that cancer may be the result of the emergence of electrical anomalies in the body. His theory of the process was outlined in his 1976 book, *Electronic Biology and Cancer*.

Another pioneer arguing for the importance of the electrical view of biological processes is Dr. Robert Becker, formerly of the VA Hospital in Syracuse, New York. He did seminal research on the use of small direct currents to stimulate regeneration of bone and tissue. He suggested that small direct currents played a crucial role in the evolutionary development of self-repair capacities of many species. A popular survey of his work is contained in his book, *The Body Electric*, co-authored with Gary Selden, (Morrow, New York, 1985).

More recently, we have read about the work of Swedish radiologist Dr. Björn Nordenström, who has put his theory concerning the importance of electrical currents in the body into practice by inserting electrodes directly into cancer tumors and attacking them electrically by creating a positive charge inside them (*Discover*, April 1986). Curiously, those writing about Nordenström's theories in Sweden seem totally unaware of Becker's work in this country and vice versa. Though far from perfected, the technique has apparently healed several patients who had been judged to be too old for surgery or too advanced to treat with normal techniques. In effect, Nordenström claims to have discovered the existence of *biologically closed electric circuits* within the body that are crucial to the healing process. As Nordenström puts it:

Injury in tissue represents a source of release of energy, which induces closed circuit transports over biologically closed electric current (BCEC) channels, leading in turn to structural modifications in tissue. These modifications are of considerable interest because they represent *a result of the process of healing*. Consequently, knowledge of BCEC mechanisms may increase our understanding of how tissues heal. Indeed, it will be shown that artificial activation of BCEC mechanisms can even lead to beneficial effects in disease.

This work, coupled with other research on biomagnetism going on in the U.S., Italy, and Japan, promises to add a significant piece to the puzzle of natural healing and self-repair.

BELIEF: THE LIGHTING ON THE STAGE

Although physical modalities are, of course, extremely powerful, nonphysical modalities can literally alter the landscape in which these physical processes play out their role. The nonphysical components of healing, such as belief, expectations, and the will to live, may be like the lighting on the stage upon which we play out our dramas of illness and healing. If there is light, even a little, there is some hope that we can observe and play out the drama; if there is darkness, then we cannot perceive and participate in what is happening. Perhaps the nonphysical components eventually will be characterized in the manner suggested by Norman Cousins in 1981, when he wrote of the special role of the belief system in health and healing:

The belief system represents the unique element in human beings that makes it possible for the human mind to affect the workings of the body. How one responds—intellectually, emotionally, spiritually—to one's problems has a great deal to do with the way the human body functions. One's confidence, or lack of it, in the prospects of recovery from serious illness affects the chemistry of the body. The belief system converts hope, robust expectations, and the will to live into plus factors in any contest of forces involving disease.

These kinds of ideas are still a source of discomfort for many of a more reductionist persuasion. Many are ultimately more comfortable with the idea that the "real" explanation for all this is at the levels of atoms and molecules alone. While it is true that the climate in this regard may be changing in the public domain, the notion that psychological states can have specific positive impacts on health is still questionable in mainstream medical circles. This situation is likely to remain so until solid research showing the preventative and/or regenerative role of positive emotional and psychological states is carried out—notwithstanding the fact that there exists a vast range of literature on the placebo effect already.

INNER MECHANISMS OF THE HEALING RESPONSE

In an effort to stimulate research in the field of healing, the mind/body relationship, and the study of our natural self-repair capabilities, the Institute of Noetic Sciences has created the Inner Mechanisms of the Healing Response Program (IMHRP). The program selects key projects in healing research and awards a series of seed grants to stimulate pilot projects. It also provides partial support for professional conferences organized around various approaches to creating a new science of healing.

Proposed Properties of the Healing System

The following premises summarize the basic assumptions around which the IMHRP has organized its activities. These premises may change or be developed in new directions by the data that emerges:

1. **The Evidence:** There is a wide body of evidence suggesting that extraordinary healing takes place, including regression of normally fatal tumors for which no scientific explanation is known.
2. **The Healing System:** This implies the existence of a healing system which appears to contain three components:
   a) a self-diagnostic system,
   b) a self-repair system, and
   c) a regenerative system.

3. **Triggers**: The evidence suggests that this kind of healing can be triggered by a variety of stimuli, diverse in nature, including signals, suggestions, and guidance from the physical, mental, and/or spiritual realms of every individual.

4. **Researchability**: This unknown healing system is describable and researchable in a manner similar, but not identical to, the way other well-known control systems in the body became known, e.g., the nervous system and the immune system.

5. **Anatomy**: The anatomy of the healing system will resemble the communications system now being uncovered in psychoneuroimmunology. The immune system does, of course, have a host of physical components, but its primary functions are revealed by its way of recognizing its environment and communicating the consequences of that recognition within itself and to the body as a whole. Similarly, the healing system will have physical components that act in concert when challenged, but its true nature may follow the model of a communications/information system rather than that of the more familiar, physically connected systems in the body.

6. **Structure**: Certain aspects of the healing system are similar to other systems in that this system can also organize and direct "lower" levels to effect specific reactions, remove unwanted substances, cleanse tissues, and restore order. So it is proposed that the healing system will also prove to be a hierarchical system with both physical and symbolic components.

7. **Meta-Structure**: Other aspects of this unknown healing system are dissimilar to other known systems in that it acts as a meta-system between the realms of mind and matter in symbolic ways that resemble the manner in which the nervous system alone normally acts, but which includes a wider realm of expression.

8. **Significance**: It will be as important to discover the healing system as it has been to discover the nervous system or the immune system. This unknown system may turn out to be a special interface between these two systems, but it operates by rules that are not identical to those of either system.

Some may argue that there is no need to complicate things by inventing yet another system in the body, but it is worth remembering that science seems to progress more rapidly when there is a clearer organizational picture of what is being examined. When the diversity of data on healing is examined with the aim of integrating it, it is hard not to come away with the sense that we have been unable to see the overall patterns in the data simply because we have not thought of healing from a systems point of view. The recent emergence of a systems perspective in several areas of medicine may accelerate our efforts to understand the healing process and along the way may uncover aspects of ourselves that have remained hidden from view for far too long. Today we seem to be poised at a unique point in history where we have not only the means to ask deeper questions about healing, but also a vital body of new researchers are willing to tackle the complex questions involved. Perhaps more than any other field, the new science of healing will not only make us see the mind, body, and spirit as a unified system, but may also unify our understanding of ourselves as human beings with capacities and potentials we have only dreamed about.

5 THE HEALING FACTOR

Steven E. Locke, M.D., and Douglas Colligan. Dr. Locke is Associate Director of the Psychiatry Consultation-Liaison Service at Boston's Beth Israel Hospital and he teaches psychiatry at Harvard Medical School. Since 1976, Dr. Locke has conducted research, taught, and published in the emerging field of psychoneuroimmunology (PNI). He serves on the scientific advisory board of the Institute for the Advancement of Health and on the editorial committee of their journal of mind-/body medicine, *Advances*. Dr. Locke has co-edited three books on PNI: *Mind and Immunity: Behavioral Immunology* (New York: Institute for the Advancement of Health, 1983); *Foundations of Psychoneuroimmunology* (Hawthorne, NY: Aldine Publishing Co., 1985); and *Psychological and Behavioral Treatments for Disorders Associated with the Immune System* (New York: Institute for the Advancement of Health, 1986). He has written (with co-author Douglas Colligan) *The Healer Within*, a popular book on mind and immunity published by E.P. Dutton in 1986. Dr. Locke maintains a private practice in Boston, Massachusetts, specializing in behavioral medicine and psychotherapy.

Psychoneuroimmunology (or PNI) is the study of the psychological effects of the mind on the immune system. It is considered by some to be the most exciting new field in medical research today. PNI increasingly is used in the treatment of cancer and pain disorders, employing such techniques as biofeedback and meditation. Research centers have been formed to explore the puzzling relationship between mind and body and to decipher whether a proper mental attitude and an ability to relax at will might make one less vulnerable to disease. If we can learn to control our immune systems through our emotions, certain traditional medical techniques may quickly become obsolete.■

Every week a group of patients gather together in a room at Boston's Beth Israel Hospital to participate in a process called mindfulness meditation. Their ailments are varied and unrelated—cancer, heart disease, diabetes—but their goal is the same: to feel better. They are seeking not merely the temporary sensation of feeling better but a genuine improvement in health.

At Penn State University, psychologist Howard Hall asks people to conjure up dramatic, sometimes violent scenes—sharks gobbling up fish, for example—and he then scans their blood for microscopic evidence that their immune cells have taken on some of the same aggressive behavior.

In San Franciso, AIDS patients are gently questioned about their lives, including the stresses they have been feeling apart from the disease, in an effort to probe the emotional undercurrents that may affect the course of the illness.

Throughout the United States in medical schools, research laboratories, and clinics, the effects of a very young and little known medical discipline are beginning to be felt. It is a field of research that has the challenging job of integrating our knowledge about how the mind, the brain, and the immune system interact to keep us healthy or, at times, to make us sick. It's a complex discipline with an equally complex name, psychoneuroimmunology, or PNI for short.

PNI researchers have been trying to answer a medical riddle that has eluded science for centuries: how do moods, feelings, attitudes, and emotional traumas (like grief) affect our health? One of the ironies of psychoneuroimmunology is that although it is a new scientific discipline, it is based on ancient ideas about how emotions and mental states determine our health. Until recently the notions that stress affects the immune system and that reducing stress can have beneficial, disease-fighting effects were considered part of medical folklore, beyond the reach of science. New technologies have given us the ability to study both the immune and nervous systems in exhaustive detail, and with these techniques we can trace the effects of the states of mind through the neural and biochemical pathways in the body.

This is a quest that has fascinated some of the most original and imaginative research talent in the country. Today it probably would be hard to find a major medical school in the United States that did not have an investigator working on a psychoneuroimmunological research program. There are psychologists, psychiatrists, neurologists, epidemiologists, sociologists, immunologists, biologists, oncologists—all bringing their respective expertise to bear on one of the most challenging areas that medical research has ever tackled.

The range and variety of work in this field is impressive. It varies from studying the performance of individual immune cells of people under stress to using imagery and relaxation techniques as experimental therapies for everything from asthma to diabetes. This work is all based on a simple premise that the body is a complex of interconnected systems, and by taking the interactions of these systems into account, we can do a better job of healing the sick. Like holistic medicine, PNI research in humans takes into consideration the whole individual, psychological elements such as personality and coping mechanisms, as well as physiology and biochemistry. Also, as with holism, PNI clinicians try to involve the patient in his own treatment.

Unlike holistic medicine, psychoneuroimmunology is a scientific approach in which clinical practices are endorsed only after exhaustive research. While PNI shares some of the spirit of holism, its proponents value the power of the scientific method to prove the efficacy of new treatments. As its name suggests, psychoneuroimmunology involves the interaction of the mind (psycho), the nervous system (neuro), and the immune system (immunology). The field originated in the Soviet Union in the 1920s. The American father of PNI research is Dr. George Solomon, a psychiatrist now at the University of California at Los Angeles. He has been one of the key figures in establishing the link between the mind and the immune system, the body's self-defense.

While at Stanford University in the 1960s, Solomon was fascinated with the disease rheumatoid arthritis (RA) and the observation that some people who had RA factor in their blood succumbed to the disease while others did not. Rheumatoid arthritis is an autoimmune disease—the body is attacked by its own immune system—and Solomon's early studies of female arthritic patients made him suspect that there were psychological dimensions to the disease. Why did some women have rheumatoid arthritis while their sisters, who also had the RA factor in their blood, escaped arthritis? One chief difference seemed to be in the personalities of the arthritis patients. They were not as well adjusted as their siblings and tended to have common personality traits. They were passive, long-suffering, and self-sacrificing to an almost masochistic degree. How could it be determined whether these traits contributed to the onset of the disease or were the result of its ravaging course?

Since personality seemed to be a factor in RA, Solomon wondered what the brain had to do with the immune system. By scientific tradition, suggesting that the immune system was responsive to the influence of the nervous system was a revolutionary idea. The immune system was believed to be self-regulating.

If you put immune cells in a test tube and release some bacteria into their midst, they attack and destroy the bacteria with the same efficiency with which they act inside the body. Evolution, it seemed, developed an autonomous bodyguard within us.

But Solomon had heard of some highly original research done in the Soviet Union that showed when a small portion of an animal's brain called the hypothalamus was experimentally removed or damaged, the immune system was weakened. He duplicated the Russian experiments and got similar results. Because this suggested that the brain (psycho) was able to influence the immune system, he termed the new science *psychoimmunology*.

By the mid-1970s psychologist Robert Ader at the University of Rochester found himself inexorably drawn into this field as a result of a series of accidental discoveries made while he was performing routine experiments. Ader was trying a simple taste aversion experiment; he wanted to teach his rats to dislike the taste of saccharin. Each time Ader gave his rats some harmless saccharin-flavored water, he also gave them an injection of a nausea-inducing substance, cyclophosphamide. (The underlying principle of behavioral conditioning was the same as the one Pavlov used to make his dogs salivate when he rang a bell.)

Mysteriously, the rats began to die. At first Ader was perplexed, since they had been healthy animals. Later, when he learned that cyclophosphamide not only caused nausea but was also an immunosuppressant, he theorized that he had conditioned not only their minds but their immune systems as well. In other words, the conditioned rats had learned to suppress their immune systems whenever they tasted the saccharin.

To test this idea, Ader and his colleague, immunologist Nicholas Cohen, injected the rats with a foreign tissue, sheep red blood cells, and watched the rats' immune systems react. Then those rats who had been conditioned by pairing the taste of saccharin with cyclophosphamide were reinjected with the foreign blood cells. The conditioned animals reacted less strongly to the second injection of the foreign blood cells if they were also given drinks of the saccharin-flavored water (despite the absence of cyclophosphamide). It appeared to Ader and Cohen that their conditioned animals had, in fact, learned to suppress their immune response. (Their precedent-setting research was later reproduced in two other laboratories with identical results.) Because his experiments proved that the nervous system—the brain, nerves, and neurochemicals—played a part in this conditioned immunosuppression, Ader added *neuro* to George Solomon's term, giving us the more accurate, if unwieldy, nomenclature *psychoneuroimmunology*.

In the 10 years since Robert Ader puzzled over his sick rats, much more has been learned about the interactions of the mind and body. To give some idea of the explosive growth in this field, when Locke and co-editor Mady Hornig-Rohan compiled a bibliography of scientific publications on PNI, they found that between 1976 and 1983 there were over 1300 scientific articles. They covered an intimidatingly complex sweep of topics: how certain behavioral factors like moods, attitudes, personality, and social support have measurable effects on immunity; what kind of interactions there are between the immune and nervous systems; how those interactions work; what kinds of influences modulate that interaction.

Experts have, in fact, found evidence of biochemical and neuronal links between the brain and the immune system. We now know there is an exchange between the immune and nervous systems. Immunologists including Terry Strom of Harvard Medical School have detected receptors for neurotransmitters on lymphocytes. Also, neuroanatomists have found nerves distributed throughout areas of the body vital to the immune system: the thymus gland, lymph nodes, bone marrow, and the spleen. Finally, studies done in the Soviet Union, France, Switzerland, and the United States have shown that selectively damaging various parts of the brain is followed by noticeable changes in immune behavior, usually the suppression of the immune system.

The evidence that the immune system also influences the nervous system includes the discovery that traces of hormone-like substances produced by the thymus, thymosins, have been found in the brain. Injections of certain thymosins into the brain can affect the activity of the pituitary gland which is usually under the control of secretions from the brain. Research in Swiss labs disclosed that when an animal's immune system is challenged, there is a definite and noticeable change in the firing rate of neurons in the brain. And one immunological researcher, Edwin Blalock, found that the immune system appears to produce an analogue of the potent pituitary hormone ACTH, which is involved in the body's stress reaction, fight or flight.

That stresses can have an effect on the body's immune system has long been the subject of controversy, but experiments with animals and, later, humans have shown that the effect is real and detectable. One of its more elegant demonstrations was done by Vernon Riley, a cancer researcher with the Pacific Northwest Research Foundation in Seattle. Using specially bred mice that develop breast cancer, he showed that by varying the amount of stress, he could produce progressive degrees of damage to the animals' immune systems. He built his basic stress apparatus using a record turntable and put the mice in a cage mounted on top of it. The mice were spun in the cages at one of four speeds—16, 33, 45, or 78 rpm—producing a variable rotational stress.

As he studied the developing breast cancer in the mice, he saw an interesting reaction pattern that correlated neatly with the four different record speeds. The cancer in the 16 rpm mice was less malignant than that in the 33 rpm mice, which in turn was less malignant than the 45 rpm mice. The 78 rpm animals had the fastest growing tumors.

But what about us as humans? As it is unethical to put people in boxes spinning 78 rpm, imaginative researchers have used safe but stressful lab experiments designed for humans. At the Karolinska Institute in Sweden, an internationally famous stress research center, scientists have been asking people to perform complicated mental tasks under stress. In one experiment, people were stressed by playing a target practice game that required continuous attention. For 3 sleepless days they were asked to hit the target on a small tank with a rifle that fired light beams. With each hit they were rewarded with a loud blast of battle noise. The combination of the sleeplessness and the demand to do precision work under the added stress of loud noise made for a complex stress situation. The Swedish researchers found that the immune system of the subjects lost some of its ability to destroy bacteria.

But laboratory stress, no matter how ingeniously designed, is not the same as the stress and strain of real life. For this reason and because it has long been believed that bereavement is dangerous to one's health, PNI research has recently focused on people who have had to face the tragedy of having someone close to them die. Common sense accounts partly for why grief could lead to illness. The widow or widower may start overindulging in unhealthy habits—drinking more, smoking more, maybe taking more tranquilizers or sleeping pills. As a by-product of their grief, the bereaved could be eating less, exercising less, ignoring the healthful needs of their bodies. This neglect and abuse could add up and take its toll, impairing the body's resistance to disease.

Even so, there was a nagging conviction that this did not fully explain the sometimes abrupt deaths of survivors. For example, in 1969 a British physician, Dr. C. Murray Parkes, and his colleagues at the Tavistock Institute of Human Relations in London published what has become a classic study on the lifespan of widowers. For 9 years following the death of the wives, they monitored the health of 4448 widowers, all 55 years or older. One of the most striking findings was that the widowers were dying at an unusually high rate—often within six months of their wives' deaths. Since many of these deaths resulted from heart disease, the researchers called their study *Broken Heart*. But this and other early studies of death and illness in grieving spouses have not explained how grief damages the body's defenses.

More detailed information about the impact of grief was provided when a team of Australian researchers decided to do a microscopic study of survivors' reactions. Dr. Roger Bartrop and his colleagues got permission to do a simple blood test on a group of 26 men and women who had recently lost their spouses. They took two sets of blood samples, one drawn 2 weeks after spouse's death and the second drawn 6 weeks later.

In the samples taken after 2 weeks there was no detectable decline in immune potency. But at the 6-week mark, the immune cells' responsiveness had diminished. Although the aftershock of the death was not immediate, its effects were profound and detectable. The study findings suggested that it took time for the damage done by grief to reach measurable levels. "This is the first time," the group announced, "severe psychological stress has been shown to produce a measurable abnormality in immune function."

These findings have inspired others to look more closely at the bereavement effect. At the Mount Sinai School of Medicine in New York, psychiatrist Dr. Steven Schleifer, inspired by the Australian research, decided to do a similar study using periodic blood tests of men whose wives were diagnosed with (and eventually succumbed to) terminal breast cancer. Every month for a year following the spouse's death they took blood samples from the group and ran them through immunopotency tests. During the first 2 months after the death, the widowers' immune systems showed a sharp drop in immune responsiveness. Gradually their systems regained strength, but even as long as a year later, the men's immune response had not rebounded completely.

Israeli scientists from the Weizmann Institute of Science and Kaplan Hospital got similar results studying a more specialized instance of bereavement. They tested a group of women who had lost unborn children either through spontaneous or induced abortions. Psychiatric tests divided the women into two groups, those who found it hard to accept the consequences of their abortions, regardless of how it happened, and those who were less upset.

The scientists noted that the emotional reaction of the nonaccepting group was very much like that of an individual grieving the death of a loved one. Also distinctive was how the immune systems of each group responded to standard laboratory tests. Those who had more difficulty coping with the loss of a child had feebler responses from their T cells, a specific type of immune cell, than did those who coped better with the loss. The nonaccepting women who were the most depressed also registered the hardest jolt to their systems.

Although a specific stress is related to a certain immune response, there are other variables that come into play. How an individual copes with that stress is another. Whereas most people do not have to face the stress of losing someone close more than a few times in life, there are other more common stresses that can take their toll on our bodies' self-protection mechanisms. In my own research with students I found that those who could be typed as "poor copers"—individuals who complained more about the standard stresses of college life—also had lower activity of natural killer cells, another type of immune cell. This discovery was also reflected in work done by psychologist Sandra Levy of the University of Pittsburgh School of Medicine. While studying breast cancer patients, she discovered that the "good" patients, those who were quiet, docile, and stoic about their disease and who seemed to be coping poorly, also showed a distinctly lower amount of activity of natural killer cells than some of the feistier patients. This diminished cell activity was reflected in the outcome of the cases. As a group, the "good" patients had lower survival rates than the others.

Since there is growing evidence that the brain and immune system are intermeshed, those studying psychoneuroimmunology have thought about using this interrelationship in a beneficial way. One approach has been to exploit the mind's ability to generate states of calm and relaxation.

A pioneer in this field is Harvard Medical School cardiologist Dr. Herbert Benson. In the 1970s he was curious about the ability of some individuals to settle into a peaceful and soothing mental state. After research and studying, he and his fellow scientists concluded that people who managed to attain a serene state of relaxation in meditation, prayer, or other mind exercise did four distinct things to achieve that state. Each practiced the exercise in a quiet place—a cool, shaded room, a temple, a church, a chapel. Each used what Dr. Benson called a mental device, an object of concentration that was either a symbol or a single sound (like the famous OM) which helped to block out distractions. Each practitioner also assumed a passive attitude; he did not worry how well he was performing. Finally, the practitioner assumed a position that was comfortable, but not so comfortable that he would fall asleep. (That, suggests Dr. Benson, is how the cross-legged yogic seated position evolved.) The result of these rituals was something Dr. Benson called the relaxation response, a natural becalming state of body and spirit that arose from within the praying or meditating person.

Joan Borysenko of Beth Israel Hospital and Harvard Medical School used Dr. Benson's method in her Mind/Body Group, a clinical program of the Division of Behavioral Medicine. Her group treats a broad variety of ages and diseases. Some patients come to the program because, as Borysenko puts it, "they have come to realize that their attitude really has an effect on their health." Others, she says, are people "who are coming because they've simply run out of other things to do. Their medical problem isn't getting better, often after years of treatment by different physicians. They come out of desperation."

The goal of the program is the same for everyone: "We are trying to help people realize that they are responsible for their body's own reactions and that they *can* learn to respond differently," she explains. In its 4-year history, over 1500 people have passed through the program with many noticeable benefits. "The most dramatic changes have been with people who have had high blood pressure for years," she says. One of the more remarkable cases was a blue collar worker who had been taking high doses of medication to keep his blood pressure down. He had come to the group at his doctor's recommendation to learn to control his blood pressure without such high doses. The man was hit particularly hard by one occasional side effect of this medicine, impotence. At the end of his 10 weeks of meditation he was able to stand up in front of his group with an important announcement: He was once again able to engage in sex. The meditation had let him cut back his drug intake to the point where some of the drug's debilitating effects had disappeared.

Psychoneuroimmunologically, she has gotten other encouraging results. In one 6-month follow-up of group participants she found lower levels of stress-related chemicals, catecholamines, in their systems. In another study done with people afflicted with diabetes, a form of which is thought to be an autoimmune disease, those who faithfully practiced the relaxation response exercises had slightly lower levels of blood sugar. Borysenko described the results as "very encouraging" but hastened to add that it was a small study and needed to be repeated with more patients.

But the relaxation response is just one of many possible ways of using PNI insights to treat the ill. At the University of California at San Francisco

(UCSF), psychologist Lydia Temoshok has been using a psychotherapeutic approach in her work with cancer patients. There are those who fit what she calls the "Type C" (for cancer-prone) personality profile. That kind of individual is cooperative, patient, passive, and appeasing to an extreme. Type C's also suppress negative emotions, particularly anger. Her claim is not that this personality dooms an individual to develop cancer, but that it may affect the progress of the disease. When she asked her psychologist collaborators to single out from 106 patients those who seemed to fit the Type C profile, the group they selected did in fact turn out to have a poorer prognosis than those judged as not having those traits. (It is also possible that the Type C group was sicker to begin with and that influenced their behavior, increasing their chances of being deemed a Type C.)

Based on these preliminary results, Temoshok has embarked on an experimental psychotherapy program for cancer patients, trying to get them to break the vicious cycle of Type C behavior. "Obviously, you have time constraints. There is only so much you can do," she says. And she certainly makes no claims that this treatment will turn a person's life around and mentally "cure" his cancer in one blow. But teaching cancer patients to be a little more assertive about their needs helps improve the quality of their lives and, if there is any basis for the idea that emotions influence the immune system, it could thereby make some difference in their healing.

It is that same belief that motivated the research of the Biopsychosocial AIDS Project now under the direction of Temoshok's UCSF colleague, psychologist Jeffrey Mandel. He has been studying the impact that psychological events have on victims of AIDS. His interviews have turned up patterns of personality traits among the patients: They tend to be stoic about their disappointments and stresses in life; they suppress their negative feelings; they feel guilty and conflict-laden about their homosexuality; and in the year preceding the AIDS diagnosis many experienced a series of stressful life events.

Where this research will lead is not clear yet, but preliminary findings suggest that one way of helping AIDS patients is to assist them in dealing with the trauma of their disease. Neither Mandel nor Dr. George Solomon, who is working with him on the project, make any promises about what it will yield, but at the very least their efforts should make life a little more comfortable for a group of patients often treated as pariahs of our society.

As for the future, the idea that we might be able to influence the immune system has stimulated speculation and inspired novel experiments. In referring to the potential of PNI, for example, Robert Ader has suggested that it might someday be possible to train patients to suppress their immune systems and thereby allow doctors to use smaller doses of toxic immunosuppressant drugs in preparation for organ transplantation, as well as for control of autoimmune diseases or even certain cancers.

Ancient techniques that may also be enlisted to modify the immune system are hypnosis and mental imagery. There has already been some intriguing research on the effects of hypnosis on immunity. In the 1950s and early 1960s British researcher Stephen Black and his colleagues did a series of experiments in which they tried to influence the way the body reacted to common allergens. They took highly hypnotizable individuals whose arms were pricked with substances to which they were allergic. While under hypnosis they were given suggestions that their bodies would not react to the allergens. Among one group of 12 people Black found a reduced allergic reaction among eight individuals. Although no one has replicated Black's experiments, author/physician Dr. Lewis Thomas has said that the experiments were important enough that someone should be trying to repeat the work done in England some 20 years ago.

Black's experiments used only local symptoms to gauge the effectiveness of his technique—the redness and swelling of a spot on the skin and the measures were *in vivo*. A more recent attempt tried at Pennsylvania State University by psychologist Howard Hall focused on the whole immune system and used more modern immuno-logical techniques to measure the reaction. He studied a group of healthy people taught to use a combination of imagery and self-hypnosis and asked them to visualize under hypnosis their white blood cells proliferating and attacking imaginary invaders. After they practiced this daily for a week he took blood samples and compared them to prehypnosis samples. He found that the younger, highly hypnotizable subjects appeared to raise their white blood cell counts significantly. These results have not yet been published, reflecting some controversy about the meaning of the findings. Nevertheless it is an innovative approach. Hall suggests that using hypnosis in this fashion could provide insight into what he calls the "psychology of healing."

Inspired in part by Black's work, my fellow investigators at Harvard's Beth Israel Hospital and I decided to use routine skin test antigens—tuberculin antigen, for example—injected into both arms of a dozen highly hypnotizable people. Enough was injected to evoke an immune reaction in presumably sensitized individuals. Thirty other nonhypnotized people were given the same injections for comparison. Under hypnosis the 12 individuals were instructed to try either to suppress their body's reaction to the antigen or to enhance its reaction *in one arm only.*

There have been a few previous reports of hypnotism having effects on the reaction of the immune system, but they have been scarce and not easily duplicated. Using newer technologies than those employed in the past we attempted to test the idea that the mind can modulate the body's resistance to disease. What we found was that of the dozen hypnotized people, a difference in the immune reaction in the arms occurred in only one person. This does not prove that it is impossible to evoke reactions on demand from the immune system. There are other possible explanations for the lack of any skin test response: It is very possible that the ability to perform this feat exists, but in a very small percentage of individuals; it is also possible that the subjects were not sufficiently trained in hypnosis techniques;

another possibility is that they should have been selected for some trait other than hypnotizability; finally, the problem could have been with the procedures used—the antigen may not have been delivered uniformly to each arm. For all these reasons, and because there is so much anecdotal evidence suggesting that hypnosis can influence the immune system, the idea should not be dismissed. What this and other studies suggest is that more research is needed.

The relationship between the mind and body is certainly unpredictable, but it is one that warrants further investigation, especially since there have been those who have shown that there are ways to exploit the mind-body rapport other than through hypnosis.

Janice Kiecolt-Glaser of the Department of Psychiatry at the Ohio State University College of Medicine demonstrated this recently with a group of healthy elderly people living in a retirement community. Earlier work she and her colleagues had done showed how stress—final exams for medical students—or self-rated loneliness was associated with diminished activity of natural killer immune cells. Reasoning that any strategy which diminished stress and loneliness might have the opposite effect, Kiecolt-Glaser and her fellow researchers divided the elderly test population into three groups. One group was visited regularly by college students for a month to combat the loneliness. A second group was taught a progressive relaxation exercise, which they were asked to practice three times a week for a month. The third group, the controls, were given no treatment or intervention.

Two blood tests were taken from each person, one at the beginning of the month and one at the end. What the tests found was a significant increase in the activity of natural killer cells among those who had practiced relaxation exercises. They found this particularly interesting, as natural killer cells are thought to be part of the body's antitumor surveillance system and they help fight virally-caused infectious diseases.

Psychologist Howard Hall, who has been experimenting with imagery's influence on immunity, talks of the day when medicine will find its way back to using the mind and the powers inherent in the psychology of healing. "You know," he observes, "the psychology of healing kept the human race alive long before the development of modern medicine. People took stuff that we now know to be pharmacologically inactive. But they believed in it, and they got better. Now we've gotten lazy. Our technology is so seductive; 'Let the pill do it.' Well, the pill can't always do it."

6

MEDITATION AND RELAXATION: AN OVERVIEW OF THEIR APPLICATIONS

Daniel Goleman, Ph.D., is the Behavior Writer, Science News for *The New York Times* and a former Senior Editor for *Psychology Today*. He is a recipient of the American Psychological Association National Media Award and the National Association of Mental Health Award. He serves as editorial consultant for the New American Library book series and the *International Journal of Clinical and Experimental Hypnosis*. He was a Harvard University Graduate Fellow in clinical psychology.

Dr. Goleman's most recent book is *Vital Lies, Simple Truths: Cognitive and Social Underpins of Denial* (New York: Simon and Schuster, 1984). He is co-author of *The Essential Psychotherapies* (with Kathleen Speeth), *Introductory Psychology* (with Trygg Engen and Anthony Davis), and *What Psychology Knows That Everyone Should* (with Jonathan Freedman). He was co-editor of *Consciousness: The Brain, States of Awareness, Mysticism* (with Richard Davidson).

For centuries man used meditative techniques to control his mind and body. In the 20th century we have spent millions of dollars creating tools, techniques, pills, and palliatives to treat our illnesses. But we've overlooked the most powerful medical tool, available to us from birth: our minds. In the 1960s we rediscovered meditation. Health practitioners are now urging their patients to use meditation as a means of relieving daily stress, lowering high blood pressure, and easing themselves through painful medical treatments, including chemotherapy. Teaching patients how to achieve deep muscle relaxation may be an important first step toward regaining their health. Dr. Goleman explains how current research into meditation may lead to new forms of medical treatment.∎

It was in 1984 that the National Institute of Health released a consensus report recommending meditation, along with salt and dietary restrictions, as the first treatment for mild hypertension, to be tried before drugs are prescribed. That official recognition of the medical utility of meditation was a benchmark in the spread of meditation and other relaxation techniques as treatments in medicine and psychotherapy. While that recognition has grown slowly and steadily over the course of the 70s and 80s, that spread should accelerate with more and better research establishing the medical utility of relaxation.

I find this recognition of the benefits of meditation and relaxation personally gratifying, since my own professional career has been bound up with these developments, especially its early phases. My own involvement with these techniques goes back to the late 1960s, a time when meditation showed all the signs of being just another passing fad. While a graduate student in clinical psychology at Harvard, I became—along with millions of other Americans—a transcendental meditator.

It was through the transcendental meditation (TM) organization that I began to hear of the emerging scientific literature on the effects of meditation, particularly the work of Wallace and Benson. And from Charles Tart's seminal 1969 collection, *Altered States of Consciousness*, I learned of the studies of Zen meditators in Japan and of Yogis in India. Intrigued, I set off for India as a Harvard Pre-Doctoral Fellow, and spent more than a year there investigating as many schools of meditation and yoga as I could.

On my return to Harvard, I did my dissertation research on meditation and relaxation as antidotes to stress reactivity. Although no longer a TM meditator myself, I used TM teachers in my study, which found that meditation lowered anxiety levels and sped the meditator's recovery from stress arousal. The clinical applications for stress disorders seemed obvious.

I was not alone in my findings. The mid-seventies saw a flood of research on meditation, particularly its health benefits. The methodological rigor of these studies was, frankly, uneven. But the thrust of the findings was clear: meditation helped, in many ways and with many things.

The regular practice of meditation, for instance, lessened the meditator's frequency of colds and headaches and reduced the severity of hypertension. Although these medical applications got some attention, the stronger initial welcome for meditation was from psychotherapists, who saw it as a way for patients to manage anxiety without drugs, to gain access to otherwise blocked memories and feelings, and as a general prescription for handling garden variety stress. Meditation was a stress management tool par excellence and—with a variety of other relaxation techniques—was vigorously marketed that way to schools, hospitals, and businesses.

Meditation and relaxation are not one and the same; meditation is, in essence, the effort to retrain attention. This gives meditation its unique cognitive effects, such as increasing the meditator's concentration and empathy. The most common use of meditation, however, is not for these benefits, but as a quick-and-easy relaxation technique.

Although the Eastern roots of meditation were quite exotic, it became apparent to investigators that, in terms of its metabolic effects, it shared much with homegrown techniques of relaxation, such as Edmund Jacobsen's progressive relaxation and muscle tension biofeedback and with European imports such as autogenic training. Although meditation differed from other relaxation techniques in its attentional components, as Herbert Benson pointed out in his 1975 best-seller, *The Relaxation Response*, much of what was so therapeutic about meditation was its effectiveness in getting the meditator into a state of deep relaxation.

As the research on relaxation techniques for the management of stress disorders has continued, the evidence for their effectiveness has become more compelling. The neuroendocrine changes brought about by becoming deeply relaxed have turned out to be more profound than was first believed by the earlier investigators, who saw relaxation techniques mostly in terms of their relief of muscle tension and mental worry. But more biologically sophisticated investigations have revealed profound effects on immune function, as well as a range of other changes with specific clinical applications.

The findings are of several sorts. Of most general import are the nonspecific effects of relaxation on immune function. Ronald Glazer and Janice Kiecolt-Glazer found that elderly residents of a retirement home who learned and used a relaxation exercise had a significant increase in the strength of their immune defenses against tumors and viruses. Medical students who used these techniques while undergoing the stress of exams showed increased levels of helper cells, which defend against infectious disease. The discovery of these changes would explain earlier reports that meditation, for example, increased resistance to colds and flus.

Perhaps the earliest and strongest medical interest in relaxation has been as an aid in fighting heart disease. Researchers working with Dr. Benson reported that meditation decreased the body's response to norepinephrine, a hormone released in reaction to stress. Although norepinephrine ordinarily stimulates the cardiovascular system, increasing blood pressure, in the meditators it did not have its usual effect. Instead, the meditators showed a diminished blood pressure increase to norepeneprhine, a response that mimics that of the beta-blockers prescribed to control blood pressure.

The clinical use of relaxation to control high blood pressure, especially mild cases, has become a well-established treatment, as the NIH report reflects. The control of blood pressure through relaxation, if practiced faithfully, can often take the place of medication or lessen reliance on drugs. For instance, in a British study, patients trained in these methods were found to have lower blood pressure 4 years after the training ended.

The benefits for heart disease go far beyond controlling blood pressure. Relaxation has been found to benefit patients suffering from angina and arrhythmias and to lower blood cholesterol levels. And Dean Ornish has shown that relaxation training enhances blood flow to the heart, lessening the danger from silent ischemia.

Diabetics, too, can benefit from relaxation. Richard Surwit found that relaxation training improved the regulation of glucose in patients with adult-onset diabetes. And Paul Lehrer, using Jacobsen's progressive relaxation with asthmatics, found that it lessened the emotional reactions that often preceded attacks and improved the flow in the airway passages that become constricted during the attacks.

For pain patients, some forms of relaxation offer particular promise. Jon Kabat-Zinn found that mindfulness meditation, coupled with yoga, lowered the reliance on pain-killers and lessened the level of pain in patients who had suffered chronic pain. The causes of the pain ranged from backaches and headaches (both migraine and tension) to the range of cases seen in pain clinics. The benefits of the training held even 4 years after the training ended for the patients.

Relaxation techniques of all kinds are being used with medical patients of many different kinds, particularly where stress plays a causative role or exacerbates the problem—and there are few cases where it does not. Some of the more promising applications are with the side effects of kidney dialysis and cancer chemotherapy, gastrointestinal disorders, insomnia, emphysema, and skin disorders. At the same time, relaxation is widely used as an adjunct in psychotherapy, where it has been accepted far longer than in medicine.

Even so, there are some problems in applying these techniques. For one, there are some people—though very few—who react to relaxation with increased tension and even panic. For these people, relaxation may need to be introduced after special cognitive preparation, or not at all.

One task ahead is to sort out the significant differences, if any, between relaxation and meditation techniques in terms of the kinds of people and problems for which they will be most effective. But, as the research evidence makes clear, these methods offer a powerful way to tap the inner capacity of patients to aid with their own healing.

7 BIOFEEDBACK: TECHNOLOGY AND AWARENESS

Dennis T. Jaffe, Ph.D., is Director of the Center for Health Studies at Saybrook Institute in San Francisco. He is the author of *Healing from Within*, which brought Dr. Jaffe a Medical Self-Care Book Award. He is a co-author of *From Burnout to Balance, The ESSI Systems Stress Map,* and *Take This Job and Love It!*

Some of our physical responses to external stimuli are conscious and some are not. We believe we can control some responses and not others. Biofeedback is a technique that enables a person to voluntarily control his internal responses. It has been used to control high blood pressure, heart rate, migraine headaches, chronic pain, psychosomatic illnesses, and nervous disorders. It has also been useful in counteracting alcoholism and drug addiction, and it has helped lifelong smokers to kick the habit. Medicine in the future may incorporate the techniques of biofeedback and meditation. These techniques have revolutionized our understanding of healing by weakening a traditional medical premise that the mind and the body can be treated separately.∎

Biofeedback is a learning process that is often confused with the monitoring apparatus that helps an individual become aware of his or her shifting internal processes. Using tiny sensors that instantaneously pick up subtle variations in bodily functions—such as temperature, muscle tension, skin conductance, blood pressure, or brain waves—a person learns how to "feel" body shifts. After receiving this form of physiological feedback for a while, the person begins to learn how to use conscious awareness to create changes in the body processes being measured. In a few hour-long sessions, a person learns to increase or decrease muscle tension, blood flow, even turn on and off alpha brain waves. The biofeedback equipment is like trainer wheels on a bike. Once learned, the person can make the desired changes without the additional information from the machine. He or she knows how it feels when the changes take place.

What's the importance of this learning? The simple physical processes that can come under conscious control are relevant to many serious and chronic illnesses. For example, headaches can often be relieved by decreasing muscle tension or blood flow, which can be learned through biofeedback. High blood pressure can often be reduced by learning to relax and by diminishing muscle tension or raising hand temperature. Achieving these results through consciousness enables one to avoid the negative side effects of drug treatment. Many serious physical symptoms, and many of the daily negative effects of excess stress, can be reduced through biofeedback training.

But the consequences are broader than symptom relief. Increasing internal sensitivity to one's physical functions is the essence of self-care. Many serious ailments can be sidetracked early if we simply become aware of early warning signs. Inner self-awareness has other positive effects. If one is able to control one's physical self through conscious awareness rather than with drugs, you feel a deeper and greater sense of self-confidence, self-reliance, and personal power, all of which have been linked to greater physical and psychological health.

Biofeedback apparatus can be thought of as a learning tool, a programmed textbook that moves a person on the road to self-awareness and self-care. Less than 20 years ago it was thought that conscious control over internal physiological functions, like blood flow and brain waves, was not possible. A person could control the muscles of the voluntary nervous system, but the involuntary, or autonomic, nervous system, connected to the endocrine system, stress response, and circulatory system, was not susceptible to conscious control. Biofeedback research has broken down that barrier, leaving health practitioners with the message that the limits to the power of the mind to influence and modify the body have yet to be reached. More recent research on the immune system, which enables the body to heal and fight off all sorts of invaders, including cancer, suggests that it also may be within our conscious control. The new tools of computers and technology bring us more instantaneous information about inner states, which we in turn can learn to shift and change at will. This chapter will explore the history, research, use, and potential of biofeedback training as a pathway to healing.

A CASE EXAMPLE

The best way to get a sense of how biofeedback can become part of a self-care learning program is to report on one person's experience. Jean, a 45-year-old woman, overweight, with many chronic pain and stress symptoms, was referred to me by her family physician, who was alarmed by the medication she was taking and frustrated by her inability to find relief. Jean seemed unmotivated to deal with her ailments, but underneath, she believed she was helpless to do anything about it. Surprisingly, she responded positively when biofeedback treatment was suggested. For many people, science and technology provoke trust and credibility that a nonmechanical approach like meditation does not. Also, Jean's insurance company would reimburse her for biofeedback as a "medical treatment," while it would not pay for meditation training, health classes, or psychotherapy. This implied to her that biofeedback had more validity as a treatment.

The biofeedback equipment was compact, like a cassette recorder with an added digital readout screen. Like other technical equipment, biofeedback equipment has become miniaturized, inexpensive, more precise, and easier to use in the past few years, and it can be linked with any small computer for complete printouts of changes during a session. In a few seconds, wires from the machine were connected with velcro binders, to Jean's fingers and forehead, and attached to her shoulders with Band-aid-like patches. These sensors monitored changes in blood flow (finger temperature), skin conductance (like the polygraph, a measure of anxiety and tension), brain waves, and muscle tension. On the digital screen or via a modulating sound, Jean could instantly see or hear a display of the tiniest fluctuations in her internal functioning.

At the beginning of Jean's first session the digital screen registered her hand temperature at 76 degrees, not uncommon for extremities but suggesting some tension. Another readout of muscle tension suggested that her shoulders and forehead muscles were unusually tense. Jean learned that when she relaxed, the blood vessels would dilate and her hands and feet would warm up.

Jean tried to relax but to her surprise and frustration her muscle tension shot up slightly, and her hand temperature went down one degree. Why had her first attempts failed? Her conscious efforts, which included bracing herself for a difficult ordeal, had inadvertently placed her body into the stress response. This was probably the way she prepared herself for other challenges in her life—by tightening up, bracing for danger. Overuse or inappropriate activation of the stress response over time leads to an incredible range of stress-related illnesses.

Jean was told not to try too hard. Instead, she should try thinking of something relaxing and pleasant—perhaps a lovely day at the beach. Within moments, her hand temperature began to inch up, and her muscle tension diminished. As she imagined peaceful times, which included memories of her pain-free past, her thoughts drifted away from trying to do anything in her body. Her temperature climbed and her muscle tension continued to drop until, 15 minutes later, her hands registered 90 degrees.

Jean was delighted and surprised. By the end of the hour she was also feeling energized and free of pain. How was she able to modify her body and relax so deeply? She succeeded by adhering to the principle of "passive volition," which is the key to modifying the autonomic nervous system. You succeed not by making anything happen, or trying hard, but by imagining that something is happening that brings your body to the desired state. Other people imagine their muscles letting go of tension like limp rubber bands or their hands dipping into a bowl of hot water. The memory is transferred into the body; the body follows the instructions provided in the mental image.

As biofeedback pioneer Barbara Brown proposes in *Stress and the Art of Biofeedback*, there are few internal processes that a person can't learn to control with the proper feedback. In a classic experiment, psychologist John Basmajian taught his patients to fire a single neuron without activating any of the other neurons around it!

Jean learned two crucial experiential skills in her session. First, she could control the workings of her body in a positive direction, even more quickly and effectively than with medication. Second, she learned she could accomplish that not by trying but by letting it happen in her body, using an image representing how she wanted to be. Her success lifted her out of her rut and eroded her sense of helplessness. She began her road to healing through self-regulation.

In the ensuing weeks, Jean pursued an extensive learning program, incorporating more biofeedback, but also practicing at home using relaxation methods and cassette tapes, as well as counseling, to modify some of the stressful situations in her life. Biofeedback was the center of the educational process, by which she learned to "read" her internal body signs, to connect them with emotionally difficult situations in her life, and to take herself out of the negative "bracing" that had been her universal response to pressure. The machinery did not become a crutch; instead, by giving her objective data on how well she was doing, it helped instill self-confidence and verified that the mental techniques she was using were indeed having the desired physical effects.

RATS AND SWAMIS: THE POSSIBILITY OF SELF-CONTROL

The detailed, instantaneous, continuous inner information that comes through biofeedback is only useful when it helps make long-lasting changes in the body. Two types of research have been useful in opening the road to voluntary self-control: research on rats, and research on extraordinary human beings who seemingly perform superhuman feats.

Following the lead of Russian psychologist Ivan Pavlov, Neal Miller and his colleagues at Rockefeller University demonstrated that autonomic functions could be changed via a learning process. Rats whose voluntary muscles were paralyzed with drugs were nonetheless able to alter their blood pressure, heart rate, intestinal contractions, and urine formation to avoid electrical shocks. The shocks were the rats' version of biofeedback, and they quickly learned to modify their physical responses in the desired direction, going against traditional medical science that had postulated that they could not.

Could people learn as well as rats? Indeed, the next line of research was to use new computer technology so that readings could be obtained from the body, without puncturing the skin, that were exact, that did not take much time, that could quickly pick up slight shifts, and that could be read and understood as easily as reading a clock. So, instead of having to wait 3 minutes for a mouth thermometer to register temperature, and then having to squint at the mercury for another minute, a person could instantly and precisely determine if his temperature—or anxiety level—was moving up or down. Many research groups developed this new technology, and people used biofeedback to learn to relax and to modify myriad negative physical symptoms that caused pain and endangered health.

Feedback is part of every control and guidance system. Consider driving a car. Your eyes receive signals telling you whether you are staying in your lane. If the feedback from your eyes says you have hit the lane divider, your hands are signalled to take corrective action via the steering wheel. Biofeedback represents the extension of that same principle to the body. If you get continuous feedback on things that are happening beneath the skin—tiny changes in tension, temperature, or brain electricity, for example—then you can begin to experiment with ways to change it. For example, you get biofeedback that the muscle tension in your forehead is high. Then you tell your head to let go. The feedback tells you that you haven't succeeded; indeed, you may see that tension has gone up a microvolt or so. The problem in learning physiological self-control is that the controls aren't as obvious as those in an automobile. There isn't an internal steering wheel or brake pedal. When you receive signals from the body, you have to use an often extensive trial-and-error mode of learning to discover what you need to do to get the desired results. That learning process, once completed, offers unprecedented power over aspects of your self that are connected to many of the common, and even most lethal, illnesses of our time.

The feedback about what is happening in the body can be offered in any form. Barbara Brown, in her laboratory in a Veterans' Hospital, hooked up an electric train so that it would run as long as a person's muscle tension was diminishing and stop if the person tensed up or remained the same. Her patients learned to relax without tensing or trying by having train races where the winner was the most relaxed. Biofeedback can take many forms. Today, there are several computer games that run on biofeedback, including one that can be run by modifying brain waves. The era of telepathy may be at hand as computer technology teaches us to extend the limits of conscious control over inner functions.

What are the limits of conscious control over the body? How much can we learn to change, or heal, with the aid of biofeedback? Elmer and Alyce Green of the Menninger Clinic, and more recently Harvard cardiologist and relaxation teacher Herbert Benson, have gone to India to study yogis who were reportedly able to exercise amazing feats of self-control. Yoga stems from a philosophy of mind/body unity, inner awareness, and self-control. The Greens invited Swami Rama, who purportedly could stop his heart, control his brain waves, and exercise almost total internal self-awareness, to come to their laboratory in Kansas. During an array of tests, he demonstrated astonishing control over his autonomic functions—heart rate, blood flow, temperature, pain receptors, brain waves, and most internal muscles. His responses were all recorded in the Greens' biofeedback lab. The Greens report in their book *Beyond Biofeedback* that, on the final day of his stay, he actually stopped his heart—a dangerous and seemingly impossible maneuver—while hooked up to their monitoring devices. He did this by making his heart muscle contract so fast (several hundred times a minute) that blood could not flow through it for 30 seconds!

Another series of feats were performed with a Dutch meditation teacher, Jack Schwartz, who was able to pass a dirty knitting needle through his arm without shedding a drop of blood or becoming infected. Both Swami Rama and Jack Schwartz have helped hundreds of people to achieve internal self-control, using meditation techniques supplemented by biofeedback.

In the 1960s biofeedback attracted attention when Joseph Kamiya reported that he had used it to train his students at San Francisco State to produce a particular type of brain wave that was associated with the high levels of consciousness reported by Eastern meditators. The press reported that people could obtain instant enlightenment as they programmed their brain waves. In fact, people could learn to produce states of deep relaxation and peace by producing alpha waves. However, there was some doubt as to whether this was the most effective way to learn to relax. Other forms of biofeedback were less difficult to measure and had much clearer results. Another research project by the Greens at the Menninger Foundation involved training people to produce another type of brain wave—theta waves—which are associated with creativity. Just before drifting into sleep, a person has a preponderance of theta waves. By training people to enter theta, they produced all sorts of creative imagery. These and other experiments with brain waves are helping researchers to map brain function and to explore some of the broader possibilities of human consciousness and creativity. But since the results of brain wave measurement are still controversial and complex (there are many areas of the brain that must be measured simultaneously and then averaged), brain wave biofeedback has become less of a clinical tool, and is now mostly used in brain research.

Even early biofeedback research such as this suggested that voluntary, internal self-regulation was potentially as powerful as drug treatment and certainly far safer. How can people learn to accomplish this? Erik Peper, former president of the Biofeedback Society of America, an organization of several thousand researchers and clinicians, notes two common factors in achieving internal self-control: 1) passive attention, the opposite of actively "trying", and 2) focusing on the process and paying active attention to it, rather than on the outcome or the goal. Adepts like the Swami and Schwartz, and others like Rolling Thunder, a native American medicine man also in the Greens' study, report that they enter a special state of consciousness where their attention is focused on what is going on in the here-and-now, not on where they want to go. When they use imagination, as Jean did in the earlier example, they imagine something happening in their body right now, as if it is going on. Achieving self-regulation involves learning to let go and to allow change, or healing, to take place. These principles form the basis for all relaxation, meditation, and self-regulation exercises.

BIOFEEDBACK AND HEALING

Biofeedback is an important clinical tool for teaching people not just how to relax, but how to control life-threatening and dangerous symptoms that sometimes cannot be treated any other way. Before it could be used as a clinical tool, researchers had to determine what happened to patients after the electrodes were removed. Whereas a patient might be able to relax in the laboratory or office, he might leave the office and have a heart attack an hour later when he ran into a stressful situation. We had to be able to learn biofeedback without machines.

One of Neal Miller's first patients was Robin, a young woman with slight brain damage complicated by dangerously high blood pressure, a body state that can lead to heart attacks. Whereas elevated blood pressure produces no discomfort, it is like a time bomb in the body that can go off at any moment. Therefore, physicians have learned that they need to reduce blood pressure, most often by using drugs that have serious and unpleasant side effects. Robin was selected to see if she could became aware of her blood pressure and learn to control it using biofeedback rather than drugs.

A complicated machine was devised to measure shifts in her blood pressure, and she began her learning process. A light flashed when her blood pressure was dropping, but would go off if it were rising or staying the same. Her task was to keep the light on. At first, the fluctuations were nearly random. Robin felt nothing and had no sense of how or why the changes were happening. Gradually, following hunches, subtle cues, and a lot of trial and error throughout 20 sessions, she began to learn how to reduce her blood pressure. She did it by inventing her own method of relaxation.

Robin became so successful that she was taken off medication. Her blood pressure increased again, but in a few days Robin brought it down again. Here's her account of how she did it:

I was determined to succeed. I felt that this was the only part of my treatment that I could do anything about at all, and I am a habitual overachiever. At first, it seemed that lowering my blood pressure was only a simple muscular trick. I thought it was only a matter of relaxing my stomach, my chest, my breathing, but none of these worked all the time. I found I could drop my pressure quickly by fooling with my muscles, but I could only sustain the drop if I relaxed my mind. It all seemed to depend on clearing my mind of all stressful thoughts. . . . Making the pressure go up is a lot easier than lowering it. The best way to get it up is to take a big breath and think angry thoughts—I may remember some real jackass I knew in the past and get mad all over again at his stupidity.

Robin found that she could recognize when her blood pressure was going up, then use her techniques to bring it down. It sharpened her awareness of internal sensations and taught her to modify them when needed. Like many successful biofeedback patients, Robin needed a periodic refresher session to sharpen her skills and reinforce what she had learned.

Many patients ask for biofeedback as if it were a new pill. They are prepared to play only the traditional passive patient role. They want the treatment done to them; they aren't really clear that they have to perform the treatment themselves. They think the machine will change them, when actually they need to learn a new skill. It demands many sessions—from 5 to 20—and daily home practice. But the rewards in the form of increased self-control and health can be enormous. It's just that they don't come easily.

There are some clear limitations to biofeedback as a healing tool. It is not effective if the particular physiological function is not easily accessible (e.g., without having to put a needle under the skin). The function must be measurable, and it must be something that the body has the capacity to control. Dilation of blood vessels or the secretion of hormones can be controlled. Biofeedback would not help a person grow back a severed finger.

The internal functions that are easiest to modify are those that are the closest to consciousness. Muscle tension, for example, is easy to detect at the skin's surface, and because muscles are under conscious control, a person can quickly release this form of tension. Chronic tension in the back, the shoulders, or the forehead leads to chronic pain. Once the back is strained or a headache has begun, it is difficult to make it go away. However, through biofeedback a person can become aware of the subtle early warning signs of increasing tension. A person can abort a headache more easily in the hour before it begins than after it has blossomed.

Muscle tension, low temperature in the hands, and low skin conductance are all signs of the activation of the stress response. Many of our chronic ailments, our days lost from work, and our more serious illnesses stem from the build-up of such tension. Often stress can build up because we are not aware it exists. Many people cope with the strain of life's pressures by ignoring their bodies. They ignore tension until it leads to a breakdown or crisis.

For example, in a training session with a group of male executives who were recovering from heart attacks, nearly all maintained that they knew how to cope with stress, that it didn't get to them, and that they were relaxed. Each one was then given the opportunity to try biofeedback. To their surprise, when they experienced themselves as relaxed, their true muscle tension was about ten times higher than a person should be at rest. Their bodies had developed the habit of not registering the real tension they were accumulating. Consequently, they were not receiving tension warnings that may have led them to slow down. The biofeedback made them aware that they were habitually carrying an immense amount of tension, and they learned how to release it.

Biofeedback works best when a specific, somewhat localized symptom troubles a person. For example, Raynaud's disease (a bloodflow constriction that leads to abnormally cold hands and feet), abnormal heart rhythms, specific muscle atrophy with no organic damage, teeth grinding, headaches, and other conditions related to chronic tension in one particular muscle group have all been relieved by using biofeedback. Such ailments can be permanently altered with biofeedback.

Bernard Engel taught patients with cardiac arrhythmia, a comparatively mild symptom that can have serious health consequences, to recognize irregularity in their heartbeats by watching light signals reflecting their heart rhythms. After a while they could sense the irregularity and control it. In a follow-up study several years later, many still maintained this sensitivity and regular heart functioning. They no longer needed medication— an impressive demonstration.

While the physiological mechanisms that produce illness generally are complex, interconnected, difficult to measure, and thus not particularly treatable by biofeedback, the number of illnesses that can be treated is increasing as technology develops. For example, Barney Alexander and his colleagues at the City of Hope Medical Center have developed several ingenious biofeedback sensors to help people with asthma develop control over their asthma symptoms and chest/lung congestion. Asthma sufferers can learn to feel the build-up of fluid blocking their lungs and they can learn to slow down this blockage or even decongest their lungs.

THE FRONTIERS OF BIOFEEDBACK

In the 20 or so years since Miller's breakthrough research, biofeedback has gone beyond the laboratory into the hospital, the clinic, and everyday life. While research has gathered momentum, many different types of illnesses from headaches to ulcers have been found to be susceptible to biofeedback control, and medical and psychological practitioners have begun offering this procedure to their patients. The Biofeedback Society of America develops clinical standards, treatment techniques, and training programs, and certifies qualified biofeedback technicians. Many companies make biofeedback machines, and more and more hospitals and medical offices feature them. Their virtue is that the treatment is relatively inexpensive. With a technician as coach and trainer, a person can come to an office and be hooked up, then work on his or her own. Checking and discussion come at the end of the session, and homework for daily practice is assigned. A person can work every day on gaining self-control.

Over the past few years, the price and size of apparatus has gone down, and a new biofeedback industry has formed. Portable relaxation machines, costing only a few dollars and as accurate as the original machines used by Miller and his associates, are sold at department stores. They come with cassette relaxation tapes and instructions, so any person can learn the rudiments of relaxation. In medical offices, these portable home machines are often loaned or sold to people who want to help their home practice. While the more serious one's medical condition, the more need there is for professional supervision, these machines are practical and helpful aids to general stress management.

Biofeedback is part of the popular culture, and that has had positive effects. Through biofeedback, many esoteric techniques such as meditation have been verified as having clear healing capacities, and the use of biofeedback has demystified relaxation and meditation for many lay people.

The frontier of biofeedback continues to expand. Every day, researchers are seeking ways to measure additional body functions. For example, if we were able to measure the degree of secretion of body hormones, or the activation of certain lymphocytes that make up the immune system, then we might be able to supercharge our body into hyperactive healing when we were ill.

We might speculate what would happen if the principles of self-regulation were made part of childhood education. Just as the child learns to control his voluntary muscles in writing and in sports, so he could begin to learn to increase internal awareness, to understand tension and stress from the inside, and to create changes in physical states at will. Imagine grade school students learning to keep their blood pressure down or reduce muscle tension. By the time they were adults, they might achieve a degree of inner familiarity and self-regulatory capacity that could go far beyond what Swami Rama and others could learn in 20 or more years of practice in their adult years. Like many skills, the earlier and the more naturally the skill is made a part of one's life, the more effective a person can use it. Self-regulation and self-healing might be the first line of defense against stress and major illnesses.

PART III

HEALTH EMPOWERMENT: YOUR ENVIRONMENT

8 **The Importance of the Social Environment for Health and Well-Being**
S. Leonard Syme, Ph.D.

9 **The Health of Cities**
Leonard Duhl, M.D.

10 **Children and Youth in Cities: The Story of Seattle's KidsPlace**
Robert A. Aldrich, M.D.

11 **Occupational Diseases**
Phillip Polakoff, M.D.

12 **Health Empowerment: An Approach to Community-Controlled Self-Care Development**
Lowell S. Levin, Ph.D.

8 THE IMPORTANCE OF THE SOCIAL ENVIRONMENT FOR HEALTH AND WELL-BEING

S. Leonard Syme, Ph.D., is Professor of Epidemiology at the School of Public Health at the University of California, Berkeley. His major research work has been in two areas: 1) the study of psychosocial factors as they influence the development of disease (with special emphasis on coronary heart disease and hypertension), and 2) the application of research findings at the community level in order to prevent disease and promote health. Dr. Syme's latest book (co-edited with Dr. Shelton Cohen) is *Social Support and Health*, published by Academic Press in 1985.

Our society affects our health. We don't yet understand why some cultures or races are more susceptible than other groups to certain diseases or why some groups tend to live longer, healthier lives than others. But there is evidence that the social environment plays an important role. We are not talking about hereditary differences or contagious elements of disease within a group of people or a geographical area. We are discussing the effects of group life upon the health of individuals. Professor Syme explains how greater awareness of this impact may prevent disease and promote better health.■

When we think about staying healthy and preventing disease, most of us think, naturally enough, that this desirable state of affairs is in our own hands. For example, to improve our health and prevent illness, we can stop smoking, eat better, lose weight, and drive more carefully. We can visit physicians, dentists, and other medical professionals to seek help in changing our behavior or to get medicines. In many cases, it is true that we can ensure health and well being only by our own behavior. In many other cases, however, our health is affected in significant ways by the environments in which we live. In this chapter we will review the impact of the *social environment* on health and well being. Since environmental factors affect our health in important ways, a better understanding of this influence is essential to the prevention of disease and the promotion of health.

DISEASE RISK FACTORS AND BEHAVIOR CHANGES

A considerable amount of medical research is aimed at identifying risk factors for disease. The rationale behind this work is that when people are informed of their risks, they will happily change their behavior to lower that risk. Although this is certainly a reasonable assumption, it turns out that things are not quite that simple and straightforward. First of all, health is not necessarily a top priority in everyone's life and, for these people, changing behavior in the interests of health may interfere with other, more important, matters. Second, the benefits to be derived from such changes rarely are immediate or obvious. Usually improvements in health take place over long periods of time and are quite subtle. Third, we all are so bombarded with information about the thousands of health hazards to which we are exposed that most of us "tune out" much of this information. This latter issue is compounded by the fact that much of the new information to which we are exposed through the media is exaggerated and, as often as not, is contradicted later by even "newer" information. For these and other reasons, simply knowing about a risk does not necessarily

ensure that people will take appropriate steps to lower it.

Even when people want to change their behavior, this is not easy to do. For example, the overwhelming majority of smokers in this country want to quit, but despite great effort very few are able to do so. Most smokers acknowledge, at some level, the health hazards associated with smoking and most wish that there were a simple and painless way to stop. Similarly, the number of people who want to lose weight is very large, but few of these people are able to do it and even fewer are able to maintain such weight losses.

Perhaps the most dramatic example of the difficulty we have in changing unhealthful behaviors is provided by the Multiple Risk Factor Intervention Trial (MRFIT). This trial was the most ambitious effort ever organized to test the hypothesis that mortality rates from coronary heart disease could be reduced if people changed their behavior. After 7 years of follow-up, disappointingly few people had made and maintained the recommended changes. These findings are of particular importance because this trial contained all the elements one would desire in an intervention program and, for this reason, one would have anticipated better results than were achieved. Three features of the trial are of special importance: First, the 6,428 men randomized to the Special Intervention group had been carefully and clearly informed of the fact that they were in the top 15% risk category in the country for coronary heart disease. They also knew that their risk was due specifically to high serum cholesterol levels, high blood pressure, and/or cigarette smoking. Indeed, before being selected for the trial, each man had agreed to change his eating and smoking behavior and to take antihypertensive medications if necessary. Thus, all of the men in the trial knew of their special risk and had volunteered to change behaviors to lower it. Second, an excellent intervention plan was devised to help people change their behavior. This plan was carefully developed to take account of individual circumstances and it used a variety of approaches, including group meetings, one-on-one counselling sessions, and opportunities to involve family members. Research findings from the behavioral literature were reviewed and, wherever appropriate, successful strategies were included in the plan. Third, the staffing pattern at each of the 22 MRFIT clinics was designed so that each participant would have close and continuing contact with well-trained professionals for the entire 7-year study period.

In spite of these unique features, the behavior changes observed in MRFIT were of modest proportions. The best achievement was that 40% of smokers had stopped smoking by the fourth year of the trial. Of those men with hypertension, 64% had controlled their hypertension by that time. But only a 6.7% reduction was observed in serum cholesterol levels. It should be noted that these results refer only to men in the Special Intervention (SI) group and not to the 6,438 men in the Usual Care (UC) group. The overall objective of the trial was to see if those in SI would have a lower mortality rate from coronary heart disease than those in the UC group. The mortality results after 7 years of follow-up in MRFIT showed no statistically significant difference between these study groups. This result was due, in part, to the fact that men in the UC group changed their behavior on their own. Indeed, they changed to such an extent that the contrast in behavior change between the two groups was much smaller than had been anticipated. Why men in the UC group changed so dramatically is an important topic in its own right; for the purpose of our discussion here, however, it is important to note that men in the SI group changed much less than was anticipated.

In an ordinary study, the results achieved in the SI group would have been quite acceptable. In MRFIT, however, they were disappointing because this trial included so many of the elements needed for a complete success: an informed and highly motivated group of participants, a superb intervention plan, excellent staff in sufficient numbers, and enough time to bring about behavioral change. That the results observed fell short of 100% is disappointing because this was probably the best program that could be devised. It would

be hard to imagine a situation better suited to complete success.

From the MRFIT example, it seems clear that wanting to change behavior is not enough; nor is it enough to provide people with lots of information and research data; nor is it enough to bring in experts in behavior change. Two lessons can be drawn from this experience: (1) we *can* achieve some success in one-on-one efforts, but (2) even under the best one-on-one circumstances, results cannot be perfect or even close to perfection.

BEHAVIOR CHANGES AND THE SOCIAL ENVIRONMENT

In spite of the fact that people find it difficult to change behavior in the interest of better health, major changes have occurred in such behaviors. For example, about 32% to 35% of the adult U.S. population now smoke cigarettes compared to over 40% smoking in 1964. Among teenagers, about 20% now smoke while almost 30% smoked in 1977. In many parts of the country, it is increasingly difficult for people to smoke cigarettes at parties or at restaurants. It would be difficult indeed to convince large numbers of men (or women) to take up chewing tobacco and to use spitoons for their tobacco juice—a practice that was widespread earlier in this century. With regard to fatness, it is not nearly as easy to be fat as it was only 30 or 40 years ago in this country. Although the reasons for these changes are complex, it is clear that behaviors are socially acceptable at certain times and less so at other times. This "climate of acceptability" is a potent force in shaping our behavior and inclination. Thus, although we think we are free agents with regard to behavior and tastes, it turns out that we are influenced to a greater or lesser extent by the social environment within which we find ourselves. We may think we act on our own, but much of what we believe and want is influenced by the customs, traditions, and values of the groups to which we belong. When we fail to take into account the importance of this social environment, we are ignoring what may be some of the most important influences on behavior.

Let us consider the case of cigarette smoking as an example of this issue. An enormous number of programs have been established since the early 1960s to help people give up smoking. Most people who participate in these programs are not able to stop; of those who do succeed, most do not abstain from smoking for any substantial period of time. In general, only about 20% to 25% of all people who try to quit permanently are successful. In all of these programs, we have viewed the problem of smoking entirely as a problem of the individual. We have carefully considered the smoker's motivations and perceptions, need for information, and disease risks. Rarely, however, have we considered the social and cultural environment of the smoker: the cultural associations between smoking and relaxation, adulthood, sexual attractiveness, and emancipation; the economic structure of tobacco production, processing, distribution, and legislation; the extensive program of advertising by the tobacco industry; the behavior of role models such as movie stars, teachers, and doctors; and the influence of parents, siblings, and peers. All of these have important influences on who starts smoking, how long they smoke, and how difficult it is to stop. To consider only the smoker and to ignore all of these environmental influences is to miss perhaps some of the most important factors of all.

THE SOCIAL ENVIRONMENT IS PEOPLE

In recent years, more and more research is being done to study the relationship between the social environment and health and disease. The first modern study on this issue was done in 1897 by Emile Durkheim, a French sociologist. At that time, Durkheim was studying the causes of suicide—a cause of death that was considered primarily a consequence of individual and private suffering. Durkheim noted that most other diseases were clearly influenced by environmental factors: For example, many diseases could be traced to impure water, food, air, and other diseases to hazardous working and living conditions. Suicide, on the other hand, was considered a product of intensely personal and intimate feelings and problems. Nevertheless, Durkheim noted that suicide rates were characteristically higher or lower in certain occupational, religious, and geographic groups and that these differences persist although individuals in these groups come and go over the years. How could it be, Durkheim asked, that groups produced the same rate of suicide among individuals, even when people in those groups were continuously entering and leaving them? Durkheim proposed that to account for this phenomenon, one must discover something about the group itself and not simply about the characteristics of individuals within the group. Durkheim's research led him to conclude that the major factor affecting suicide rates was the degree of social integration of groups. He suggested that the extent to which the individual was integrated into group life influenced the likelihood that the individual would be motivated to commit suicide. In addition to Durkheim's substantive contribution regarding the causes of suicide, however, is the important observation that systematic patterned differences in disease rates between groups must be explainable in group terms.

Since Durkheim's work, a substantial body of research has accumulated showing that people with fewer social ties have higher rates of disease than people with more ties. In one study of 7,000 adults done in Alameda County, California, people who were unmarried, had few friends and relatives, and who did not belong to social groups or churches died two to three times more frequently during a 9-year follow-up period than those with more social connections. This finding was observed for all age groups and for both sexes. Another study done in Techumseh, Michigan, came up with basically the same results as were found in California. Since those studies were done, projects in Durham, North Carolina; Evans County, Georgia; and North Karelia, Finland, have confirmed these findings.

The important thing about these findings is that in virtually every study, the link between social connections and disease is independent of other major disease risk factors. Thus, the higher rate of disease seen among those with few social ties is not simply due to the fact that these people smoke more, are more overweight, are sedentary, drink more alcoholic beverages, and so on. After these factors are taken into account, people with few social ties continue to have disease rates about two to three times higher than those with more ties.

In the search for another explanation for these findings, several researchers have suggested that people with fewer social ties are more likely to be sick at the time they participate in research projects; if this were true, it is argued, these people would have fewer social relationships *because* of their illness and they would, of course, also be more likely to get sicker and to die later on. In this scenario, it is the fact of *sickness* that causes fewer social ties and not vice versa. This possibility has been studied carefully in Alameda County, in Techumseh, and in North Karelia and found not to be true. Thus, after taking account of health status at the beginning of these research projects, social ties still strongly predict subsequent disease events.

It also is important to note that social networks influence a wide range of conditions and diseases, not just one or two. Thus, higher rates have been seen among lonely people for heart disease, cancer, arthritis, mental illness, childhood infections, complications of pregnancy and delivery, and low self-esteem and depression. In addition, the absence of social networks has been observed to affect recovery from a variety of diseases. Unfortunately, little is known about how social networks "get into the body" to affect so many different diseases and the conditions of many organ systems.

One idea that has been suggested is that the absence of networks somehow depresses the immune system so that the body's defenses are weakened. In this view, any number of disease agents can subsequently cause disease. The absence of social networks, therefore, affects whether or not one becomes ill, but it does not influence the type of disease that occurs. Another suggestion is that the presence of social networks provides people with information and assistance,

so that they can take better care of themselves. And when they are not well, these people can get good advice about medical care. Yet a third idea is that people frequently behave like other members of their networks. If people have ties to others who do not smoke or drink to excess, who are physically active, and who eat sensibly, they may be influenced to behave in similar ways simply to maintain their friendships.

Research evidence is available to support all of these possibilities, but their relative importance in explaining the causes of disease is not yet clear. What *is* clear is that a link does indeed exist between social networks and disease.

MAKE FRIENDS TO PREVENT DISEASE?

If social networks are helpful in preventing disease, is it reasonable to suggest that people develop more and deeper friendships? Are several friends more helpful than one or two? Is it important to really *like* people or is it enough merely to have people around? Is it better to *receive* help and advice from others than it is to *give* help and advice to others? The answers to these and similar questions are important for anyone trying to enhance health and well being. Unfortunately, few answers are available for these questions. The latest evidence, however, suggests that the crucial ingredient in social networks is whether people are available to help in specific circumstances. If you need a ride, is there someone you can count on to give you one? If you need to borrow money, is there someone you can count on to loan it to you? The evidence also suggests that a variety of people may be needed in one's network to cover a variety of situations.

Here again, the importance of the social environment cannot be overlooked. It is not reasonable to urge people to make friends when the environments in which they live and work are designed to make this difficult. At work, the provision of coffee rooms or lounges makes it easier for people to meet; the absence of such areas discourages social interaction. Similarly, work groups that make it easier for people to work together on tasks have been shown to be more efficient and congenial than in offices where workers are isolated from one another. In residential areas, it is often possible to provide places where people can meet or pass one another so that interactions are facilitated. These types of environmental designs are not intended to *force* people to be sociable but rather to enhance the opportunity for interaction if it is wanted. The point is that the social environment is important to health and it can be designed to facilitate or hinder healthful living. To burden people with advice about sociability when the environment is a negative force is not only inappropriate but also unfair.

THE ETHICS OF ENVIRONMENTAL INTERVENTION

There are three ways to bring about behavior change. People can decide to make such changes on their own, their environment can be changed to facilitate such changes, and laws can be passed to prohibit unwanted behavior. Each of these is appropriate depending on the circumstance. The isolation of people with certain contagious diseases is required by law and is probably the best way to enforce that behavior, as is the law that drivers stop at red traffic lights. Introducing environmental interventions such as safer highways and designing safer cars with passive restraints built into them is probably more effective in saving lives than teaching people, one at a time, to drive more safely. On the other hand, many believe it is each individual's responsibility to choose a dietary pattern, drink alcoholic beverages in moderation, avoid obesity, avoid smoking, and be physically active. Serious questions have arisen about the appropriateness of introducing environmental interventions to bring about such healthful behaviors. This kind of manipulation easily can be seen as dictatorial and paternalistic.

This is a complex issue that deserves careful thought. No one would argue against laws that protect us from people with contagious diseases or from unsafe drivers. Nor would one argue against environmental interventions that provide safer water, food, and air for all. Many would argue, however, that such behaviors as eating, smoking, and exercising are private and not in the public domain. With regard to these private behaviors, it is argued, people should be able to make their own choices, and others should not attempt to manipulate them.

"Manipulation" is, of course, relative. Researchers who have studied the smoking behavior of junior high and high school students report that many of these children are under so much pressure to smoke that it often is easier to do so than to refrain. The tobacco companies have been extraordinarily effective in helping to create a "climate of acceptability" regarding smoking and they have managed to make cigarettes highly visible and easily available everywhere. Are children who begin to smoke under these pressures truly making a free choice? One could argue that by mounting a campaign against the tobacco companies, this current imbalance would be equalized and, as a result, children would have a freer choice than they now have.

Similarly, when one shops at the supermarket, it is easy to see that unhealthy foods are generally placed at eye level and are cheaper than healthy foods—which one may find on the bottom shelf. Does the average consumer have a free choice in this circumstance? Would it not be appropriate to redress the balance by an environmental intervention whereby healthy and *unhealthy* foods are placed on the same shelf and are priced competitively? It can be argued that commercial interests have effectively made their case to the public but that those interested in health have not. It can further be argued that environmental interventions to provide a truly free choice are therefore neither dictatorial nor paternalistic.

A CASE EXAMPLE: BUS DRIVERS IN SAN FRANCISCO

An illustration of the importance of the social environment is provided by a research project we are now doing among bus drivers in San Francisco. We had been told that these drivers had very high rates of hypertension, and our task was to make recommendations to help them. The

usual approach—an individually-oriented one—
would be to provide medical treatment for those
drivers with hypertension and to help all drivers
to change their behavior in specific ways. Thus,
drivers could be counselled in developing better
eating habits, getting more exercise, and coping
more effectively with stressful situations encountered while driving. Although these activities are
useful and should be implemented, it is important to recognize that many drivers will not change
their behavior and that new drivers will continually need to be counselled over the years as they
arrive on the job.

An environmental approach to this problem
consists of identifying those factors in the work
environment that are causing the hypertension
so that they can be modified or eliminated. We
are now studying such environmental factors as
exposure to noise, vibration, and carbon monoxide fumes. But we are paying particular attention
to the social environment of drivers. Early on,
the "tyranny of the schedule" was brought to our
attention. Drivers must keep to a specific schedule, but in almost every instance this schedule is
arranged without realistic reference to actual road
conditions and, in fact, cannot be met. The instant
the bus driver sits down in his bus, he is behind
schedule and he is continually reprimanded for
this.

In preliminary work with drivers, we were
struck by their social isolation and loneliness.
Most drivers work a very long shift without an
opportunity to talk meaningfully to other people
all day long. In spite of this long, lonely work
day, many drivers do not immediately go home
after work. Instead, they remain at the bus yard
for 1 to 3 additional hours to "wind down." By
the time they do arrive at home, it is very late
and they usually go directly to bed. Many drivers
with whom we have talked say that they have
very limited interactions with their spouses, children, or friends. In addition to loneliness, we have
observed that driving a bus often provokes inappropriate coping responses. In particular, we have
observed hostile and impatient behavior being
stimulated and provoked in situations that involve

limited personal control, unpredictability, deadlines and tight schedules—a behavior sometimes
referred to as "type A" behavior.

If we can identify characteristics of the job
of bus driving that are associated with disease,
we may be able to introduce interventions, not
merely among bus drivers but directly on those
environmental factors associated with the job. For
example, perhaps by changing the way in which
schedules are arranged, the bus company will be
able to earn more money as a result of reduced
rates of absenteeism, sickness, accidents, and, in
particular, employee turnover. In addition, rest
stops might be located in or near central cities so
that drivers would be more likely to meet other
drivers from time to time, instead of the current practice of locating rest stops at remote and
lonely places on the outer edges of a city. Further,
it might be possible to arrange work schedules
so that more time is available for drivers to be
with their families and to participate in outside
community activities. One of the most important
results might be to initiate a campaign to inform
the public of the difficult circumstances faced by
drivers. As the situation exists now, bus drivers
feel themselves to be the objects of considerable
negative feelings from passengers, car drivers, and
the media, and they feel they are blamed for problems that are not of their making.

CONCLUSION

No one would argue that, as individuals, we are
responsible for our own health. In the final analysis, we are the only ones who can change our
life style in the interests of better health. We are
the only ones who lift fork to mouth, who inhale
smoke, who plant feet on the sidewalk. And we
are the only ones who can *decide* to do these
things. It is important to recognize, however, that
we do not live in a vacuum. Whether we like it
or not, our thoughts, ideas, wishes, and behavior are influenced and conditioned by the people
around us, by the environments in which we find
ourselves, and by the customs, traditions, fads, and
fashions to which we are continuously exposed.
Some of us are able to behave more indepen-

dently of these environmental forces than others. But all of us, to some degree or another, are influenced by them.

To change behavior, we need information. But facts rarely are sufficient to ensure that behavior change will occur. We must *want* to change. In addition to information and motivation, we must recognize the difficulties we face when the environments within which we live provide more obstacles than enhancements. Effective behavior change, therefore, requires not only that we do our best as individuals but also that we work with one another to create more healthful and supportive social environments. In a very real sense, no man is an island. We need to be more aware of this, and we need to be ready to help each other in the interests of better health.

9 THE HEALTH OF CITIES

Leonard Duhl, M.D., is a professor of public health, city planning, and psychiatry at the University of California at Berkeley and San Francisco. He is concerned with policy planning, social and personal change, and sociological troubleshooting. His work with the World Health Organization on Healthy Cities is the focus of his research.

When Dr. Leonard Duhl was commissioned in the Public Health Service, he rattled his colleagues by requesting an assignment to the Department of Housing and Urban Development. What did urban development have to do with health? A lot, as it turns out. A city must meet the needs of its inhabitants if they are to lead full lives. This requires strong communications, careful neighborhood planning, education, and better use of a city's human resources. Dr. Duhl discusses the interrelationship between man and his environment and suggests ways in which urban planners and policymakers can protect the health of their communities.■

"Since it has taken more than five thousand years to arrive at even a partial understanding of the city's nature and drama, it may require an even longer period to exhaust the city's still unrealized potentialities."

This insight, expressed by Lewis Mumford in his classic text, *The City in History* (1961), is as true today as it was then. However, we are just beginning to realize the urgency of finding these potentialities. In his history of city life, Mumford begins with a city that symbolically was a world, and he closes with a present-day world that has become in many practical aspects a city.

Today's cities are indeed where most things happen—or at least where it is easiest to see what is happening. Only in the recent history of men coming together in cities has anyone asked whether cities are doing what men expect of them. As long as the cities were economically viable and the people were reasonably healthy and uncomplaining, few questions were asked. Usually those who considered the health of the city thought in terms of the prevalence of disease. And when they thought of health, they thought of the absence of disease or they remembered crisis situations. These attitudes persisted despite the fact that the Hippocratic school had outlined the holistic approach to public hygiene in a treatise, *Air, Water, and Places*, almost 2000 years ago.

Today we question the holistic idea of the Hippocratic school, which dealt with what could be seen. We also question the ideas of the 19th century epidemiologist John Snow, who dealt with one of the worst cholera epidemics in history (originating in London's Broad Street sewage system). We now accept that environment impinges upon man as he impinges upon it. We also see that health includes "everything under the sun" and that the context of health and social activity are critical to the health of the individual.

Basically what we need to know is: What is a healthy city? What characteristics does it possess? How can the city work to the maximum benefit of its inhabitants? And how can an unhealthy city be redirected to work for the people who live in them?

A city is an interrelated system whose separate functions ideally act in concert with one another. When one part of the city falters, the city as a whole suffers. In looking at a city, one usually first sees things of the obvious infrastructure: the streets, transportation system, communications, disposal systems, schools, fire and police services, and the like. However, these parts are only the beginning of a process. There is also the *soft* infrastructure—the rules by which we play—and it is probably here that individual cities are unique.

In the healthy city, certain elements of effective management are either in place or are the goal. The presence of these qualities is an indication that the city's health is good.

A city must have the ability to meet the bottom-line needs of its various citizens, and it must be able to set the climate within which people can live their own lives. To accomplish this, the city as a whole must understand the needs of its diverse parts and must be imbued in others' ways of being, putting aside prejudices, preconceptions, and firmly-held points of view. To do this, people must talk to one another.

All of the functions of life must be able to take place in the city. There must be places to be born, to grow, learn, work, and die. There also must be places to play, to waste time, to be in the company of our loved ones—a place to nurture the spirit. These areas are complex in terms of resource allocation. The city is made up of complex pleasures as well as the bottom-line basics. People must be able to deal with the varied activities that make up human life; these include the aesthetic, artistic, and sporting experiences in which people can participate actively or passively. This is an important part of the nurturing process of the city organism.

In cities where all kinds of functions take place, people become interconnected and willing to talk to one another about their particular interests, and they tend to gradually develop their local concerns into big-issue concerns. It isn't easy to combine economic and social development in a city, but when it occurs, it makes for strong realities.

If one is in the housing, transportation, or health care business, one has to face multiple issues. For instance, housing involves more than the buildings themselves. People are born, live, and die there. Buildings and their inhabitants impinge on each other and on the surrounding community as it impinges on them. The person designing the building should know how to create a community that will allow everything to intersect.

Probably the best way to see the implications of a lack of multidimensional activities is to study the development of a single-industry town, for example, a mining town. While such a town is being developed, does one plan housing only around the miners—a one-dimensional policy? Or should the designer ask, "I know that this town is primarily for mines, but shall I design the town for families? Shall I design communities?" Populations build up quickly. Very early in planning, a multidimensional system must be foreseen. In addition, a city must be connected to its surroundings and to its hinterlands.

Healthy cities are heterogeneous. The modern city is a crucible for people and ideas. Contributing to this is the surge of immigrants into large American cities in recent years. Ghettos have always been places where people learn from their elders how to cope with city life. Ghetto dwellers also learn their life style from the streets and businesses in their neighborhood. In this way the city educates its citizens.

Although there were mass immigrations into the United States at the beginning of this century, most of the European immigrants' ways were not radically different from those of their new world. Today's immigrants come with experiences and cultures that are quite different from those in the world they are entering and even from one another, and they must learn new ways of doing and being. Hopefully the culture already in place will be flexible enough to encompass them without engulfing them, to learn from new inhabitants, and to allow them to retain the richness of their origins.

As these changes take place, another kind of migration is occurring. The middle class and many of the poor who move into middle-class status are shifting to the suburbs, leaving the cities

to the poor, the new migrants, and the affluent singles. Because of their great differences, many of these groups are fragmenting the cities as they move away from being part of the whole. Certain groups are oppressed, whereas others form special interest groups.

To be healthy, a city must have room for families in all their forms, as well as for the entrepreneurship and creativity that allows people to express their unique skills and cultural heritage. The importance of individual development and the involvement of the family in the process of making the city a better place cannot be underestimated. Meeting the needs of children and families is as important to individual and collective growth as is a hospitable atmosphere for families.

Basic needs and places, cultural enrichment and activities alone cannot make a city healthy. Connecting linkages are required that are different at different times. Linkages include people talking with each other in their neighborhoods, offices, shops, and schools.

The ability of individuals to connect in a network of extended family and community has been accepted as having an effect on decreasing morbidity and mortality. People who are sick or who face critical events in their lives recover faster, are less apt to die prematurely, and manage their crises better when they have the support of family or friends.

The characteristics of a healthy city cannot be studied separately. Each has within it elements of another and they all impinge upon or complement others. Clearly what we are dealing with in a healthy city is an environment that can best be dealt with in ways that are sensitive to what can be called the social ecology of the city.

Intrinsic to the social ecology model is the concept of reciprocal maintenance: If I take something out of the system, I must put something back. In *Lives of a Cell* (1974), Lewis Thomas observed that, "We do not have solitary beings. Every creature is, in some sense, connected to and dependent on the rest."

Aristotle believed that no city should be larger than one in which a cry for help could be heard on all of the city's walls. This observation probably was not meant as a comment on the logistical consideration but on an organic one. In such a city, people would reasonably be expected to know and to assist one another, making the city functional as a social entity.

The concept of reciprocal maintenance is integral to a healthy city. Physicist Fritjof Capra expressed this central association when he wrote that "the more one studies the living world, the more one comes to realize that the tendency to associate, establish links, live inside one another, and cooperate is an essential characteristic of living organisms."

One way of dealing with an ailing city is one that has long been used in medicine, though not always to best advantage—that of responding to the symptoms. Sometimes this reaction can be very effective, particularly as an immediate reaction to a perceived wrong or injustice, when it carries a lot of energy along with it. At other times there may be a rising awareness of what needs to be done. Although symptoms reaction may not always get at the root of the problem, it is important, and clearly many programs would not have occurred without it.

A particularly compelling example of this is the formation of Mothers Against Drunk Driving (MADD), a response of a mother to the death of her daughter. The program has spread throughout the country and spawned offshoots, including Students Against Drunk Driving. Responses to more complex issues tend to be slower, but a provocative situation or event can cause people or governmental bodies to move more quickly. Such issues could be the changing taste and quality of drinking water, the need for security on dark and unpopulated streets, traffic inconveniences and dangers, aesthetic considerations, eroding soil, chemical contamination, and nuclear waste.

We have all become a society of victims, or potential victims, but we are all trying to decrease our helplessness and increase our ability to meet our needs and pursue our values. We have seen that people who have control over their lives are healthier and better able to cope with stress. It is the same with cities.

A time comes when victimization leads to polarization and fragmentation. It is here that dealing with underlying issues of the city is imperative. The patient can't be cured unless the etiology of the disease is understood and addressed. In the city, the issues are interconnected, complex, and multidimensional. It is the interconnectedness and relationship between the parts and the sense of community that is essential to making a city healthy. Toward that end there is a need to develop new approaches, to utilize a new kind of management of organizations and people, and to recognize that justice involves meeting the essential needs of the community, both by allocating resources and by involving people in the search for answers to problems that affect them.

Corporate management has had the imagination to try new ideas, some of them from other countries and cultures, which may have application in our cities. These ideas include increased participatory management and even ownership by employees.

An interesting current management phenomenon is the "new populism." As U.S. business has looked for ways to resist external control by government and institutions, it has come to accept the opposite concept, "exerting control over our own lives." In corporate decision making, this has extended to greater participation on the part of employees at all levels, including top executives and managers, as well as by public interest groups. Companies are encouraging people within the organization to participate more fully in management.

There are new concepts and trends in our cities today, and how we deal with them can be important. In every city there are people from all parts of the city who are "in touch" and who know how to accomplish things. A healthy city finds these people and creates a context for success.

One consideration almost seems superficial but can play an important part in contributing to a context for success: the healthy city probably has a focal point that attracts people. A good downtown should have people in it 24 hours a day. Something physical should be going on most of the day and the space should be available for many kinds of activities to take place. Ideally housing, work places, and areas for learning, worship, and play should not be isolated.

Finally, there also should be a visual concept that identifies the city. It is difficult to relate to, let alone take pride in, something that one can't visualize. If things are brought to the center of the city, the city's rituals help to embody symbolic things. If this happens, it indicates a physical infrastructure that probably works well.

When suggestions are made about some of the ways that cities can redirect their energies to achieve a greater degree of health, inevitably the theme that prevails is that as the city becomes healthier, the people living in the city have a better chance of reaching their greatest potential in health and spirit.

As in Lewis Mumford's city-world, we see that if all the things that impinge upon the health of the individual are added up, we are talking about the city. If we are interested in improving our lives and the lives of those close to us—the lot of man, his total health and functioning—we see that to have healthy people, we must have healthy cities. They cannot be separated, and what improves one improves the other.

The World Health Organization defines health as "a state of complete physical, mental, and social well being, not merely the absence of disease or infirmity." This definition clearly has implications for the citizen of the healthy city.

10 CHILDREN AND YOUTH IN CITIES: THE STORY OF SEATTLE'S KIDSPLACE

Robert A. Aldrich, M.D., was the first director of the National Institute of Child Health and Human Development. He chaired the Department of Pediatrics at the University of Washington. He now serves as Vice President for Health Affairs at the University of Colorado. Dr. Aldrich has written on human development, life span, child ecology, and the future of children. He has been an active participant in international child health programs for 30 years and is one of the few pediatricians knowledgeable in anthropology and urban planning.

It's no surprise that Bob Aldrich and Leonard Duhl are good friends and colleagues. In his many important roles in the health field, Bob has always pushed the boundaries of health care wider. In the previous chapter, Leonard Duhl concentrated on the health of cities. In this chapter, Bob focuses on children in cities. He is a pediatrician, and he has always been vitally concerned with kids and their health. He has also been impatient with the limitations placed on pediatric medicine. In recent years, through the KidsPlace Project in Seattle, Bob has been able to fuse his health and urban planning interests into one dynamic model that he believes can and should be reproduced everywhere.■

The growth of modern cities and their rapid urban development, especially after World War II, have neglected the basic needs of children and youth. If we believe that a good quality of growth and development for children and youth in an urban environment is essential to a society's future productivity and health, then we should concern ourselves with what is happening today in our cities.

The phenomenon of rapid urbanization can be observed in nearly all developing and developed nations. It does not appear to be related to political ideology, nor is it favored by any of the major religious faiths. Urbanization is a man-made condition, and as such, mankind should be resourceful enough to make those changes that will improve the living circumstances for children, youth, and their families.

BEGINNINGS

I first became acquainted with Spyros A. Doxiadis, M.D., a Greek pediatrician, while we were flying from Athens to Ankara, Turkey en route to the Eastern Mediterranean Pediatric Congress of 1958. Little did I suspect the consequences of this journey for my future career interests. They were to change greatly in the next years, resulting directly from this encounter. Spyros is the youngest of four brothers. It was his brother Constantinos, an urban planner and architect, who suggested we visit a secluded place in the Bay of Naflion.

The bay is on the western side of the Peloponnesus not far from the ancient ruins of Myacenae. A tiny island fortress stands alone in the center of the bay across from the town of Naflion. One can reach the island through the services of Greek boatmen who are readily available beside the quay at the village. Towering above the village are ruins of a Venetian castle whose rulers at one time had need of a hangman's services. Today it has become a pleasant place to stay on holiday.

As the boatmen maneuvered his craft alongside the wharf that serves the island, we were greeted by Constantinos Doxiadis, who led us up the stone stairway to a comfortable patio where we were served fruit juices, and we started a conversa-

tion which proved an electrifying experience for me. Constantinos Doxiadis was one of the world's leading urban planners. His book, *Ekistics*, is a text on cities for people. Its chapter manuscripts were carefully distributed among the rooms of the island fortress. Even then I noted his sense of organization of which I was to learn much more in coming years. But the impact of the short visit that morning has never dimmed in the slightest. For here was a man who knew how man-made environments can shape human development, a subject of major pediatric importance. My medical training was focused upon individuals, diseases, their diagnosis and treatment. Environmental influences received very little attention. Doxiadis's *Ekistics*, has become one of the classics on human settlements. The title derives from the Greek root *ecos*: ekistics is the science of human settlements. It seemed to me that shaping the growth and development of children and youth through designing characteristics into the man-made environment that favored them was a little known subject, with almost nothing in world pediatric literature. If one uses the Greek root for child, plus ekistics, then the term *pedekistics* emerges, meaning the science of children in human settlements. Child ecology has a similar meaning, but pedekistics is an urban focus.

It was evident from reading issues of the journal *Ekistics* that nearly all of the literature was focused on adults in cities and that there was an enormous, unmet need for research to learn more about pedekistics. This has the potential for a new dimension of training that combines a medical background with urban planning, architecture, and some cultural anthropology. There will assuredly be a market for such men and women who could become the urban clinicians capable of diagnosing and treating "sick" cities, especially on behalf of children.

STEPPING STONES

"The Child in the World of Tomorrow—a Window Into the Future" was a lively symposium held in Athens during the first week of July 1978. A marvelous book with this title was published in 1979 by Pergamon Press. The symposium attracted over 500 participants from every type of political system, scores of cultures, and a wide variety of professions and disciplines. The meeting preceded the International Year of the Child by 2 years and served as a major international effort to seriously address the future of all children on this planet.

An international symposium, "The Child and the City," was held in Tokyo in April 1981. It was organized by Dr. Noboru Kobayashi, President of the International Pediatric Association. Dr. Kobayashi, a pediatrician, was then Director of the Department of Pediatrics at Tokyo University. He and I collaborated on designing the program content and selecting speakers from East and West. The primary focus of the 3 days was urbanization and its impact on children. Since urbanization as a phenomenon has dominated cities in many developed and developing nations during the latter part of this century, we wanted to learn what the East and the West might tell each other. Attendance during the symposium grew with each day. Japan's business community was greatly concerned and attended in large numbers.

THE ORIGINS OF "KIDSPLACE"

In 1983, civic leaders in Seattle participating in a project called "Seattle in Transition" identified the decline in the number of children in Seattle (1970-80 census data) as one the city's most distressing trends. This important indicator led to a joint proposal by the Junior League, Metrocenter YMCA, and the Seattle City Government to launch a broadly conceived program that would re-establish their city as "a great place for kids." The initiative came first from the private sector and was quickly perceived by city government as benefitting from a combined effort.

In 1984, approximately forty men and women representing Seattle's children and youth agencies, community organizations, schools, government departments, businesses, industries, and universities created a project that became known as KidsPlace. This name was selected by children. The mission of KidsPlace was to be "a kids' lobby for a vital Seattle." Convinced that children and

their families are an essential part of Seattle's present and future, they adopted the following goals:

1. Place children and their families high on Seattle's political, economic, and cultural agendas.
2. Attract more families with children to the city.
3. Support and hold more families with children living in the city.

PROGRAM INITIATIVES BY KIDSPLACE IN 1984

This year set the stage for future activities and saw the first major project completed, a survey of 6000 school-age children, who were asked what they liked and disliked about the city and its neighborhoods. When the survey was designed, it was assumed that a survey of this kind had been widely used in city planning. The big surprise was that this was not true.

Children took the survey very seriously. They want a clean, beautiful safe city with more things for children to do and places to go. They are environmentalists who are also sensitive to safety needs. Their high rating for parks and the Seattle Center (former 1964 World's Fair site) had a strong impact on the adult community, resulting in major improvements that are presently underway. One part of the survey was a question inviting them to apply for "Mayor for a Day." Selection was based upon the originality of their responses about the first thing they would do for children if they were mayor. The winner of the competition, a 12-year-old girl, impressed the media at a conference starting her day as mayor. Her poise and sophistication before the reporters from the press, TV, and radio were reflected by their editorials and reports. Public awareness of the capabilities of this age group began to rise. In addition to completing the survey, research was initiated on the demography of children and their families. The committee decided to create an action plan, hold a major national conference, establish a youth board, and initiate an annual celebration in recognition of Seattle's children.

Significant highlights of these programs are considered below.

KIDSPLACE PROGRAM EXPANSION IN 1985

During 1984, there was a visible increase in citizen participation. The numbers of men and women engaged in projects grew rapidly, rising to several hundred volunteers, many of whom brought with them professional skills, experience, and connections of immense value. One of the main objectives of this program, to raise public awareness, was going well. In 1985, the following programs emerged:

- *KidsBoard*, a youth leadership program to help middle school and high school students provide leadership in the community on behalf of Seattle children and teenagers. Proposed city policies were brought to them for review by the Mayor.
- Publication of *A Closer Look*, a collection of eight studies concerning the city's children. The individual research titles included "Seattle's Changing Child Population," "Needs of Seattle Single Parent Families," "Downtown Day Care," "Teen Activities," and "Family Responsibility and the Workplace."
- A national conference, "Looking at the City with Children in Mind," was held in April.
- The first annual KidsDay was celebrated April 27th when thousands of children enjoyed free or reduced price activities throughout the city.
- Publication of the *KidsPlace Action Agenda* challenged the city to implement thirty positive, measurable steps on behalf of children, youth, and their families by 1990. This far-reaching achievement was prepared by more than 250 volunteer citizens representing different ages, sexes, races, and neighborhoods.

KIDSPLACE ACTION AGENDA IN 1986

When more than 250 volunteer citizens spend 6 months working on task groups and selecting priority projects to benefit children and youth in their city, that is newsworthy. It may be informative and stimulating to readers who are considering a similar program where they live. For this reason, I have used much of the space available in this essay to briefly describe each of the thirty items on the 1986 *Action Agenda* and their present situation.

1. **Adopt a Kids' Art Group** Metrocenter YMCA and the Seattle Arts Commission created ARTSMATCH, a project matching 11 youth arts organizations with supporters of the arts. Forty percent of the arts organizations participating in "ARTSMATCH" represent minority youngsters.

2. **Bicycle Route Network** Mayor Charles Royer has directed the City Engineering Department to begin planning interconnected bicycle routes. Children and youth have urged this measure to facilitate visits to friends who live in other neighborhoods.

3. **City Child Advocate** This position in city government was recommended by the Mayor in his budget for 1986. The City Council elected not to fund this request at the present time.

4. **Day Care Systems**
   - The Human Resources Coalition, involving city and county governments and the private sector (United Way), has appointed a task force to plan a comprehensive day care system.
   - New downtown day care sites are being prepared as the result of building and fire code changes, plus incentives for builders or developers.
   - A school levy passed which enables construction of in-school day care space in 14 Seattle elementary schools.
   - The Seattle City Council allocated $270,000 of city funds to immediately help develop day care facilities at two elementary schools.
   - A Child and Family Resource Center has been established to regularly provide information and training to day care providers and parents.

5. **Downtown as a Safe Place** The Seattle Police Department has assigned staff and

started identifying downtown businesses that are willing to serve as safe places for children and youth who may need assistance. The City Attorney, Douglas Jewett, is evaluating liability issues. It is apparent that some retail businesses are able to undertake this role while others have liabilities that may be restrictive.

6. **Early Childhood Development** With the strong leadership of Seattle citizens assisted by lobbyists, significant progress was made at the State level, resulting in an allocation of $2,900,000 to establish early childhood education and assistance programs. Major strength in this field is in the University of Washington faculty where both educational and research programs are well staffed. The complementary relationships among local resources are growing.

7. **Effective Schools** Research has shown that leadership abilities of school principals are key factors in the performance of all students. The Mayor and the City Council will be launching new groups to seek additional ways to assist the public schools.

8. **Fight Adult Exploitation** The Office of Women's Rights started a media campaign aimed at reducing the numbers of customers of teenage prostitutes. The Police Department added a detective position specifically to address exploitation of children and youth by adults.

9. **Health Advocates for Low-Income Children**
   • Increased funds were allocated by the City Council for dental and medical care for kids.
   • Funds were also allocated by the City Council to build a new and expanded family and children's health clinic.
   • KidsPlace Board is considering appointing Health Advisory Committee.

10. **High School Vocation/Technical Classes** Action is planned for each school year.

11. **Information for Kids and Families** The KidsPlace Teen Activities Task Force is seeking funding for a teen activities telephone hotline and a teen newspaper. Pacific Northwest Bell Telephone will be asked to provide "Kids Pages," a child-oriented telephone directory, and a telephone information clearing house in 1986-7.

12. **Kids Friendly Downtown** On April 25, 1986, the Project for Public Spaces, Inc., hosted a one-day conference, bringing together leaders from cultural institutions as well as planners from the Art Museum, Convention Center, Westlake Mall, and Metro Tunnel projects to assist those major downtown developments in being "kid-friendly."

13. **Kids Arts Fund** This proposal is to be reviewed by the Seattle Arts Commission as a part of their overview and evaluation of arts funding.

14. **Kids at Risk**
   • A new summer day camp was established in 1985 by the Parks Department. It serves older kids living in the Mount Baker Apartments.
   • The United Way Organization allocated $41,000 in additional funds for 1986 to support kids who were at risk living in Seattle Housing Authority garden communities.
   • Student interns were hired by the Parks Department through an allocation of funds by the City Council.
   • The City Council allocated $188,000 in new funds for street youth services coordinated by the Atlantic Street Center. The "street kids" situation in Seattle has been documented in a film and in publications. Seattle is a city with major attractions for homeless and runaway children.
   • Additional community service officers were added to the Police Department staff for the prime purpose of aiding "street kids."
   • Project Self-Sufficiency was initiated and funded to give single-parent families access to more convenient resources.

- The Human Resources Coalition started a child abuse treatment project funded by the city, county, and United Way.
- Development of a 12-hour or 24-hour "drop-in center" has been proposed.
- A Police Department task force was formed to select the most effective strategies for helping street kids. University of Washington faculty have completed authoritative research on the origins of street kids and are a practical resource for the city.

15. **Marketing the Public Schools** An attractive brochure concerning Seattle public schools was completed by city staff and volunteers from KidsPlace.

16. **Metro Fares and Safety**
- Metro buses now carry KidsPlace logo stickers which state, "This is a KidsPlace." Drivers have two-way communications on their buses and they are encouraged to help kids in need of assistance.
- Youth agencies, schools, and Metro are discussing reduced bus fares for children and youth. No conclusions so far.

17. **Multicultural Education** Proposed funding reductions in multicultural programs of the Seattle public schools were opposed by effective lobbying of citizens and community agencies.

18. **Multicultural Activities for Kids** No action has occurred.

19. **One Percent for Kids** At its 1986 budget planning retreat, the City Council began examining a broad range of children's issues. The One Percent concept may not be workable at this time, although there is evidently an increasing commitment to kids.

20. **Pacific Arts Center** The Seattle Arts Commission and the Seattle Office of Management and Budget did not approve this item for inclusion in the funding allocation, but they did reaffirm their support for youth activities at the Pacific Arts Center. The Pacific Arts Center is located at the Seat-

tle Center and has prime space allocated to youth activities.

21. **Places to Play**
- The Parks Department extended the number of hours for summer day camp.
- Community recreation center hours were extended by the Parks Department.
- The Mayor's proposal to add Sunday and holiday hours to the recreation center schedules was not funded.
- The Seattle Center has established a new children's complex that includes the Children's Museum and the Children's Theater.

22. **Playground Design for All Children**
- Burke-Gilman Park opened. It is specially designed for disabled children.
- The plans for Westlake Mall and Park were reviewed, and many suggestions were made by members of KidsBoard and KidsPlace.
- A two-day seminar was held to develop guidelines for parks and playgrounds in Seattle. The seminar was attended by playground designers, child development professionals, and kids. The improvements recommended will be achieved through a successful bond issue, "Seattle 1, 2, 3."

23. **Playground Programs**
- Eight playgrounds were reopened by the Parks Department.
- The Parks Department has added youth interns to its staff, as approved in the 1986 budget.
- Funding was achieved for adult staff to supervise summer playground activities.

24. **School Councils** The School Board adopted a new goal to increase decision making at the local school level. Individual schools now have the opportunity to participate in a state school-based management pilot project. Twenty-three schools considered participating, and seven applied to establish school-site councils.

25. **Student Business Internships** A Seattle business organization called Private Initia-

tives in Public Education has expanded its support and the numbers of student internships for the 1985-6 school year.

26. **Support Existing Arts Programs**   The Arts in Education program received substantial additional funding from the Seattle Arts Commission.

27. **Teacher Employment and Professional Standards**   No progress has been made on this item.

28. **Teen Activities**
    - A curfew proposal developed by the KidsPlace Teen Activities Task Force is under public consideration. Major differences of opinion center on the age of those affected and the hours for the curfew.
    - A series of teen dances have been proposed by the same task force. They would be held in the recreation centers, the YMCA, Girls Clubs, and Boys Clubs.
    - The Seattle Center, in collaboration with KidsPlace, has developed guidelines for policies for teen dances to be held in this popular place for kids.

29. **Teen Peer Counseling Center**   This KidsBoard program was made possible by funding from Soroptimists.

30. **Working Parents and Personnel Policies**   The City of Seattle has changed its personnel policies to allow sick leave time, in order to promote better parental support for children. This has recently been emulated by several nonprofit organizations (e.g., YMCA, Family Services of King County).

By listing all of these items and the progress (or lack of progress) for each one, I have illustrated the specific approaches made in this city so far. An effective mechanism is in place that has already accomplished some desirable changes. Other metropolitan communities may undertake similar projects with those modifications essential for their particular culture and other characteristics. Children of future generations require a higher priority.

PREPARING FOR 21ST CENTURY CHILDREN

The East and the West will soon enter the 21st century together. We share many of the same problems brought about by rapid growth of cities in which the needs of children have been neglected. This is particularly true of those factors that can interfere with children's growth and development. All of us working in child health have the common goal of improving the health and well-being of children worldwide.

Let me propose the formation of a strong and enduring alliance between East and West to share each other's knowledge about children and their health, especially focusing on the impacts of urbanization on growth and development. We must hasten to bring into our research and educational programs those who are in disciplines relevant to the design and function of cities. Architects and urban planners will be essential for training future "urban clinicians" who can practice pedekistics in our troubled cities. I would like to see a small number of men and women trained in pediatrics, urban planning, architecture, and cultural anthropology become the pedekisticians of the new century.

This approach can improve productivity and the quality of life in a nation and make the future of children and youth flourish. We need to have more experiments like Seattle's and more laboratories in which to learn and be trained. Much remains to be done on a larger scale, but making a start is a compelling challenge to mankind.

11 OCCUPATIONAL DISEASES

Phillip L. Polakoff, M.D., is a principal member of Integrated Health Management Associates in Berkeley, California. He has worked for 20 years in the area of health care delivery at the work site. He presently serves as senior consultant to the California Senate on issues concerning workers' compensation reform and human productivity in employment. He also maintains an active clinical practice in occupational medicine, and is a national syndicated columnist.

It has always been difficult for Dr. Phil Polakoff to separate health issues from politics. That's one of the reasons that he recently entered the mayoral race in Berkeley, California. For Phil, occupational health is an area that allows the proper dynamic merger of health and political interests. With the current fascination with health promotion and wellness programs for employees, it is easy to forget that occupational health has been a central issue in society for more than a century. Phil describes the status of occupational health programs in the United States today.■

How many Americans get sick every year with an occupational disease?

If you could set your car on cruise control at 55 miles per hour and drive steadily from Boston to San Francisco some 3,000 miles away, every two seconds you would whiz past a sickbed containing a man or woman lying ill with an occupational disease.

That's the depressing picture in human terms behind the U.S. Department of Labor's estimate that every year there are more than 100,000 new cases of occupational diseases in the United States.

How many Americans die annually of occupational diseases they may first have contracted years ago?

If you glanced out the other side of your car during that imaginary cross-country journey, you would pass a headstone every two seconds as you drove from Boston to San Francisco at 55 mph.

That's what it means when the statistics tell us that another 100,000 Americans die each year of occupational diseases, some of which have a long latent period before the final toll is exacted.

And those numbers account only for the sick, the dying, and the dead. You would also have to find space along that sorrowful route for the nearly 5,000 workers killed in job accidents and for the 2.5 million a year who are disabled by occupational injuries—80,000 of them permanently.

We cannot put a dollar figure on all this suffering and loss. But the direct and indirect cost of occupational accidents alone has been estimated at nearly $25 billion a year.

Job-related accidents and diseases are not new phenomena, visited upon us by the advent of 20th century technology. They have been around for a long, long time—since mankind has labored. No doubt some Stone Age man was blinded by a shard of flint from the weapon or tool he was making. No doubt many of the first fire users got burned.

From ancient written records we do know with some certainty that Greek and Roman slaves toiling in the mines fell victim to such toxic metals as lead and mercury. In the 16th century, an occupation gave its name to an affliction—"grinder's dis-ease"—brought on by inhaling silica dust generated by sandstone wheels.

Other early medical accounts describe symptoms of lead poisoning among medieval scribes. The likeliest explanation is that they ingested metallic ink solutions as a result of shaping their quills with their teeth.

The Mad Hatter of *Alice in Wonderland* could have had many real-life counterparts outside Lewis Carroll's vivid imagination. In 19th century hat factories, workers were exposed to mercury fumes while treating fur to make felt. Some of these workers suffered such extensive brain damage that they appeared to be mad.

Some accounts of factory conditions in the early days of the Industrial Revolution are true horror stories. They tell of barred windows, not to keep out marauders but to prevent deranged workers from jumping out.

Much earlier, as far back as 1700, Bernardo Ramazzini, the first occupational health specialist, had suggested that various precautions be taken to safeguard workers in various trades. He also recommended that doctors taking a case history inquire about the patient's occupation.

That was nearly 300 years ago, yet such obviously useful information is still not routinely recorded.

That lag, however, is not as shameful as a specific incident in America's annals of occupational disease. As early as 1914, life insurance companies in this country denied policies to asbestos workers and uranium workers. The underwriters, checking their mortality tables, knew that workers in those occupations ran a far greater risk than others of early death from lung disease and cancer. These risks, which the insurance people knew about, were not told to the workers by their employers. Even today, generations later, we are still seeing tragic consequences of such unsounded warnings.

Overall, however, the picture is getting better. Workers, physicians, scientists, employers, government officials, the public generally—all are better informed about the massive and continuing problem of occupational diseases.

Not only do today's workers know more about their jobs—about the processes and materials they come in contact with—but now they have a legal right to such information and to a safe and healthful workplace. This protection is guaranteed under the Occupational Safety and Health Act of 1970, which states that employers have a "general duty" to provide a workplace free of hazards. To fulfill this obligation, they must comply with standards issued by the Department of Labor's Occupational Safety and Health Administration (OSHA).

The Act also created the National Institute for Occupational Safety and Health (NIOSH) within the Department of Health and Human Services. NIOSH conducts research on job hazards and recommends new standards to OSHA.

These are not the only government agencies charged with safeguarding American workers. Others include the Mine Safety and Health Administration (MSHA) which oversees working conditions for mine and mill workers; the Nuclear Regulatory Commission (NRC) which sets standards for workers exposed to radioactive substances and conditions; the National Cancer Institute (NCI) which gathers information about cancer hazards, along with NIOSH; and the Environmental Protection Agency (EPA) which has perhaps the broadest mandate of all: to control air, water, solid waste, noise, radiation, and toxic substance pollution.

Before the turn of the century, and well into our modern era, we could with some justification associate occupational diseases and injuries with the typical manufacturing plants that blighted the major "factory towns" of America—crowded, multistoried, grimy, noisy.

In comparison with today's "clean," campuslike industrial parks, they were brutish, both in their technology and in the damage they inflicted. Then came exotic chemical compounds, electronics, sophisticated instrumentation, and all the other refinements of our modern industrial complexes. And as the technology became more rarefied, the injuries and illnesses became subtler.

American workers today are still exposed to the same high-visibility risks of the older factory environments—crushing blows, slips and falls, all sorts of contact injuries, inhalation, and ingestion. Now another factor is entering the occupational disease picture: technological stress. This is not the same as the job stresses that probably have always been with us, such as resentment toward a boss, worry about being laid off, and so on. The new stress-potential technology, largely based on computers, robots, and a whole array of electronic servo-mechanisms, literally is changing the nature of work for the first time in history.

Work has become "machine-dependent." The worker/operator may begin to feel that he or she is serving the machine, rather than the other way around. The "information-intensive" nature of the new style of work creates a voracious appetite by the machine for information which must be satiated by a diet of arcane data. Whole new interpersonal relationships among workers must be formed to make the system work—networking, instead of individual effort. All of these are stressful factors.

Physically, the human body responds to stress in a number of predictable ways. Resistance to infectious disease is lowered. Adrenaline is released as the body gears up its defense mechanisms. The heart rate speeds up. Blood pressure rises. Digestive secretions increase.

If this state of readiness is prolonged, scientists believe it can lead to chronic illnesses—cardiovascular disease, ulcers, kidney ailments, perhaps even allergies, arthritis, and rheumatism—all caused by the body's repeated attempts to adapt to stress.

Occupational stress has been under study for 20 years at the University of Michigan Institute for Social Research. Out of those studies have come some suggestions for restructuring the workplace to reduce stress on the job. They include:

- Training workers to do their jobs efficiently, using shortcuts wherever possible.
- Rotating people in high stress jobs that cannot be restructured.
- Making sure each person understands his or her responsibilities.
- Distributing work according to workers' capabilities, and giving some people the right to delegate more work.

- Setting up clear lines of communication between workers and supervisors, and reducing the levels of hierarchy within the organization.
- Giving employees a voice in decisions that are rightly theirs to make.

The occupational risks—physical, neurological, psychological— have long outgrown the confines of the old red brick factories belching smoke and fumes, noisy and dangerous with the clank of gears and the slapping of belts. The risks have marched right along in step with the workforce into light industry, the service sector, the office (once the supposedly safe haven for "nice young ladies"), and out to the great outdoors where pollution is a growing concern.

Here are the major categories of workplaces and the hazards to be found there:

- **Heavy industry**, including mining, smelting and other raw processing; materials handling, forging, stamping, assembly, etc.
- **Light industry**, including chemical, electrical, radiation, benchwork, etc.
- **Office**, including electronics, services, warehousing, etc.
- **Outdoor/environmental**, including agriculture (one of the most dangerous occupations in America), construction, transportation, transmission-line stringing and repair, forestry, etc.

This span of work in America is so broad, the composition of the workforce so varied, it would be extremely difficult to sort out who is most at risk and where. However, the National Institute of Occupational Safety and Health (NIOSH) has compiled a list of the ten leading work-related diseases and injuries in the United States.

In drawing up its lists, NIOSH used three measurements: how often the diseases or injuries occur; how severe they are, and how amenable the causes are to change for the better. Here is the list (note that it includes only selected examples of disease and injury type):

1. **Occupational lung diseases**: asbestosis, byssinosis, silicosis, coal workers' pneumoconiosis, lung cancer, occupational asthma.
2. **Musculoskeletal injuries**: disorders of the back, trunk, upper extremity, neck, lower extremity: injury-induced Raynaud's phenomenon. (This condition, affecting the fingers, may be brought on by the use of vibrating tools.)
3. **Occupational cancers (other than lung)**: leukemia, mesothelioma, cancers of the nose, liver, and bladder.
4. **Amputations, fractures, eye loss, lacerations, and fatal injuries.**
5. **Cardiovascular diseases**: hypertension, coronary artery disease, acute myocardial infarction.
6. **Disorders of reproduction**: infertility, spontaneous abortion, birth defects.
7. **Neurotoxic disorders (nerve poisoning)**: peripheral neuropathy (often characterized by weakness, muscle shrinkage, or numbness and tingling), toxic encephalitis, psychoses, extreme personality changes related to toxic exposure.
8. **Noise-induced hearing loss.**
9. **Dermatologic (skin) conditions**: dermatoses, scaldings, chemical burns, contusions.
10. **Psychologic disorders**: neuroses, personality disorders, alcoholism, drug dependency.

It is utopian to expect that we can create situations where no worker ever gets hurt on the job and no one becomes ill with an occupational disease. But it is possible to make work and workplaces safer and healthier than many are today.

Engineering controls offer the most effective and permanent way of reducing hazards. Personal protective equipment, because it does not get at the root of the problem, is the least acceptable, although it is useful in a supplementary role. Between these two extremes are various methods of modifying the flow of work, shifts, lighting and colors—all of which can contribute significantly to the overall atmosphere of wellness and safety-proneness.

The three main types of engineering controls are substitution, isolation, and ventilation. Here are examples of each of these techniques:

1. *Substitution* is the technique of choice

with safety engineers, whenever possible, because it can be applied to machines, materials, or processes—three chief sources of problems.

Diesel forklifts produce high levels of carbon monoxide. Propane-powered trucks run much more cleanly. Replacing the diesel fork lifts with the propane-driven equipment would be an example of mechanical substitution.

Vinyl chloride was being used as a propellant in paint aerosol cans until it was discovered that it caused liver cancer. Carbon dioxide was found to work just as well—an example of material substitution.

Another plant was spray painting metal sheets after fabrication, creating an inhalation problem with the mist and vapors. The hazard was substantially reduced by precoating the sheets in a permanent, well ventilated dip tank—an example of process substitution.

2. *Isolation* means putting some kind of barrier between yourself and the hazard. It could be anything that does the job—wood, glass, wire mesh. Distance is one of the most effective barriers against noise, for example. Sound is a form of energy, and this energy can be dampened by "engineered isolation." There are a number of ways of doing this:
   - Putting sound-absorbing material around a noisy machine.
   - Isolating a machine by putting it on resilient vibration mountings to absorb energy before it is transformed into noise.
   - Isolating workers in soundproof booths.
   - Setting up the work station at a safe distance from the noisy machinery. (A safe distance is a location where the noise level is less than 80 decibels.)

   Other types of isolation might include splash guards, housing for dangerous moving parts of machinery, and electronic light beams that shut down equipment when crossed.

3. *Ventilation* means moving contaminated air away from the breathing zone of the workers. Air contaminants include dusts, mists, gases, fumes, and vapors. There are two kinds of ventilation: general or dilution, and local exhaust.

   General or dilution ventilation provides a constant exchange of air in a room, diluting contaminants that may be present. This type of ventilation is sufficient in offices and other work areas where the air needs to be exchanged to make it fresher. However, if offers little protection when the air contains toxic materials.

   Local exhaust ventilation is the only way to control air contamination at the source. Properly engineered, it can capture the contaminants before they enter the worker's breathing zone.

Engineering controls are mandatory in the case of some chemicals for which exposure limits have been set by the federal health standards.

Respirators come under the category of personal protective equipment mentioned earlier as one means of hazard reduction. They are required on some jobs, and they serve a vital function. But like other items of personal safety—from hard hats to steel-toed shoes, from goggles to gloves—they place the burden of responsibility on the user. They do not get to the root of the problem.

Good workplace design, following the principles of *ergonomics*, is also a part of risk reduction. Ergonomics—from the Greek *ergon* (work) and *nomos* (law)—simply means making jobs fit people, not making people fit jobs. One aspect of ergonomics is *biomechanics*, which deals mostly with the way we use (or misuse) or arms, legs, and backs.

Good designs for tools and equipment should permit workers' hands and wrists to be approximately in the same position they would be if they were hanging relaxed at the sides. If the tool, or the position required to use it, bends the wrist, for example, that's bad design. Where possible, jobs should be designed so that the arms don't have to be raised above shoulder height on a regular basis.

Jobs should also be designed to allow workers to work with their backs straight. A major share of the blame for back injuries— probably the leading cause of job-related disabilities—lies with poor workplace design that requires people to work with bent spines. Standing still for too long can put excessive strain on the spine and the back muscles, causing pain and even permanent damage to body tissues. Such a simple solution as a foot rest at the work station—like the old saloon brass rail—lessens stress on the back.

There are so many sources of potential occupational diseases and injuries that to explore them in detail is outside the scope of this overview.

Toxic effects have been reported for some 50,000 chemicals used in manufacturing; more than 2,000 of these chemicals are suspected of causing cancer in humans.

Every year, one out of every nine workers in private industry will suffer an occupational injury. How can we sift through all the clues and pinpoint the cause of an adverse health condition as being work-related instead of something the patient is doing off the job—smoking, drinking too much, overeating, not getting enough sleep, or similar unwise personal habits?

A good way to start is with an occupational history. If your doctor doesn't ask for one, suggest it. Here are some questions from my book, *Work & Health* (Press Associates, Inc., 1984), that you should be prepared to answer. Not all of them will apply to every situation. This is just an outline to guide your thinking about your job and how it might be affecting your health. The range of these questions suggests the extensive and complex nature of occupational diseases.

What exactly is your job? Is it maintenance or production? What is the product? What materials (chemicals) are involved in the process? Do you have some idea of how the process works?

Is a list available of plant chemicals that you're exposed to? Are material safety data sheets available to you? Do you understand them?

Are you exposed to airborne substances that you might inhale? Can the suspected materials be absorbed through the skin? Can you ingest them,

get them in your mouth from your hands when you eat or smoke?

Are excessive heat and/or noise a part of your work environment?

Have air samples or other measurements been taken? If so, when and by whom? Is the data available?

What, if any, ventilation is provided where you work? Can you describe it—type, location, etc.?

Are work rules and practices to control health hazards posted where you can see them? Are they being observed?

What personal protective equipment is provided? Is it being used?

Is there a pattern to your disease or discomfort? Does it occur only during work and clear up on weekends or on vacation? Does the problem show up more frequently among workers in a particular area of the plant or only among those doing a certain job? How many people are exposed? How often? For how long? How many shifts are there?

Besides your own immediate problem, are there any health complaints by your co-workers that you know about? How many complain? How often? Have they sought medical treatment? (A list of these names and the dates of treatment is useful for the medical sleuth.)

Are medical tests performed regularly where you work? Are the records available?

It is also useful to know whether the patient's health complaint has been brought to the attention of the union shop steward or safety and health representative, whether the information was discussed with the company, and whether the company is doing anything about it.

It seems fitting to conclude with a brief mention of workers' compensation. It brings us back to that row of sickbeds and gravestones—100,000 of each, spaced every 158 feet for 3,000 miles— mentioned in the beginning of this article. For these victims of the industrial age, "compensation" is a misnomer. How can you "compensate" a worker for the loss of a hand or foot or the destruction of his or her lungs?

This, by no means, is to downplay the importance of money. Adequate financial assistance is essential for workers who have suffered some job-related impairment or for the families of those who have died. It is essential, not only for the bolstering of individual dignity and appropriate productivity but as an expression of our collective national compassion.

These noble sentiments are behind the current compensation structure. But the system doesn't work as well as it should. The process of getting help is not as clear and simple as it ought to be. Workers and their survivors have difficulty filing claims for occupational illness or death benefits when they don't know which hazardous substances may have been responsible. It's hard to treat sick workers effectively when they don't know the trade names of chemical with which they work or their toxic effects. In some cases, companies using industrial chemicals aren't required to pretest substances and make the test results available.

These problems pinpoint the pressing need for more job hazard information for workers, more toxicological data for professionals, a stricter testing system for industry to ensure the safety of substances before they are introduced to the workplace or to the market.

Along with more information and accountability, there are two other areas that need to be strengthened.

1. Rehabilitation must become an integral and more effective part of the workers' compensation program. This will give disabled workers the chance to be productive again.
2. Occupational health and safety must come out of the dark and be better understood. This will benefit doctors and other health professionals, as well as workers and employers. Such heightened awareness can lead to more and better testing, more effective monitoring, keener evaluation of results, wider sharing of essential information, and so on.

Also necessary are adequate federal and state compensation laws, job retraining, and a better overall appreciation of occupational health and safety. This potent combination, meshed and working together, could finally initiate true worker's compensation.

But although taking care of the ill, the hurt, and the grieving will remain among our concerns, we must also recognize that occupational disease is primarily a *preventable* disease.

12

HEALTH EMPOWERMENT: AN APPROACH TO COMMUNITY-CONTROLLED SELF-CARE DEVELOPMENT

Lowell S. Levin, Ph.D, M.P.H., is professor of public health at Yale University. He is a strong advocate of self-care and collective action to restore consumer control over the professional health care system. He is chairman of The People's Medical Society, the largest health advocacy organization in the United States.

Pity the people at the Yale School of Medicine. Somehow they have allowed—and even tenured—an underground figure into their midst. Lowell Levin's ideas about self-care don't confront the listener as much as they envelop him in a web of logic from which it is difficult to escape. It is tempting to see self-care simply as individuals ministering to their own illnesses. But Dr. Levin asks us to expand the concept of self-care to the neighborhood or the city and see it as a community-wide proposition.■

Lay medical populism is a pervasive trend in American society. Traditional distinctions between lay and professional roles in medical care are being blurred by substantially improved public access to health information, advances in appropriate medical technology, and a fundamental shift in disease patterns that favor more nonprofessional involvement in medical care. Medical populism, as part of a broader social trend for individuals to seek more personal control in their lives, is further fueled by widening public concern about the limits, hazards, and costs of professional care. What has emerged is a social phenomenon, too diverse in origin and concept to be called a movement or fad, that has taken off on its own with a push from the government and professional medical community.

The popularization of health and medical care gained added impetus through the women's health movement. A central feature of the movement was the emphasis on body ownership and the prerequisites of knowledge and skill necessary to regain and maintain control of professional and medical services that were demeaning, inappropriate, and often physically harmful. This highly focused challenge to the care system and the pro forma limits of lay versus professional roles was a lesson certainly not lost on the public as a whole. It became clear that concepts such as medicine, medical diagnosis, treatment and rehabilitation were not the exclusive domain of a relatively small, professionally trained elite. Lay access to knowledge and skills related to these concepts is, of course, a First Amendment right. Indeed, although state medical practice acts prohibit lay people from providing medical services to others "for gain or reward, expected or received" (among other restraints), there remains substantial latitude for individuals to diagnose and treat their own illnesses. The practices associated with home treatment rarely have been challenged in the courts, even though the home treatment repertoire has expanded considerably beyond the traditional remedies of teas and chicken soup.

Of course self-care in health is nothing new. It has deep historical roots, tapping into traditional American values of individual self-reliance, common sense, and antielitism. But the 1970s and 1980s have seen an explosion of interest in health generally (note the buzz words of prevention, promotion, wholism, high-level wellness) and in lay medical care (including mutual aid groups, religious healing, health crisis hotlines, etc.)

It is no longer valid to think of the health care system in strictly professional terms. Studies of health practices in the United States, Canada, and Western Europe conclude that by far the largest proportion of health and medical care (65 to 90 percent) is provided by lay people to themselves. The lay resource in health and medical care represents, in effect, a hidden health care *system* with supplementary professional care. Note the emphasis on system, given what appear to be substantial differences in health care functions among the various lay components, e.g., individuals, families, extended families, friends, religious healers, and mutual aid groups.

Although research and development proposals were made as early as 1975, up to that time there were only a few isolated efforts beyond women's health centers to organize medical self-care education programs for adults. One such program, the Activated Patient Program, received national press attention and ultimately appeared in a best-selling book. This early program stimulated the development of over 2,000 similar efforts at strengthening lay skills in treating common illnesses and injuries, in using medications, in symptom recognition, and in home testing. Many programs emphasized skills in dealing with the health care system, especially the doctor-patient relationship. Packaged (and marketed) self-care education programs began to appear, making it possible for a wide variety of sponsoring groups to get involved. Hospitals and health maintenance organizations were especially active in offering self-care education to their patients and community.

Although there are some variations in content or focus, self-care education has tended to adhere to orthodox allopathic values, emphasize a set curriculum, use a standard teacher-learner format, and (where it happens at all) apply professionally determined measures of benefits. This approach is primarily aimed at raising (or changing) the level and quality of lay health practices to conform to, or mimic, professional values and practices. Most programs assume that it will be necessary to wash out folk customs that are judged ineffective or harmful. Furthermore, health and medical care follow a clinical model (aspirin for headache) rather than a social model (going for a walk). Local culture, customs, and beliefs about health and medical care are by and large considered impedimentia. The above characteristics of self-care education have made such programs more attractive to middle class people who share the sponsor's values than to groups committed to substantially different experiences and beliefs. This has proven to be a serious limitation in reaching groups who are especially vulnerable to health hazards (the poor, minorities, the elderly), including the hazards of professional care.

In consideration of these limitations of organized medical self-care education, an effort was made to demonstrate an approach that would have as its overriding goal the strengthening of an individual's sense of health integrity and his ability to control his health destiny. The Yale-Kellogg Self-Care Education Demonstration Program in New Haven, Connecticut tried to provide access to health and medical knowledge and skills to all social groups, and to do this in a way that would place the community in charge of the whole process. This meant that content, methods, and benefits would all be determined by the client participants. Nothing was to be predetermined by staff consultants, or "enablers," whose task it was to facilitate the organizing process and provide the personnel, physical resources, and supporting administration. Overtones of educational anarchy were clearly discernible in both the rhetoric of the funding grant and the style of development that ensued. There was, for example, a commitment to an emphasis on problem-*posing* rather than on problem-*solving*, based on the notion that he who defines the problem controls the range of solutions. Personal experience was to be honored as the primary source of knowledge and skills in health and medical care. Mutual learning among all participants was to be the main educational method, where participants and staff shared perspectives, information, and technical skill on an equal footing.

The challenge to those who initiated this project was to share power, a process once described as sometimes requiring that we "give up our principles and do the right thing." Even among those who were aware and determined to do so, it was not easy to overcome professional instincts to lay claim to unique expertise, to seek converts to their perspective, and to manipulate circumstances to fulfill their expectations. It required nearly 6 months of the 3-year project for the staff to overcome the latent constraints of their professional education. The obvious pain of this process was eased substantially by the patience, understanding, and feedback of the community participants. A growing respect for the participants' informal knowledge of health and their pragmatic approach to health problem solving was the key to reducing the we-they dichotomy. Respect returns respect. And it is a relief to do the "right thing." As one of the program staff remarked, "Working as a self-care oriented health professional is liberating. Without the burden of making people do 'what is good for them,' you can stop acting like a remote professional robot and can finally be human."

The Yale-Kellogg project in self-care education answered many questions and in fact raised new questions of even greater relevance to public empowerment in health. The goal was to establish a model of self-care education that was truly empowering and firmly fixed in the community, its values, its style of problem solving, and its economic diversity. How does one go about enlisting clients in the program, encouraging client control, using client-preferred methods, and applying client criteria to measure effectiveness? There were also questions about the program's impact on the local sponsoring agencies and on the wider community. Although this represented respectable academic curiousity, the program staff were unprepared for the questions that participants and *their* constituencies posed on the program and its process. The client-community questions demonstrated how close the project came to the community's construction of reality, priority, and benefit.

The Yale-Kellogg project was sponsored by four health care facilities in New Haven, Connecticut and environs. One sponsor was a community hospital serving several small industrial towns with large ethnic populations of blue-collar workers suffering high unemployment. An inner-city neighborhood health center sponsored a self-care education program for a black and Hispanic population, economically depressed and living in marginal housing. The third sponsor was a private health clinic serving Italian and Puerto Rican families, as well as two elderly housing projects. An HMO, providing medical care to the Yale University community of students, staff faculty, and retirees, became the fourth sponsor. Three of the sites were staffed by family nurse practitioners. A public health educator was responsible for the university-based project. Additional consulting staff at Yale provided coordination and data collecting services. The demonstration, covering the years 1980–1983, was fully funded by the W.K. Kellogg Foundation.

There was no grand strategy for the program beyond a commitment to client control and full access to all residents of the respective communities. No large campaigns were planned. There was no blitzing of the communities with health promotions or promises of salvation from disease or from the high costs of medical care. The plan was simply to announce the availability of the self-care resource and to emphasize its intention to support individuals and groups in achieving their health interests. Very early on it was clear that the term health education had to be avoided. It conjured up too many associations with unpleasant educational experiences of the inner-city and blue-collar adults. Few in the present communities wanted to relive that kind of put-down. For them, education meant control by others, not the nurturance of self-control.

In attracting people to the self-care resources, it was obvious that relatively few people had the requisite motivation, energy, and discretionary time to take advantage of the available self-care development resources. People who had tremendous needs for self-care skills often were too exhausted by the daily struggle for survival to undertake anything beyond those activities necessary to keep functioning. Even for those who were somewhat above this level of struggle, access to self-care resources had to blend optimally into existing patterns of social life. People sought to work with long-established social resources in the mainstream of community life, including churches, clubs, senior centers, day care centers, employee groups, and recreation facilities. Although all four self-care programs had bases of operations, the learning activities were diffused throughout the communities. This happened as a result of co-sponsorship, often merely a process of blending the self-care program resources into existing activities of a given social group. The ideal began to emerge as a noteworthy strategy, where the central function of self-care program staff was one of facilitating connections between established community groups, clarifying common interests in health, sharing resources, and finally (only finally) adding an increment of administrative or technical help. One conclusion definitely can be drawn about this approach: it minimizes harm to the communities' integrity while strengthening their potential to generate new problem-solving options wholly owned by the community. What is sacrificed is speed of change and the community's acknowledgement of the contribution of the so-called change agent. The issue of slow change is only a problem if health skills are linked to an urgent need. Most self-care skills, in the context of the goal of gaining more control over health, have long-term implications. The community's failure to acknowledge the role of the change agent helps in establishing self and community ownership of change and avoiding the usual dependency that accompanies the expert-to-amateur model of education (or medical care, for that matter). Tolerance for long-term, incremental, and relatively slow change and acceptance of an animating role in the change process are often difficult for community developers and educators to accept. We have come to expect the quick fix and its rewards, as measured by quantifiable outcomes and feedback from appreciative consumers. Staff in this program had to find substitutes for these sources of gratification and reinforcement in the form of mutual support through frequent staff discussions of their progress. Neither the high level of stress involved in staff review sessions nor their essential contribution to maintaining the program's integrity should be underestimated.

When the community defines its interests and priorities in health empowerment, it should come as no surprise (although it did) that these were often based on a social rather than a strictly physical definition of health. Nearly 75% of those involved in the second year of the self-care program described their overall well-being in subjective terms (e.g., contentment, satisfaction with work and social life, self-esteem). Those who construed their health in physical terms were usually over 60 years of age and were more concerned about the immediate potential for heart disease, cancer, and other ailments associated with their age-risk categories. So although there were areas of staff-client congruence with regard to the content of the self-care curricula, the social dimension of self-care clearly dominated. Social self-care skills ran the gamut from stress management to organizing voter registration, from personal coping skills to community action promoting better housing conditions.

The reality is that, unlike health professionals and academic theorists, people and community groups seeking more control in health do not stop to debate the issue of personal versus social responsibility. Health is a seamless issue for them. Personal behavior in prevention and treatment of illness is seen as an important skill, not only their responsibility but also their right. At the same time, people are aware of the social and political constraints placed on their health potential and the necessity to gain control of forces that influence health at the community level.

People who participated in the self-care program were remarkably practical in their learning interests. They carefully balanced the time and effort necessary to learn a self-care skill with perceived benefits. This meant that people selected skills that could be learned in a rela-

tively short period of time. A second criterion was utility. There was little interest in learning skills that would be used only infrequently. Fifty-two percent of the participants sought more expertise in specific health care skills in areas similar to the coverage of packaged self-care programs described earlier. But a substantial proportion of participants (31%) indicated their primary interest was in gaining control over their health. This included specific skills in assessing health information, making decisions, and using health care resources more effectively. The experience of the Yale-Kellogg program put to rest a recurrent elitist myth about low-income earners and self-care—namely, that low-income earners would have little interest in self-care, and where interest existed, it would be limited to a rather narrow band of skills (e.g., first aid). The level of sophistication in learning choices among low-income participants was certainly equal to those of middle- and upper-income groups. Indeed, it would be fair to say that low-income choices for self-care skills were often survival skills, hardly frivolous or exaggerated.

Participants in the Yale-Kellogg self-care program used the program's resources in a self-determined rather than a predetermined way. Throughout the program, participants perceived benefits in the process itself, especially benefits in a learning situation which affirmed their sense of competence. Program staff took their place in a circle of mutually competent adults who shared their views and practices in managing illness and in promoting health. All experiences were pooled in a way that defined professional expert opinion as one of several alternatives, not the mandated choice. Home remedies and folk benefits took their place alongside a variety of allopathic and nonallopathic approaches, as well as social and medical approaches. The standard hierarchy of values—from professional to lay, from allopathic to "alternative," from clinical to social—was avoided. Participants made informed choices based on input from the whole group. It was clear that the well advertised conflicts between health belief systems was of greater significance to health professionals in their jurisdictional disputes than to lay people in their struggle to achieve the best possible health benefits from the resources (personal and community) available. An eclectic, pragmatic, integrated approach to health problem solving was the result. Ordinary people move quite assuredly among the various schools of thought in health, settling as often as not on their own family experience as a reasonable solution to the illnesses most commonly experienced. The most serious issue here is not the alleged mindlessness of lay self-care practices, but rather the possibility that professional efforts would substitute medical solutions for existing effective solutions. Participant control of the self-care program helped dilute, if not wholly prevent, this possibility.

People who participated in the Yale-Kellogg program were highly selective with regard to what they wanted and how and when they wanted to be involved. Their loyalties were not to the program but to their own requirements. This would disappoint those who measure program success in terms of low "drop out" rates. Participants sought what they wanted and they withdrew when they achieved their goals.

The empowering approach of the Yale-Kellogg program accelerated its diffusion in the community. Many participants discovered that their interest in self-care went beyond their own personal needs. They also enjoyed their contribution to the organizational and facilitating process. As a result, a second generation of self-care facilitators emerged, sometimes taking over from the staff in networking with new community groups.

An analysis of the self-care network in one community revealed a striking diversity of social institutions involved. In addition to community health care agencies, the network included churches, day-care centers, senior centers, social clubs, libraries, social service agencies, voluntary associations, and mutual aid groups. These organizations represented diverse constituencies such as the elderly, the working poor, young adults, and members of various racial and ethnic groups. So broad was the spread of sponsorship that by the end of the second year of the 3-year program, it was apparent that, for many groups, the original role of the Yale-Kellogg initiative was forgotten or unknown.

CONCLUSIONS OF SPECIAL IMPORTANCE

A careful and continuous observation of the Yale-Kellogg program showed variations in learning expectations by age, sex, economic status, and race. This was expected, but the proportionate spread of interests for all groups were rather evenly distributed over three categories: personal and family health, specific concerns associated with a health problem, and fitness. Similarly, there were variations in learning method preferences, but the overwhelming majority preferred some form of active role.

Based on structured interviews with a random sample of participants, 92% of participants reported that they were better able to deal with health problems ordinarily found by themselves and their families. Eighty-seven percent said that they actually used knowledge and skills learned from their participation, and 74% had shared what they learned with family and friends. Thirty-five percent felt more assertive, more comfortable, more in control in their interaction with health care professionals. About 16% said they were less inclined to seek professional care for concerns they felt they could now manage themselves. However, 48% of those interviewed noted that they chose to increase use of their respective sponsoring health clinic because of a new awareness of services available and of the facilities' community involvement.

The program also confirmed that strengthening the community's self-care resource is primarily a matter of removing barriers of access to information and skills and doing so in a way that builds on the existing base of lay knowledge. It is an enabling process, but not a passive process. Education in health when organized on the horizontal axis of community participation involves networking and bartering resources rather than the traditional "top-down" vertical organization of professional control. The active role of professionals is focused on locating or mapping community resources and providing an effective nexus for their exchange. This is an extremely delicate process that succeeds through existing organizational structures with a minimum of new bureaucratic organization. There is no such thing as an unorganized community; the trick is to identify the pattern of relationships and work through those connections. The Yale-Kellogg program staff found they had to develop quick response planning skills, taking advantage of community interests as they emerged, often interests associated with quality-of-life issues like street rowdiness, housing relocations, and child safety. Ironically, the inability of the staff to do long-term planning helped preserve the integrity of community control over the program.

Anyone who sponsors a self-care development program can color the extent and character of its impact. The Yale-Kellogg program was based in four health care facilities, a situation that tempted a definition of the community as a "service area." This, in turn, initially suggested attracting participants through familiar methods of reaching patients. Further, the clinical mindset of the sponsoring agencies often tended to be at variance with the social definition of self-care espoused by the program staff and certainly by the community. What, after all, are clinics doing in the business of encouraging voter registration as a health education activity? Sharing power with lay people (who may not even be patients) is not part of the medical care ethic. From the community's side, their health care facility is not ordinarily viewed as a source of health empowerment. Indeed, as noted earlier, the clinic's community involvement came as a reassuring surprise to those who were exposed to the self-care program.

Certainly, clinic sponsorship provided some obvious technical benefits and their participation helped people use the facilities more appropriately. A secondary benefit to the clinics was improved community relations. But the Yale-Kellogg experience left no doubt that self-care development need not be restricted to clinical sponsorship. Libraries, churches, social clubs, and other community groups can provide sponsorship that is uninhibited by the medical model

of health. There is no shortage of health experts that lay sponsors can call upon for consultation as required. Social sponsorship of self-care development contributes to wide diffusion of self-care as an integral part of community life, affirming the belief that the lay health resource is the effective, legitimate, and essential base of the health care system.

Evaluating a community-controlled self-care program has three primary dimensions. The first is identifying and adhering to client defined criteria of outcome; however, these may vary from professional beliefs about benefits. As noted earlier, client criteria often include evidence of improved self-esteem, better self-management of personal health care, and better control over the professional system. But lay criteria often include evidence of improvement in the community's health environment, as defined in physical, economic, and political terms. Many of these changes can be described only in anecdotal, highly qualitative terms. Quantitative evaluation methods are often cumbersome and time consuming, requiring highly trained observer-analysts.

A second dimension of evaluating community-controlled self-care programs is a matter of accounting for the process of diffusion. Network analysis reveals the pattern and sequence of community involvement and can help allocate staff efforts to facilitate access by all citizens. Also needed is analysis of self-care knowledge and skill diffusion through the more intimate networks of family members and friends. Interviews with participants in the Yale-Kellogg program suggest a powerful multiplier effect.

Finally, we must look at the impact on the attitudes, knowledge, and performance of staff involved in a community-controlled self-care program, using staff expectations of outcomes as criteria. Although the Yale-Kellogg staff approached this aspect of evaluation on an *ad hoc* basis through staff observation of each other and frequent feedback sessions, there was ample evidence of personal and professional growth. It was clear that the staff's previous professional education was substantially supplemented by knowledge of health and health care as learned from community participants. Staff also learned (indeed, invented) educational approaches that stimulate citizen empowerment in health. As noted earlier, however, achievements in staff development did not happen quickly or without sometimes painful soul-searching. It is not easy to overcome or broaden role expectations that are deeply inculcated, even in the case of staff who conscientiously seek to achieve these changes in themselves. In balance, one cannot escape the conclusion that strengthening the community's self-care capacity might be more rapidly and easily achieved through efforts other than those by health professionals.

The Yale-Kellogg program broke away from major elements of traditional health education—predetermined objectives, professionally determined content and methods, and professionally defined outcome criteria. The objective was to enhance the power of lay people in health in a way that would contribute to a lifelong learning process. To do this, the program attempted to remove artificial barriers to learning. In this sense, community participants became the teachers of the program staff. The curricula that emerged derived from clients, and educational methods followed their preferences. Analysis of the program experience indicates the wide social appeal of this approach and the integration of the program within other aspects of community life. In this sense, the program became a productive way of facilitating (and often mobilizing) community interests in health.

An important lesson of the Yale-Kellogg program for those professionally involved with health development is an appreciation of the essential contribution of the existing lay health resource and the normative nature of that resource. Health is a social idea with psychological, cultural, economic, political, and biological aspects. People view health in holistic terms and seek to enhance their health roles using community resources that are nonpaternalistic, respectful of lay experience, and empowering at a very pragmatic level. We have ample evidence of the public intent to gain control over their health destinies. The task before us now is to ensure equity of access to the necessary knowledge and tools of control, particularly for those groups who remain highly vulnerable to professional dependency in health—the poor, the elderly, minorities, and women. The Yale-Kellogg program was a beginning effort to learn how to go about this.

PART IV STRESS AND STRESS MANAGEMENT

13 **Stress: What It Is and How It Affects You**
Ken Dychtwald, Ph.D.

14 **Stress and Coronary Heart Disease—New Concepts**
Dean Ornish, M.D.

15 **Stress and Organizations: Reducing the Stress of Community Life**
Paul Rosch, M.D.

16 **Burnout: Renewing the Spirit**
Dennis T. Jaffe, Ph.D., and Cynthia D. Scott, Ph.D.

13 STRESS: WHAT IT IS AND HOW IT AFFECTS YOU

Ken Dychtwald, Ph.D., is president of Age Wave, a communications and consulting firm, and of Dychtwald & Associates, an executive seminar and training company. Dr. Dychtwald also lectures at several colleges and universities on psychology, gerontology, and health-related sciences. He has appeared on national television and radio shows, including Good Morning America, The CBS Morning News, and The Merv Griffin Show. His books include *BODYMIND, Millennium: Glimpses into the 21st Century, Stress-Management: Take Charge of Your Life, Wellness and Health Promotion for the Elderly,* and *The Age Wave.*

Stress is a daunting subject. We all think we know what it is, although no two people seem to define stress in exactly the same way. Yet we all agree that it plays a critical role in the human condition. Because stress is a common experience and its consequences can be measured scientifically, it serves as a common meeting ground for proponents of traditional medical care and advocates of new holistic approaches to health care. We asked Ken Dychtwald to give us a simple, straightforward exposition of this universal experience. He describes the symptoms and origins of stress, its effect on our behavior, and some positive aspects. ▪

THE RISE OF STRESS-RELATED PROBLEMS

America is experiencing a major epidemic today. Unlike epidemics of the past, it is not a disease transmitted by bacteria or viruses. This epidemic is an increase in diseases and problems related to stress, and it touches all of our lives.

In 1900 the average life expectancy in this country was 47, and the major killer diseases included tuberculosis, pneumonia, influenza, cholera, typhoid, and smallpox—infectious diseases which struck people of all ages, regardless of their lifestyle. Today, on the other hand, life expectancy has been extended to 74, thanks in large part to the conquest of the acute infectious diseases through improved sanitation, better distribution and storage of foods, and the introduction of immunization and antibiotics. People today are dying of different diseases than they did at the turn of the century, and the principal causes of death today are heart disease, stroke, cancer, cirrhosis of the liver, and diabetes. These non-infectious, chronic diseases have been shown to be directly related to the way we live, and one of the dominant factors in their development is stress—an element of modern life which is taking an increasing toll on our physical and mental well-being.

THE STRESS RESPONSE: AN ANCIENT MECHANISM FOR SURVIVAL

Technically speaking, stress is a physiological state of the body, a state of arousal in response to a perceived danger or threat. We are all familiar with the physical signs and symptoms of the stress state. Think about how you felt that last time you had to swerve to avoid a collision while driving: your heart raced, your palms became sweaty, your muscles tensed, and your stomach knotted. Such a combination of sensations is the result of a complex physiological chain reaction which occurs in your body in response to a threat. These changes are universal and predictable, and they happen to everyone. Our prehistoric ancestors, upon encountering a dangerous animal in the wild, would have felt exactly the same response as their bodies switched into a stress-induced "high-gear" to deal with the emergency.

THE FIGHT-OR-FLIGHT RESPONSE

Physiologist Walter Cannon, back in the 1920s, labeled this reaction the *fight-or-flight response*. Triggered by the brain and operating through the hormones secreted by the endocrine system, this heightened state of arousal prepares the body for action in the following ways:

- *The heart rate quickens* and *blood pressure rises* to provide more fuel and oxygen to the brain and muscles.
- *Breathing becomes rapid and heavy* to distribute more oxygen and eliminate carbon dioxide.
- *The muscles tense in the arms and legs* in preparation for increased exertion.
- *Digestion ceases* so that the blood can be diverted to the brain and muscles.
- *Perspiration increases* to prevent the body from overheating.
- *The pupils dilate*, allowing more light to enter, and *all senses are heightened*.
- *Attention narrows* as the mind attempts to focus on the problem at hand.
- *The hands and feet become cold* as the circulation is diverted from the extremities to protect against bleeding.
- *Adrenaline is released into the body* to promote peak functioning.
- *Stored sugars and fats pour into the bloodstream* to provide fuel for quick energy.

As the term implies, the original purpose of the flight-or-fight response was to prepare the body to respond either by fighting the enemy, or by fleeing. Whether the primitive hunter succeeded in killing the mountain lion or in running away from it, the result was the same: once the threat was resolved, the body could relax, eventually returning to its normal baseline functioning.

Interestingly enough, situations which provoke the fight-or-flight response are not necessarily unpleasant ones. Pleasant experiences, if they are sufficiently intense, can produce the same combination of physiological symptoms. When your boss tells you that he's recommended you for a promotion, you are most likely experiencing some the same physiological responses that you experience when you swerve to avoid a traffic accident: sweaty palms, racing heart, changes in breathing. Pleasant or unpleasant, it's the *intensity* of the experience that produces the stress.

EUSTRESS/DISTRESS

Dr. Hans Selye, an endocrinologist whose ground-breaking research was a major contribution to our understanding of stress, defined stress as the non-specific or general response of the body to any demand made upon it to readjust. Selye emphasized that stress is not necessarily something to be avoided. It is a natural part of our lives; any normal activity, pleasant or unpleasant, produces some degree of stress. As Selye said, "The absence of stress is death." Just as stress prepared primitive man to confront and fight his enemy or to run away, so in modern life it helps the athlete to achieve peak performance or the executive to meet impossible deadlines. Under such circumstances, stress can be a very useful response, contributing to heightened achievement and a greater sense of personal satisfaction. When stress is associated with such a positive experience, Selye called it *eustress* (sometimes also called *prostress*); when it becomes unpleasant or damaging, it is called *distress*.

THE STRESSORS OF LIFE

Events that provoke stress are known as stressors. It's easy to identify many such triggers of stress in our daily lives. Some sources of stress can be classified as environmental: weather changes, temperature, noise, air pollution, crowding, and uncomfortable living or work space can all have an influence on your stress level. A major source of stress in our modern world is change; more than ever before in history we are forced constantly to adapt to rapid change in many important aspects of our lives—changing values, family structure, and sex roles, the decline of religious faith, and the changing nature of work. Interpersonal stressors emerge from your relationships with other people—your boss, your fellow workers, your family and friends. And a significant source of stress in many of our lives today is work stressors—the structure of your employer's organization, your position within it, your interaction with

other people, and your feelings about your job are all factors that can contribute to raising your overall stress level.

You may have noted that many of the stressors we have been describing don't actually represent threats to your physical survival. Rather, they are psychological or social in nature. Imagined threats to your self-esteem or security can arouse the fight-or-flight response just as readily as an attacking mountain lion or an oncoming car. Moreover, our psychological and emotional reactions to stressful situations, such as anxiety or guilt, can actually become potent stressors in their own right.

What arouses a high level of stress in one person may not be perceived as threatening to another, for our individual perception of the stressor is what ultimately makes the situation stressful or not. We are all different in our biochemical make-up, physical strength, psychological and emotional characteristics, values, attitudes, habits, and social roles. And all these factors influence our interpretation of events and, therefore, the way we respond physically and psychologically to them.

As a primitive survival mechanism, the fight-or-flight response served our ancestors well as a means of mobilizing the body's defenses in times of emergency. Why, then, has stress become such a problem in modern life?

THE STRESS RESPONSE
IN THE MODERN WORLD

In the case of the primitive hunter, once the danger had been dealt with by fighting or fleeing, the problem was resolved and the stress was relieved. However, if we look around us today, we notice that the options of fighting or fleeing are rarely appropriate in our modern world. For example, if you have an argument with your boss, you may feel all the symptoms of stress—tense muscles, rapid heartbeat, rapid breathing—but you can't relieve your stress by striking out at him, nor would it do to run away. And so the level of anger and arousal persists in the absence of a socially acceptable outlet, and at the end of the confrontation you still feel as if you want to fight someone or run away. The fight-or-flight response has now become an internalized feeling that you carry about with you, like a ticking time bomb.

If the fight-or-flight response is activated without being used to its intended purpose, it can become a major source of distress. If it is fired off too often, or persists too long, the body will remain in a state of continual alarm or mobilization, and the potent hormones released in the stress response can actually damage the body's vital organs, nervous system, and immune mechanisms. Ironically, it appears that the stress response, which was a vital survival mechanism for our remote ancestors, may in fact be killing us today.

GENERAL ADAPTATION SYNDROME

To explain how prolonged, unrelieved stress damages the body, Hans Selye in 1936 described a general pattern that animals and humans manifest in response to a stress-producing situation. He called this pattern of response the *General Adaptation Syndrome*, or GAS, and broke it down into three phases:

1. **Alarm.**   The first phase is the alarm stage, when the body's defenses are mobilized to deal with the stressor (the fight-or-flight reaction).
2. **Resistance.**   If the stress persists, we enter a second stage wherein our resistance to the stressor that triggered the response is increased, although the body's resistance to other types of stressors may simultaneously decline. As the body adapts to the presence

of the stressor, the physiological signs of the alarm reaction virtually disappear.
3. **Exhaustion.**   If exposure to the same stressor is prolonged, however, the body eventually enters a final stage of exhaustion. The signs of the alarm stage reappear, and the body suffers damage or, ultimately, death.

MULTIPLE STRESSORS

According to Selye, the body is capable of returning to a normal state after stressful episodes, provided it has time to rest and recuperate. The problem is that in our modern world we are often exposed to prolonged and multiple stressors that permit us no time to recover. Not only are the choices to fight or flee often inappropriate in today's world, but the very characteristics of modern stressors are often such that it is virtually impossible to relieve the stress they trigger. Many stressors, such as excessive noise, are prolonged by their very nature; all our body can do is to attempt to adapt to these long-term stressors. Furthermore, many modern stressors are not external and physical at all but arise from our own imagination. Our own fears, guilt, and anxieties, our fantasies about what might be going wrong, can trigger the fight-or-flight response just as if the feared event itself were occurring. In such cases, however, there's no enemy out there to fight with or run away from.

Finally, many of the stressors in modern life are impersonal in origin. In our dealings with faceless bureaucracies, institutions, and corporations, we often experience frustrations and stress, but when a computer makes an error or we come up against "corporate policies," there's no appropriate outlet for our fight-or-flight response.

Thus the stressors that we all experience tend to persist over the long term, and the stress they arouse is often not effectively relieved through socially acceptable channels. Yet the persistent triggering of the stress response can produce mentally and physically damaging results. The greater the frequency of stressors, or the longer they persist, the greater the risk that you will develop stress-related problems and diseases.

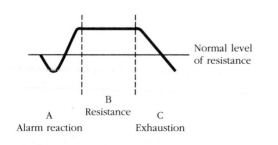

Normal level of resistance

A
Alarm reaction

B
Resistance

C
Exhaustion

STRESS BUILD-UP

For too many of us, there is no relief from the build-up of stress throughout our work days. For example, let's say you wake up late one morning and must rush to get to work. Your stress level is already high before you are out of the door. Then you must sit in bumper-to-bumper commuter traffic, worrying about whether you'll have time to prepare for an important meeting. When you arrive at work late, you get a reproving glance from your boss, which raises your stress level even higher. You try to rush to get your work done, but you are constantly interrupted by the phone or by people dropping into your office. You fumble through a meeting and worry about your performance later. You decide to skip lunch to try to get some work done, and just drink several cups of coffee rather than get a good meal; the coffee reduces your tolerance for stress even further. In the afternoon you blow up at a subordinate, then stew about your outburst. You leave the office late and arrive home late for dinner, which results in an argument with your spouse. Your stress level has remained elevated all day, and the only chance you have to recuperate is when you collapse in bed at night.

STRESS-RELATED ILLNESS

It's precisely because of the day-to-day buildup of unrelieved stress in modern life that we are experiencing an epidemic of stress-related problems and diseases. Many of our common minor disorders may, in fact, be early warning signs of excessive stress. How many of the following have you experienced?

Aching neck and
  shoulder muscles
Allergies
Anger
Arthritis
Asthma
Chest pain
Clenching of the jaw
Cold hands and feet
Colds or flu
Colitis

Constant sadness
Crying easily
Depression
Diarrhea
Difficulty getting
  along with people
Difficulty making
  decisions
Dizziness
Excessive daydreaming
  and fantasizing

Constipation
Excessive drug con-
  sumption (pre-
  scription or
  nonprescription)
Excessive or irrational
  mistrust of associates
Excessive sweating
Eyelid or facial twitch
Faintness
Feeling apprehensive
Feeling blue
Feeling hopeless about
  the future
Feeling low in energy
  or slowed down
Feeling no interest
  in things
Feeling tense or
  keyed up
Frequent accidents or
  injuries
Frustration
Grinding of teeth
Headaches (tension,
  migraine)
Heart palpitations
Heartburn
Hemorrhoids
High blood
  pressure
Hyperventilation

Increase in drinking or
  smoking habits
Indigestion
Insomnia (sleep onset,
  early morning
  awakening)
Irritability
Loss of appetite
Loss of sexual interest
  and pleasure
Low back pain
Low grade infections
Lump in the throat
Menstrual distress
Mind going blank often
Nervousness
Nightmares
Overeating
Peptic ulcer
Prolonged periods of
  brooding
Restlessness
Shortness of breath
Skin problems
Stomach problems
Tight muscles
Trembling or shaking
Trouble concentrating
Trouble remembering
  things
Weeping
Worrying

Hardly anyone could honestly say that they haven't experienced some of these complaints. However, these signs and symptoms of stress are very important and can be helpful warning signs. Your headache, your irritability, and even your indigestion are all messages your body and mind are sending to indicate that your stress has reached an excessive level. It's unwise to ignore these warning signals. If the generator light comes on in your car, you don't disconnect the light and expect the problem to go away. In just the same way, if you suffer from recurrent headaches or backache, it does no good to ignore them or to try to mask them with alcohol, aspirin, or other medications.

If you allow your stress level to remain high, these physiological warning signs will eventually progress from being acute to chronic. Then, instead of having occasional high blood pressure when you become very nervous, you may develop chronic high blood pressure; instead of feeling an occasional gnawing in your stomach when you are under stress, you may develop a chronic ulcer. In the case of the cardiovascular system, for example, the stress reaction causes an elevation of blood pressure, increased heart output, and changes in blood chemistry, which can ultimately damage the walls of the blood vessels. The result in the long term can be heart attack or stroke.

According to Hans Selye, we are all genetically different in our ability to tolerate stress. Selye says we have two kinds of adaptation energy. One kind, which he calls superficial, is readily replaced if we are able to recuperate after stressful episodes. But another kind of adaptation energy lies in deep reserves, and Selye says that this reserve is finite. Hard-driving individuals who experience constant, unrelieved stress may use up all their superficial adaptation energy without allowing themselves sufficient time to recuperate; they then have to dip into their finite reserves, and once used, this reserve cannot be replaced. As we tap into these genetic reserves, we become increasingly susceptible to illness with each successive episode of prolonged stress.

According to Selye, stress is also a major factor in aging. Each stressful episode leaves behind irreversible physical scars; stress produces wear and tear on the body. Aging is the sum of all the stresses, or wear and tear, to which the body has been exposed during a lifetime. As a species, our potential life span is 120 years, and we all have the capacity to live many more years than the present average of 74. Stress is one significant factor that can prevent us from realizing our full biological potential.

But is stress always bad? Must stress always produce a negative effect on our lives?

No. Although too much stress can clearly produce physical and psychological illness, it's important to remember that we all require a certain amount of stress in order to feel good. It is stress in this positive sense, or eustress, which makes for challenge and vitality, and adds to the vibrancy of life. For example, you've most likely had the experience of doing a job better than usual because you had to meet a tight deadline, or of going slightly beyond your normal limit in athletic performance under the pressure of competition. The pressure of deadlines, the challenge of competition, or the self-generated drive to do a little better can often boost our performance to a higher level.

HOW STRESS AFFECTS PERFORMANCE

In the figure on page 92 you will see that mental and physical performance is directly related to the degree of stress in a bell-shaped curve. Without stress, performance is low because arousal is low, as shown on the lefthand side of the curve. Then there is an optimal level of stimulation, or stress, between high and low, where performance will reach a peak. However, once we pass this optimal stress zone, performance begins to deteriorate rapidly. Thus, both understimulation and overstimulation result in lower than optimal performance.

We can readily observe how this curve affects performance in the workplace. Workers who are under too much stress will tend to perform poorly, making frequent errors, becoming ill, and not getting along easily with their fellow employees. By the same token, workers who are not presented with enough challenge are also likely to perform poorly and to display boredom, high rates of absenteeism, low motivation, and negative attitudes. Underload can be as much of a problem as overload. Overloaded, overstimulated workers tend to "burn out" on the job, never having time to recover from the excessive levels of stress generated during the day. Those who are understimulated tend to "rust out," owing to lack of challenge, variety, and change.

MAKING STRESS WORK FOR YOU

Stress need not be a negative experience; in fact, well-managed stress can represent a mechanism for transformation and growth. The Chinese language contains a clue to the two sides of the stress cycle; the Chinese character meaning "crisis" is

STRESS AND PERFORMANCE

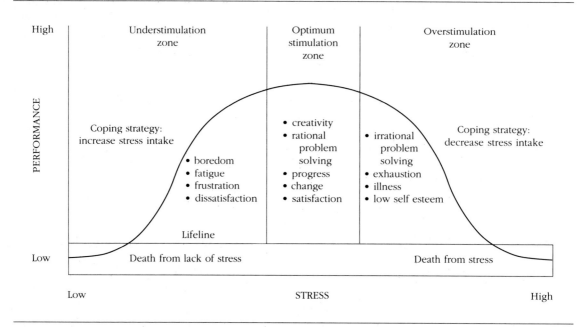

High

Understimulation zone   Optimum stimulation zone   Overstimulation zone

PERFORMANCE

Coping strategy: increase stress intake

- creativity
- rational problem solving
- progress
- change
- satisfaction

- boredom
- fatigue
- frustration
- dissatisfaction

- irrational problem solving
- exhaustion
- illness
- low self esteem

Coping strategy: decrease stress intake

Lifeline

Low   Death from lack of stress   Death from stress

Low   STRESS   High

composed of the symbols for "danger" and "opportunity." Although stress can be damaging, it can also challenge us to grow. Thus in the positive stress cycle, when we are confronted with stressors, we respond to the stress in a way that promotes growth, reinforces the development of effective coping mechanisms, and leads to even greater strength when we are confronted with new stressors. The sense of elation and accomplishment that comes from dealing effectively with stress enhances our own self-confidence and makes us more capable of dealing with stressors

in the future. In this way, the stress of modern life can ultimately become a source of challenge, richness of experience, and enhanced mental and physical vitality.

With each day that passes there is every indication that the quantity and complexity of the stress in our lives will continue to increase. Our job is not to run from stress, but to learn methods and strategies for coping effectively with it and harnessing the energy and excitement it unleashes to our best advantage.

14 STRESS AND CORONARY HEART DISEASE— NEW CONCEPTS

Dean Ornish, M.D., is executive director of the Preventive Medicine Research Institute in San Francisco and author of *Stress, Diet, and Your Heart* (Henry Holt and Co., 1982). Dr. Ornish is also Assistant Clinical Professor of Medicine at the University of California at San Francisco, where he is directing a 3-year study to determine whether heart disease can be reversed by changing the patient's lifestyle.

One of the editors of this book once surveyed a cross-section of employees at a large pharmaceutical company concerning the stress in their lives. Every person surveyed, from the executive vice president to the groundskeeper, declared that stress was a major problem in his life. Upon further discussion, however, virtually no one surveyed could link stress to some specific problem, disease, or limitation. Still, most people think that, aside from being just generally debilitating, stress must be linked to the health of the heart. But in what specific ways does stress compromise cardiac well-being and, more specifically, coronary heart disease? Dean Ornish summarizes his research on the subject.■

Coronary heart disease is still the number one cause of death in this country and in most of the industrialized world. The impact of lifestyle on coronary heart disease—for better and for worse—is becoming increasingly well understood. State-of-the-art, expensive, high tech advances are now making it possible to assess the effectiveness and power of ancient, inexpensive, low tech approaches.

In particular, the mechanisms that explain why emotional stress leads to coronary heart disease (CHD) are becoming clearer. In this context, understanding how emotional stress affects the heart can serve as a model for studying how stress and lifestyle contribute to other illnesses.

While evidence is accumulating that lifestyle factors are powerful determinants of health and illness, the limitations and costs of high tech medicine are becoming more apparent. Later in this essay, I will explore some of the resulting health policy issues, focusing on coronary artery bypass surgery as both example and metaphor of the consequences of "bypassing" health problems rather than addressing the underlying causes.

Let's begin by examining how cardiologists have viewed the role of emotional stress in coronary heart disease. Although the general public tends to take it for granted that emotional stress plays an important role in CHD, many cardiologists do not, because it has been difficult to measure, quantify, and observe the effects of emotional stress on the heart.

Because of this, scientists and physicians have tended not to study the role of emotional stress or stress management training in cardiovascular disease. Instead, they have focused on what *can* be measured more easily—blood pressure, cholesterol levels, EKGs, coronary angiography, and so on. As Abraham Maslow once wrote, "If the only tool you have is a hammer, you tend to see everything as a nail," like the man who lost his wallet in an alley but searched for it under a streetlamp because the light was better over there.

In 1977, perhaps heralding a new era in cardiology, Bernard Lown, M.D., a renowned cardiologist and recent Nobel laureate, stated in an article published in the *American Journal of Cardiology* that, "To date, research has been focused exclusively on the heart as the seat of deranged function. In fact, the focus should be shifted from the heart as target to the brain as trigger. . . . The therapeutic implications are profound."

Until very recently, however, scientists and cardiologists have not had the tools to measure the effects of the brain on the heart. New technology—such as positron emission tomography of the heart (PET)—is beginning to demonstrate that emotional stress may cause immediate and profound reductions in blood flow to the heart. These changes can be observed and measured. PET has the unique capability of noninvasively constructing a three-dimensional model of the heart, allowing measurements of very small changes in coronary blood flow.

Thus, for the first time, the effects of emotional stress on the heart now can be measured directly. Recent work by John Deanfield, M.D., from the Hammersmith Hospital in London and Andrew Selwyn, M.D., from Harvard Medical School has demonstrated that even mild emotional stresses such as mental arithmetic may produce reductions in blood flow to the heart that can be detected by PET. For example, simply asking a heart patient to perform serial subtractions of the number seven (100, 93, 86, 79, etc.) may cause measurable reductions in coronary blood flow.

New technological advances such as PET can profoundly alter our view of the world, accelerating shifts in concepts and even paradigms. In the 17th century, Galileo used a different technological breakthrough, the telescope, to challenge the prevailing worldview of his era. Using the telescope, people could see for themselves that the Earth was not the center of the universe. During the 1960s, the technology of space travel gave astronauts a new vantage point, allowing them—and us—to see the Earth as a whole. In an analogous way, new technologies such as PET may help to bridge the gap between mind and body that has existed for so long in Western medicine.

WHY IS THE HEART AFFECTED BY LIFESTYLE FACTORS SUCH AS EMOTIONAL STRESS?

The heart pumps blood to organs throughout the body, but it first pumps blood to itself through blood vessels called coronary arteries. Blood carries oxygen, the main fuel of the heart, which is bound to hemoglobin molecules. Love may inspire the heart, but it is oxygen that the beating heart most requires. Because the heart is always beating, it requires a continual supply of blood and oxygen.

In coronary heart disease, blood flow to the heart becomes reduced. If this oxygen deprivation is for a brief time, then angina (chest pain) results. If blood flow to part of the heart is reduced for more than a few minutes, then that area of the heart which is deprived of blood may die. This is called a myocardial infarction (heart attack).

During the past 100 years or so, cardiologists have tended to view coronary arteries from a plumber's perspective—as rigid pipes. For much of this century, reduced blood flow to the heart was thought to be due to only one mechanism, clogged coronary arteries. Most of what was known about coronary heart disease was learned at the autopsy table, where examination of people who died of heart attacks revealed that their coronary arteries were clogged by cholesterol and other substances in the blood that had become deposited on the inner walls of those vessels.

These blockages build up over a period of many years, like rust building up in a pipe. Autopsies performed on soldiers who died in Korea and Vietnam demonstrated that most men in their early twenties had some blockage in their coronary arteries. More recent studies have revealed that even young children who died in accidents and who had high levels of blood cholesterol also had some blockages in their coronary arteries.

During the late 1970s, a different picture of coronary heart disease began to emerge, one that is much more dynamic. A series of research reports showed that other mechanisms can also reduce blood flow to the heart. These discoveries have revolutionized our understanding of coronary heart disease.

In particular, these mechanisms help to explain why lifestyle factors can cause coronary heart disease, help to prevent it, and in some cases reverse the disease process. In short, the ability of lifestyle factors to harm or heal can be mediated via these mechanisms.

The most important of these mechanisms are known as coronary artery spasm and platelet aggregation (clumping). Diet, emotional stress, too much or too little exercise, nicotine, caffeine, and cocaine—each can powerfully affect the heart via these mechanisms.

Although blockages in coronary arteries may take many years to build up, coronary artery spasm and platelet clumping are much more dynamic, leading to rapid variations in coronary blood flow, sometimes within seconds.

Coronary arteries, like other arteries throughout the body, are not static and unchanging. The arterial walls are lined with smooth muscle that can go into spasm (constrict), reducing or shutting down blood flow.

Platelets are specialized cells that promote blood clotting. During injury, platelets clump together and form blood clots, thus helping to stop the flow of blood. However, platelets also may form clots inside coronary arteries, which can lead to a heart attack.

These three mechanisms—blockages (plaque), coronary artery spasm (constriction), and platelet clotting—can work in concert to reduce blood flow to the heart. If an artery is, say, 80% blocked with plaque, then only a relatively small amount of coronary spasm and/or a relatively small blood clot may completely shut off blood flow to the heart, leading to chest pain or a heart attack.

Emotional stress can cause both coronary artery spasm and platelet clumping. These effects seem to be mediated via (1) the sympathetic nervous system, and (2) the release of stress hormones. This helps to explain why people sometimes experience angina or heart attacks during times of emotional stress.

Part of the nervous system is divided into

two components, the sympathetic and parasympathetic nervous systems. During times of emotional stress, the brain stimulates the sympathetic nervous system more than the parasympathetic, causing the heart rate to increase and the arteries to constrict.

These changes are controlled by cellular switches, or receptors, that are located on the heart and in the arteries. During times of stress, nerve endings located near the heart's receptors release packets of hormones called catecholamines, which include norepinephrine and epinephrine (adrenaline). Catecholamines also are produced by the adrenal glands, located near the kidneys.

When released, these hormones bind to the receptors and turn them on, causing arteries to constrict and platelets to become stickier, forming blood clots more easily. These hormones also cause platelets to release another hormone, a prostaglandin called thromboxane A_2. Both thromboxane A_2 and catecholamines are potent constrictors of arterial smooth muscle and powerful endogenous stimulators of platelet aggregation.

This stress-induced stimulation of the sympathetic nervous system is known as the "fight-or-flight response," a series of physiological changes that prepare us either to fight or to run. As part of this response, heart rate, blood pressure, rate of breathing, muscular tension, and general metabolism all increase.

Some of these changes have evolved because of their survival value. In ancient times, if a tiger suddenly joined someone on his morning walk, the fight-or-flight response would help him to run away more quickly. If he decided to stay and fight, increased muscular tension would offer more protection and "body armor" during the fight. If the tiger mauled his arm, stress-enhanced arterial spasm and platelet clumping in his arm would stop the bleeding more quickly. Once the danger was over, his body would return to normal.

In modern times, however, the stresses are more relentless, so the fight-or-flight mechanisms are more chronically activated. We wake up, listen to bad news on the radio, fight traffic, go from hectic meetings to anxiety-producing phone calls, negotiate a deal over lunch, fight more traffic on the way home—on and on and on. It is easy to remain oblivious to the early warning signals of stress until illness forces us to slow down.

Twentieth-century stresses are usually emotional rather than physical, but the body reacts in the same way to emotional stresses as it does to physical ones. Running from danger and doing battle are the physical actions for which the fight-or-flight response has prepared us, but in the modern world we usually do not take this kind of action, even though our bodies are geared to do so. Thanks to our imposed social and behavioral restraints, fight-or-flight has become grin-and-bear-it.

When the fight-or-flight mechanisms are chronically activated, mechanisms which have evolved to protect us can themselves become lethal. Rather than help us to survive danger, the chronically activated fight-or-flight response may create it by causing arteries to constrict and platelets to form clots in the coronary arteries (rather than just in the peripheral arteries), which can cause heart attacks.

Caffeine also stimulates the sympathetic nervous system. So does nicotine, but much more so, and this is one reason why smoking cigarettes is a major cause of coronary heart disease. Indeed, cigarettes cause more people to die from heart disease than from lung cancer.

Cocaine and amphetamines stimulate the sympathetic nervous system even more than nicotine or caffeine. The recent deaths of world class athletes—basketball star Len Bias and football star Don Rogers—are tragic testimonies of the power of cocaine to cause sudden cardiac death in otherwise healthy people. While neither had blockages in his coronary arteries, cocaine probably induced heart attacks by intensely stimulating the sympathetic nervous system, causing coronary artery spasm and platelet clumping, thereby reducing blood flow to the heart and disrupting the heart's rhythm. It is also important to note that both deaths occurred during times of intense emotional stress—Len Bias had been drafted by the

Boston Celtics the day before his death, and Don Rogers died at an all-night bachelor party the day before he was to have been married.

Cholesterol levels, while affected by diet, also are affected by stress. A remarkable breadth of stressful situations can raise cholesterol to a significant degree, ranging from taking exams, going into battle, watching suspenseful or erotic films, or arguing with a spouse. Conversely, stress management training can lower cholesterol levels independent of dietary changes.

Even a single high-fat, high-cholesterol meal may cause acute enhancement of platelet reactivity. These changes may result from increased thromboxane A_2 production; some evidence supports this. Cholesterol-enriched platelets release more thromboxane than cholesterol-depleted platelets. In animals with atherosclerosis induced by high-cholesterol diets, platelets synthesize thromboxane A_2 in increased amounts.

Emotional stress also increases blood levels of free fatty acids (FFAs), one of the breakdown products of fats. FFAs cause the heart to require more oxygen. Also, a diet that contains a large proportion of animal products results in high blood levels of FFAs. The opposite is true with diets low in animal products, probably by shifting from non-carbohydrate to carbohydrate energy sources during physical or emotional stresses.

Emotional stress has been linked to the development of atherosclerosis in monkeys as a factor independent of diet or blood cholesterol levels. In adult male cynomolgus monkeys fed a moderately atherogenic diet, Dr. Jay Kaplan found that social stress tended to promote atherosclerosis. Stressed monkeys fed a low-fat, low-cholesterol diet developed more extensive coronary artery atherosclerosis than unstressed controls, although not to the extent of stressed monkeys on a high-fat, high-cholesterol diet.

We are living in a modern society with minds and bodies that evolved for a much different environment. There has not yet been enough time to evolve ways of coping effectively with the chronic stresses of modern society. The stresses faced by our ancestors may have been more intense, but they probably were not as chronic.

Stress management techniques can help. These include stretching, breathing techniques, meditation, visualization, and progressive relaxation. Their purpose is to gain progressively more awareness and control over body and mind. Although simple, these techniques are powerful. (Besides its physical benefits, exercise also helps to reduce stress.)

Stretching slowly helps to loosen up and remove chronic muscular tension due to stress. Sometimes we may not be aware of how stressed we have become until a sore back or stiff neck at the end of the day reminds us—the result of unwittingly tensing our "body armor," waiting for the blow that doesn't come. Stretching increases flexibility and the awareness of areas that become tense, making it easier to recognize symptoms of stress at an earlier stage. Taking heed of these early warning signals may prevent more serious problems later.

Breathing is a link between the body and the mind—it both reflects and affects your state of mind. During times of stress, breathing is shallow and rapid. When relaxed, breathing is usually slow and full. Likewise, how you breathe affects your internal state. When feeling stressed, you can become more centered and focused simply by reminding yourself to breathe more slowly and deeply. (Almost any basketball player, for example, takes a slow, deep breath when shooting from the foul line.)

Meditation is focusing awareness on a particular sound or activity. When energy is focused, it increases. By analogy, a laser emits focused, or coherent, light—the same light found in a regular light bulb, but with much greater power because it is focused.

Whenever awareness is focused, the mind's effect on the body increases, for better and for worse. Meditation brings awareness into the present. In contrast, for example, while driving down the highway, your mind may be thinking about a variety of things—remembering what you forgot to do, planning the rest of the day—unless someone veers in front of you causing you to slam on your brakes. Then your mind becomes very focused. To paraphrase Samuel Johnson:

"Anger wonderfully concentrates the mind."

During moments of anger, concentration is profound, so the mind has a profound effect on the body, but because the thoughts are negative, the effects may be harmful. Blood pressure, heart rate, and tension increase substantially. By redirecting your awareness to something neutral— (breathing, for example) you can break negative meditations and begin more positive ones.

Have you ever found yourself during the afternoon humming a song you had heard that morning on the radio? Similarly, a few minutes of meditation in the morning continues subconsciously throughout the day and raises your threshold for what causes you stress. Your fuse gets longer.

Visualization is directed meditation using mental images. The body responds to pictures in the mind.

Like meditation, visualization may have both healing and harmful effects. Dr. Louis Sigler, a New York cardiologist, described one of his patients who was forced to witness the murder of seven of his comrades in a Nazi concentration camp. Visualization of this horror produced severe irregularities in the patient's heart even though it was 30 years later. Conversely, visualization can produce positive changes.

In 1977, when I was a medical student, I conducted a pilot study to assess the short-term effects of these stress management techniques and dietary changes in treating patients with documented coronary heart disease. It was a small, 1-month study of 10 patients (no control group). I was encouraged by the degree of subjective and objective improvements that we measured, including improved blood flow to the heart demonstrated by exercise thallium treadmill testing.

In 1980, my colleagues and I conducted a larger, randomized trial of the effects of lifestyle changes in treating coronary heart disease. In that study, patients with coronary heart disease were randomly divided into two groups. One group lived together in a controlled environment and received the program of lifestyle changes, while the other group received only their usual medical care. After 24 days, there was a 91% reduction in the frequency of chest pain in patients whose lifestyle had changed, and many patients were able to return to full-time employment, some after many years out of work.

Also, we measured clear objective improvements in these patients. Blood pressure and cholesterol decreased, while exercise capability and psychological status markedly improved. Over one half of the patients were able to reduce or discontinue cardiac and blood pressure medications. Using nuclear cardiology tests, we demonstrated that the heart began to pump blood more effectively and to contract more uniformly— objective evidence that the disease process was improving. All of these differences were clinically and statistically significant when compared to the nonintervention control group.

However, many questions remain unanswered. Can people with coronary heart disease be motivated to change their lifestyles while living "in the real world" instead of in a controlled environment? What are the best strategies for doing so? What are the long-term effects of these lifestyle changes? Most important, does atherosclerosis (blockage) within the coronary arteries improve after lifestyle change—that is, can the disease process be halted or reversed? Do people who practice stress management techniques have more blood flow to the heart (as measured by PET) during times of stress than before learning these techniques? We are conducting new research designed to help answer these questions.

WHY ARE STRESS MANAGEMENT TECHNIQUES EFFECTIVE?

There is a tendency to think of stress as something "out there" that happens to us. Some situations seem inherently stressful, while others do not. But how we *react* to a situation determines how stressed we feel. In this context, stress management techniques can be useful in helping us learn to react to potentially stressful situations in ways that are less harmful.

Some situations do seem to be inherently stressful, from asking the boss for a raise or dealing with an angry client to walking on the moon or performing open heart surgery. Yet many of the best heart surgeons are relaxed while in the midst of a complex, life-and-death operation, because that is what they are trained to do. They love to operate. And according to an Apollo astronaut who walked on the moon, "Life in the business world has been much more stressful than anything I did during the space program." Being blasted into space would seem to be one of life's more stressful experiences, yet the astronauts were trained in simulations, over and over, to react more calmly to hostile environments.

Air traffic controllers also have jobs that can be highly stressful. Dr. Robert Rose of the University of Texas Medical School studied 416 air traffic controllers for 3 years. He assumed that most air traffic controllers would show signs of stress-related illnesses. Surprisingly, he found that the incidence of illness, both physical and emotional, was directly related to the attitude they had toward their work. In other words, the intensity of stress is dependent on the way it is perceived.

If this is true, then the implications are important. Our behaviors are a result of our motivations. Our motivations, in turn, are a result of how we perceive the world. Therefore, it is not sufficient to change only behaviors, such as Type A behavior. It is necessary to change perceptions.

I believe that perceiving oneself as isolated, separate, and alone leads one to behave and react in ways that are stressful. This perception is very common among patients with coronary heart disease.

Our prior studies provided me the opportunity to live together with heart patients for a month at a time. They were a diverse group of men and women from a wide spectrum of socioeconomic and educational backgrounds. After a few days, people who ordinarily would not have spent much time together began to trust one another and to discuss how they viewed themselves and each other.

To a lesser or greater degree, beneath the surface differences, there were shared ways of viewing the world. In general, people viewed themselves as apart from rather than a part of the world, isolated and fragmented, alone.

These perceptions of isolation led to feeling lacking: "If only I had _____, then I would be happy, then I would not feel stressed." More money. More power. More prestige. More love. And so on.

In the process, stress-inducing cycles were established:

1. Because they viewed themselves as lacking, they often drove themselves relentlessly in an attempt to fill the void they felt. Drs. Ray Rosenman and Meyer Friedman termed this behavior pattern as "ceaseless, Sisyphean striving." The resulting stress contributed to their illness.

2. Their self-esteem and identity often were invested in the outcome of what they did. Events took on an exaggerated importance because their net worth as human beings was on the line. Competition became keen because the stakes were so high: to fail at a task was to be a failure until proven otherwise by the next success.

Seen in this way, coronary heart disease can be a catalyst for helping an individual transform his values and sense of identity. For example, one of the participants in our research as a world-class runner and national champion. One day, while running, he developed chest pain. Subsequent testing confirmed the presence of severe coronary heart disease.

He underwent balloon dilation (angioplasty) of his coronary artery blockage, but a few weeks later the artery reoccluded. He could no longer run without chest pain.

The result was a crisis in values and identity: "Who am I? I can no longer be what I defined myself to be." Many heart patients experience a similar crisis in values and self-perception, to a lesser or greater degree, and emotional depression often follows. The chest pain is only the tip of the iceberg. The emotional pain is usually even more profound. But within this crisis and pain are the seeds of personal transformation.

First, in our studies, the group support was a

powerful way of breaking through this perceived isolation. In a real sense, patients became both healer and healed. Instead of setting themselves apart, they began to help one another, making an effort to understand and to share feelings and perceptions that, in the past, they would have kept to themselves.

Beneath the seeming differences, they shared many of the same hopes and fears and were grappling with similar problems. For many, it was the first time they felt loved and respected *for who they were*, not for what they did or what they had. In other words, the boundaries that had separated them from each other and from themselves began to crumble. The physical chest pain became a window through which we could work on the emotional pain, a way of reaching the rest of the iceberg. When the angina diminished, our credibility and effectiveness correspondingly increased.

Second, we presented the stress management techniques as tools to quiet the mind and body enough to enable them to experience an *inner* sense of contentment and well-being. We emphasized that these techniques do not *bring* contentment; rather, they help to identify and remove disturbances that keep one from feeling at ease. For example, at the end of each meditation, we reminded participants that their increased sense of well-being came not from getting something from outside themselves. It came from quieting the mind enough to experience the inner peace they already had when they didn't disturb it by striving to obtain what they thought they were lacking.

This is not really farfetched or simplistic, and it helps to tie together a number of research findings.

For example, the journal *Science* published Dr. Robert Nerem's study of rabbits who were fed a high-cholesterol diet and who were individually touched, talked to, petted, and played with on a regular basis. Compared to a genetically identical control group of rabbits who were given the same diet and normal laboratory animal care, the experimental group showed more than a 60% reduction in arterial blockages, even though blood cholesterol levels, heart rate, and blood pressure were comparable.

The counterpart also may be true: People who have pets have a lower incidence of sudden cardiac death than those who live alone. Having a pet—or being petted—may help to break through a perceived sense of social isolation, even in animals.

In the 1960s, Drs. Stewart Wolf and Helen Goodell found that rural Italians living in the Roseto community in Pennsylvania had a low death rate from coronary heart disease, even though their diet was rich in fat and cholesterol. At that time, those families were stable, closely knit, and relatively secure with strong community ties. With increasing urbanization and disruption of the family, the sudden death rates increased and now approach those of the general population.

Dr. Leonard Syme found similar data in his study of 7,000 residents in Alameda County near San Franciso. Over a 9-year period, people with fewer social connections had increased coronary heart disease incidence and mortality compared with residents who were married, had close friends, belonged to a church or synagogue, and so on. Other studies in Evans County, Tecumseh, and Finland have found social support to be a powerful determinant to health and disease.

In related work, Dr. Larry Scherwitz discovered that the more frequently patients used personal pronouns (I, me, mine) during a structured interview, the more severe was their coronary heart disease and the more likely they had suffered an earlier heart attack. Self-references remained a significant correlate of heart disease, even when controlled for age, blood pressure, cholesterol, and Type A behavior.

Why? An exaggerated focus on the self may be the behavioral manifestation for self-perceptions of isolation and separation, as well as for aspects of Type A behavior. That is, if you see yourself as separate and lacking, and if you believe, "If only I had _____, then I'd be happy," then ambition, competition, hostility, and time urgency (characteristics of Type A behavior) logically follow. The world is then perceived as a zero-sum game: "The more I get, the happier I'll be. The more other people get, the less there is for me. This is a dog-eat-dog world." Finally, after years of striving, the heart whispers, "You stop now."

Unfortunately, this zero-sum world view (like most world views) tends to be self-reinforcing. When someone looks out for #1 at the expense of others, he tends to respond in kind, reinforcing his belief and perception that he lives in a dog-eat-dog world. Friendships may be harder to sustain and tend to have what Martin Buber termed and "I–it" relationship, in which oneself is symbolically involved but the other is not. In short, self-involvement at the expense of others leads to increased social isolation which, in turn, can lead to greater self-involvement in a vicious cycle.

WHAT ARE THE HEALTH POLICY IMPLICATIONS OF THESE IDEAS?

Someone once described coronary heart disease to me as "the big stick. It gets your attention." He went on to explain that illness should motivate us to ask, "Why did I get sick? What are the causes?"

Unfortunately, doctors usually do not take full advantage of the opportunities for education that illness provides. Most of us go into medicine because we want to cure people. "Doc, it's my heart." "Here, take these pills"—or better yet, "We'll have to operate"—and presto! He's cured. The patient goes home and the doctor rides off into the sunset.

But pills don't cure heart disease. Neither does bypass surgery. For most people, the disease progresses relentlessly and inexorably over time because the causes are not addressed. So pills usually have to be taken for the rest of one's life, often in ever-increasing dosages. And bypassed arteries tend to reocclude.

Now, don't get me wrong. Drugs and surgery can be lifesaving. When someone comes into the emergency room with crushing chest pain, I don't feed them vegetables and teach them to meditate. I use whatever is needed—often drugs, and sometimes surgery—to help the person through a life-threatening crisis.

Once the danger has passed, I have the patient's full attention. Instead of just sending him home with cardiac medications, we talk: "Ok, now the real work begins. How did you get in this situation, and what can you do to begin healing yourself?" We review his lifestyle in detail. I usually prescribe a very low-fat, low-salt, low-caffeine, vegetarian, or "fishetarian" diet (there is no cholesterol in plant-based foods), stress management techniques, smoking cessation, a walking program, and limited alcohol consumption (no more than 2 ounces per day). We talk about other sources of stress—job, relationships, etc.—and what can be done. I often refer patients to a psychiatrist or clinical psychologist, a nutritionist or dietician, and a certified yoga instructor.

Implicit in this discussion is the fact that I believe the lifestyle factors described here are the major causes of coronary heart disease. Of course, genetic factors play a role, but for the vast majority of people, lifestyle factors seem to be of overriding importance. For example, one's ability to metabolize dietary fat and cholesterol may be genetically influenced. A cheeseburger may raise one person's blood level of cholesterol much more than another's, but if both people eat a low-fat vegetarian diet, both are likely to have low levels of serum cholesterol and a correspondingly reduced risk of developing coronary heart disease. While heart disease tends to run in families, so do patterns of eating, smoking, exercise, alcohol consumption, and responses to emotional stress.

On the other hand, coronary bypass surgery does not address these causes of heart disease—it literally and figuratively bypasses the problems. Treating heart disease in this way in analogous to busily mopping up the floor around an overflowing sink without also turning off the faucet.

Since bypass surgery does not address these causes, the disease process tends to recur. Recent studies have shown that two thirds of bypass grafts become partially blocked or completely occluded after 10 years; further, the blockages frequently worsen at an accelerated pace in the remaining coronary arteries that were not bypassed. This progression of disease is directly related to life-style factors.

A major benefit of bypass surgery is a dramatic reduction in angina (chest pain). Because patients feel so much better following surgery, they tend to believe they are cured—a belief all too often reinforced by their surgeons—and thus feel little motivation to change their lifestyles. But the chest pain is there for a reason, and treating the pain without addressing the causes is somewhat like clipping the wires to a ringing fire alarm without putting out the fire. According to legend, ancient Romans killed messengers who brought bad news. In contrast, we found in our studies that changing lifestyle abolished chest pain in most of the patients, improved coronary blood flow, and reduced risk of subsequent disease progression.

Last year, over five billion dollars were spent on coronary bypass surgery. At current rates of growth (which the economy cannot sustain), bypass surgery would be a $100 billion per year industry within 15 years.

Despite this, bypass surgery prolongs life only slightly and only in the most severe form of coronary heart disease in which all of the major coronary arteries are blocked. This fact has been confirmed in all three of the large-scale, randomized, controlled studies of bypass surgery: the Veteran's Administration Collaborative Study, the European Cooperative Study, and the Coronary Artery Surgery Study. These studies compared survival of heart patients who underwent bypass surgery with patients who were treated only with drugs. No study has yet compared the effectiveness of bypass surgery combined with altered lifestyle.

I am aware of six ongoing clinical trials to determine if coronary heart disease can be reversed. Four of these studies are evaluating cholesterol-lowering drugs (University of California, Harvard, University of Washington, University of Southern California). At Stanford, scientists are evaluating a program of moderate lifestyle changes plus cholesterol-lowering drugs. My colleagues and I are studying the effects of intensive lifestyle changes without additional

drugs. If these studies show that heart disease can be reversed, the need for bypass surgery may be greatly reduced. (If not, then we will have to rethink our assumptions.)

Recently, cardiologists have developed a new procedure, coronary angioplasty, in which a small balloon is directed by catheter into a partially blocked coronary artery and inflated, squishing the blockage against the arterial walls, thereby dilating the artery and reducing the blockage. While this procedure is an important advance, there are problems. In approximately 5% to 10% of patients, the coronary artery ruptures, requiring emergency bypass surgery. In 10% to 20% of patients, the artery reoccludes within a few months. As with bypass surgery, angioplasty does not address the lifestyle factors which lead to coronary heart disease. It is too soon to know if the long-term rate of reocclusion will be similar to that of bypass surgery, but I suspect that it will be.

How physicians are paid for their services is a powerful determinant of how we practice medicine. If I perform bypass surgery on someone, his insurance company will pay the costs of approximately $30,000. If I perform coronary angioplasty, his insurance company will pay approximately $7,000. If I teach a patient to change his lifestyle in a cardiac rehabilitation program, his insurance company will pay only a very small fraction of what it would pay for a bypass or angioplasty. And if I counsel a patient to change his lifestyle to *prevent* heart disease, his insurance company usually will not pay me at all. While these discrepancies are perhaps easiest to see with heart disease, they apply to other illnesses as well. As pressure to reduce health costs continues to grow, I suspect that these issues will assume increasing importance.

One can argue that physicians are not the right people to be teaching lifestyle changes, anyway. After all, we do not learn much about these areas in medical school. Yet I believe that physicians are in an ideal role. We know our patients' medical histories. We have great credibility with them. Perhaps more important, we can help them sort through the hyperbole and outright quackery of, for example, some nutritional therapies, and form networks of responsible resources to whom they can be referred. Patients are seeking "alternative therapies" in increasing numbers, so they might as well have the benefit of lifestyle counseling that is scientifically based.

In summary, the limitation and costs of high-tech medicine, exemplified by coronary bypass surgery, are becoming apparent, while evidence is accumulating that lifestyle changes can help to prevent—and perhaps reverse—coronary heart disease. The number one cause of death in this country may be largely preventable, but to do so will require major shifts in health education, medical training, and public policy.

15 STRESS AND ORGANIZATIONS: REDUCING THE STRESS OF COMMUNITY LIFE

Paul J. Rosch, M.D., F.A.C.P., is president of the American Institute of Stress and past president of the New York State Society of Internal Medicine. He has received numerous awards, including the Outstanding Physician's Award of the New York State Medical Society. Dr. Rosch has worked and published with Dr. Hans Selye, the founder of the stress concept, and with Dr. Flanders Dunbar, who coined the term psychosomatic. Dr. Rosch is a clinical professor of medicine and psychiatry at New York Medical College and adjunct professor at the University of Maryland.

Job stress has been estimated to cost American businesses at least $150 billion each year. The skyrocketing price of illness, coupled with the growing awareness that stress and illnesses are frequently linked, is causing many businesses to seek ways of alleviating stress among their employees. The results of stress reduction programs are anecdotal but testify to the effectiveness of various techniques. Employers have reported an impressive reduction in sick leave and accident compensation as a result of stress management programs in the workplace. Dr. Rosch draws upon his 35 years of stress research in explaining the most recent advances in identifying and alleviating job-related tension.∎

Annual health care expenditures in the United States rose to approximately $420 billion in 1986. That sum represented almost 11% of the gross national product and was 9% higher than costs for the previous year. The Health Care Financing Administration estimates that in 1987 and 1988 health care costs will grow even more rapidly than the general economy. Heart disease, cancer, strokes, and accidents are major contributors, and there is increasing evidence that such problems are related to stressful lifestyles and behavior. Seventy-five to eighty percent of all visits to primary care physicians are for stress-related symptoms such as headache, backache, insomnia, anxiety, depression, gastrointestinal disturbances, etc. Over the past decade, a variety of studies have supported the contention that job stress represents the most significant health problem for the middle-aged working population, as well as the most rapidly rising major expense for American corporations.

Job stress has been estimated to cost American industry $150 billion annually as assessed by absenteeism, diminished productivity, compensation claims, health insurance, and direct medical expenses. Put into perspective, that's more than 15 times the price tag for all strikes combined. A Metropolitan Life Insurance Company study indicated that an average of one million workers are absent on any given workday largely due to stress-related disorders. An American Association of Family Physicians' study of six occupational groups confirmed that job stress was considered to be the greatest factor leading to adverse health habits. Several studies have also linked stressful working conditions to an increased incidence of heart attacks. While it is difficult to put a price tag on the loss of an individual who has succumbed to a heart attack, the Xerox Corporation estimated that it costs approximately $1,000,000 to $1,500,000 to replace a top executive, and $200,000 to $500,000 for a lower echelon manager. In addition to the major illness categories cited, other stress-related behaviors take their toll. Alcoholic employees and smokers exhibit twice as much absenteeism and have significantly diminished productivity. Stress-related workers' compensation claims are rising so rapidly that they threaten to bankrupt the system in some states. In general, claimants tend to be younger, rewards are larger and increasingly represent claims that involve gradual on-the-job stress complaints. These trends are bound to escalate as scientific research validates mechanisms of stress-related illness that support such claims.

As a consequence, American industries, particularly large corporations, have become increasingly involved in developing methodologies to identify and measure stress in the workplace, as well as techniques and programs to remove or reduce stress or teach employees how to deal with stress. A variety of approaches have been used with varying success. Obviously, specific programs vary depending upon the size of the company and the population to be served, as well as goals, resources, or other specialized considerations. Evaluating the success of such interventions is difficult in most cases because of a lack of control groups, long-term follow-up studies, and objective parameters to prove efficacy. In addition, stress reduction programs are frequently minor components of much larger ongoing employee assistance that encourage exercise or offer conseling on nutrition, smoking cessation, alcohol and substance abuse, marital problems, etc., all of which can have stress-reducing effects. Consequently, it is difficult to define the benefits derived from a formal stress reduction program per se when it is offered in conjunction with other efforts. However, enthusiastic anecdotal reports abound concerning improved employee health and productivity, better quality of life in the workplace, and cost effectiveness for each dollar spent in such activities. In a few instances, well designed studies do provide information that corroborates such claims.

Moreover, there is growing evidence linking job stress to illness. As indicated previously, concern about reducing stress in the workplace has received increased impetus because of recent evidence demonstrating mechanisms of stress-related illness and implicating stress in the workplace as a major source of such complaints. Type A coronary-prone behavior has now been shown to be as predictive as any other known, controllable risk factor for future heart attacks. Furthermore, reducing such stressful behavior currently represents the most successful strategy for preventing recurrent heart attacks, and programs specifically designed to reduce harmful Type A behavior are steadily being introduced in worksite settings. The important influence of stress on blood pressure is evidenced by the latest National Heart, Lung and Blood Institute's recommendations for the treatment of hypertension and its emphasis on nonpharmacological measures as an initial treatment approach. To a considerable extent, these new guidelines also reflect a growing acknowledgement of the efficacy of stress reduction strategies such as meditation, progressive muscular relaxation, and specific biofeedback techniques in treating hypertension.

Clearly industry has also shown great interest in this approach. A recent study of 160 corporations indicated stress management programs to be their first health priority. There were four times as many projects in this category as the next two largest segments, physical fitness and nondrug treatment of hypertension. At the present time, a 3-year program is underway, sponsored by the University of California School of Medicine, Bank of America, and several major corporations in California to develop and evaluate behavioral approaches to hypertension treatment utilizing stress reduction techniques that can be implemented at worksite settings.

In addition to effects on heart attacks and hypertension, there is growing appreciation of the role of psychosocial stress in the development or course of various infections ranging from the common cold to herpes, as well as certain malignancies. Verification of such relationships comes from the rapidly emerging discipline of psychoneuroimmunology, which clearly confirms the ability of stress to reduce immune system defenses against cancer, as well as bacterial and viral infections. Stress can also cause altered gastrointestinal secretory and motility patterns that predispose to peptic ulcer, various types of colitis, and the very common irritable bowel syndrome. Similarly, the aggravating effects of stress on a vari-ety of allergic phenomena that affect the skin and lungs provide additional insight into understanding the role of emotions in dermatologic, allergic, and pulmonary disorders such as emphysema and asthma. Further understanding of the nature of stressful stimuli that can provoke such responses increasingly implicates work-related problems as a potent factor.

Recent research has linked particular stressful working conditions with an increased incidence of heart attacks. The common denominators in such situations appear to be increased responsibility without commensurate decision-making capability, an inability to express true emotions or to get things off your chest, or a general sense of lacking control. Many occupations that fall into this category primarily involve women and certain subsets of working mothers appear to be at particular risk. More and more women are also subjected to further stress due to their increased migration into a male-dominated work force that has not fulfilled the promises of the Equal Rights Amendments or the Women's Liberation Movement. One study at Stanford University indicated that four times more female MBAs than male controls seek psychological counseling and have more frequent functional stress-related complaints. Working females also seem to be exhibiting more male Type A coronary-prone behavior traits and a concomitant substantial increase in heart attacks.

Conversely, it appears likely that "positive" stimuli and emotions may confer health enhancement benefits. The availability of strong social support networks, a feeling of being in control, pride in what one is doing, and the ability to express one's true feelings without fear of recrimination or reprisal all seem to fall into this category. Such considerations are particularly relevant for the successful design and implementation of stress reduction and employee assistance programs.

IDENTIFYING THE CAUSES OF STRESS IN THE WORKPLACE

Job stress can have many roots and causes. Some may be obvious: annoying physical and environmental problems such as crowding, noise and air pollution, or exposure to potentially hazardous substances. Others may be due to the nature of the job. The common denominators here are being placed in situations which demand considerable responsibility without commensurate authority or decision-making capability, or customer service jobs where it is impossible to express true feelings. Dull, dead-end, assembly line work which does not permit full use of one's talents or potential, or jobs in which constant deadlines do not permit enough time to finish the work to one's satisfaction may be particularly stressful, especially for individuals in middle management positions.

Stress at work can also be the result of the individual's own personality. A good example is the Type A executive who is continually frustrated by self-imposed, unrealistic goals that are inflexibly pursued. Such individuals may themselves be vectors of stress in the workplace as their aggressive and hostile behavior produces adverse repercussions on co-workers and customers. More often, it is not the individual or the job per se but rather a mismatch between the two in terms of basic goals, needs, and values, leading to continuing problems. Stress at work may also have its real roots outside the workplace—family or financial problems that lead to alcoholism, depression, or anxiety affect performance on the job. Some common factors that contribute to job stress are:

1. Inadequate time to complete the job to one's satisfaction.
2. Lack of clear job description or chain of command.
3. Absence of recognition or reward for good job performance.
4. Inability or lack of opportunity to voice complaints.
5. Lots of responsibilities but little authority or decision-making capability.
6. Inability to work with superiors, co-workers, or subordinates due to basic differences in goals and values.
7. Lack of control or pride over the finished product.
8. Job insecurity due to pressures from within or a possibility of merger.
9. Prejudice and bigotry due to age, sex, race, or religion.
10. Unpleasant environmental conditions caused by smoking, crowding, noise and air pollution, exposure to toxic chemicals or carcinogens, or commuting difficulties.
11. Concerns related to responsibility for employees.
12. Not being able to utilize personal talents or abilities effectively or to full potential.
13. The FUD factor (fear, uncertainty, doubt).

STRESS MANAGEMENT TRAINING PROGRAMS AT THE WORKSITE

Evaluating the efficacy of stress management training programs is difficult due to a general lack of objective criteria. Most efforts consist primarily of educational programs designed to acquaint workers with the role of stress in health and illness, causes of stress, nature of stress-related symptoms, or informational material illustrating various stress reduction techniques that can be employed. In some instances, these are delivered in the form of lectures, symposia, or workshops lasting several hours or several days. Vendors offer packaged programs that utilize slides, descriptive material, case histories, and audio or video cassettes. Most commercial programs attempt to provide participants with individual stress profiles based upon responses to questionnaires or standardized psychological assessment instruments. On occasion, specially constructed questionnaires are designed to focus on a particular occupation or location.

Formal stress management training usually includes meditative or autogenic techniques to induce general relaxation and, to a lesser extent, behavioral and cognitive approaches. In some instances, biofeedback services are available. Encouraging jogging, aerobic exercise, dancing, and participation in athletic activities represent the most common approach.

PHYSIOLOGIC TECHNIQUES

Most standardized stress management programs utilize procedures designed to assist the individual in dealing with environmental demands that cannot be avoided. One example is progressive muscular relaxation, which is achieved by contracting and then relaxing various muscle groups in a progressive and systematic fashion. The goal here is to produce a level of deep muscular relaxation. The original technique described by Jacobsen has been modified in many ways so that attention is also often directed to accompanying such exercises with relaxing thoughts and images and a tranquil breathing pattern. Other forms of autogenic training place a particular emphasis on creating feelings such as limb warmth or heaviness, utilizing visual imagery in conjunction with physical relaxation.

A variety of meditative measures are also frequently employed. These range from specific Eastern techniques to the simplified relaxation response, which merely utilizes a repetitive deep breathing pattern and an associated focus on some word or phrase with each expiration. It has been suggested that this induces a suppression of "fight or flight" arousal responses. Individuals practicing meditation seem more adept at resisting intrusive stressful thoughts or unpleasant external stimuli throughout the day as well as during the procedure. In rare instances, transcendental or Siddha meditation or yoga have also been taught. A brief technique, known as the quieting response, consists of a combination of deep breathing and muscular relaxation combined with visual imagery for 10 or 15 seconds. It is easy to learn and can be used several times a day, especially when stressful situations are anticipated or encountered.

In sites where biofeedback is utilized, individuals learn to develop self-control over a number of physiological activities previous thought to be entirely involuntary. The most frequent training techniques utilize frontalis muscle tension, fingertip temperature, and electrodermal response. Special electronic sensors located at appropriate anatomical sites generate a signal that is converted into electrical activity. This input is then transformed into either an auditory or visual cue which varies correspondingly with the degree of activity. By receiving such information on a continuing basis, individuals quickly become aware of body processes which were previously unknown and can recognize stimuli or feelings which produce consistent changes in a certain direction. By repetitive training and reinforcement of measures which reduce muscle tension or raise fingertip temperatures, a state of relaxation can be induced. These techniques can be learned and practiced to reproduce such benefits at will. Biofeedback does require specialized equipment and trained personnel and generally requires individualized instruction. Consequently, it is not as cost effective as meditation, muscular relaxation, or autogenic training, which can be taught to groups of individuals.

COGNITIVE TRAINING

Behavioral modification is another method used to reduce exaggerated or inappropriate responses to stress. One example is assertiveness training, which is designed to provide individuals with more effective control over their activities. This approach emphasizes the development of appropriate assertive techniques to facilitate communication of personal needs and requirements. It is particularly useful in dealing with difficult interpersonal relationships, such as a need for a new job assignment, since it reduces the anger and anxiety often associated with such situations. Other behavioral techniques are directed towards improving skills and communication, time management, and career development to more fully utilize potential skills and talents. Increased use of techniques to reduce coronary-prone behavior can be anticipated as soon as training programs and methodologies become standardized. In general, behavioral modification utilizes role-playing, observation, self-report feedback, and other behavioral therapy techniques which can be taught effectively in group settings.

Improving cognitive skills may also provide important stress reduction benefits. This approach is based on the assumption that harmful stress responses often result from the individual's past experiences in terms of appraising threatening situations. Frequently, it is not the external event itself but rather the individual's perception of it that causes problems. Cognitive training is designed to assist individuals in learning how to reappraise stressful situations by logic and reasoning rather than emotional reactions that have been ingrained by past habits. Often this involves emphasis on improving one's self-esteem and personal worth.

PHYSICAL FITNESS

Physical fitness is far and away the most popular method used to deal with stress in the workplace. This may take various forms ranging from lunch hour or other company-sponsored walking and jogging groups, aerobic dancing or exercise classes, or the use of community or in-house fitness facilities where specialized equipment is available.

Proponents of jogging claim that regular running dissipates the buildup of stress-related hormones and provides a period of quiet time for personal reflection, free from the intrusion of external noxious stimuli. In general, physical fitness programs require comparatively little expenditure of funds or specialized personnel and can be adapted to a variety of situations and occupational resources.

Reduction of psychological stress through the use of counseling services that deal with weight reduction, cigarette smoking, alcohol and substance abuse, and financial and family problems are also benefits provided by many corporations or unions. Other employee programs are offered that sharply reduce costs for legal assistance, medical and dental care, and drug treatment or provide expanded insurance coverage. The increasing use of flex time, in which personnel have more latitude in determining working hours, and baby-sitting services available for working parents with preschool children are other types of stress reduction benefits. In addition to reducing workers' anxiety and expenses, they also improve employee-company relations by fostering a sense of caring and concern.

ILLUSTRATIVE PROGRAMS

The Johnson & Johnson "Live for Life" program offers stress management and information on lifestyle activities that can promoted successfully at the work setting. In 1985, 75,000 employees were involved in action programs in the United States, Puerto Rico, and Europe. Employee participation is voluntary and services are provided free of charge.

Upon entry, a "health screen" allows individuals to rate their current lifestyles. Following this, the concept of the program is explained in depth and a variety of action programs are offered to assist with smoking cessation, stress management, exercise, nutrition, weight control, and general health knowledge. These are all integrated closely with established medical programs such as hypertension detection and control and other employee assistance activities.

A 2-year epidemiologic study was designed to evaluate the success of the program using several criteria evaluated annually. These included biometric, behavioral benefits and attitudinal observations. Approximately 4,000 employees were involved. Preliminary findings on the employees who completed both the baseline and 1-year health screen did suggest an ability to achieve significant and meaningful improvement. Obviously, programs such as "Live for Life" require a major commitment on the part of the employer as well as personnel, equipment, and other resources frequently not available to many organizations.

However, stress management techniques that can be utilized in almost any industrial setting have also been studied and determined to provide significant benefits. One such program was conducted at the New York Telephone Company for some 160 volunteers who reported high stress. Upon entry, the subjects completed several stress evaluation questionnaires, which were used again to measure progress at the end of 6 weeks and again after 5½ months. Thirty-eight subjects were assigned to one of three treatment groups utilizing clinically standardized meditation, Benson's Relaxation Response, and progressive muscular relaxation. A control group of 40 received no specific instruction. The techniques were taught through audio-taped instructions with supplementary reading material which the participants reviewed at home. The techniques were practiced twice daily for 15 to 20 minutes. At the end of 2 weeks, psychologists taught additional, shorter relaxation techniques that could be utilized throughout the work day.

All four groups, including controls, showed improvement after 5½ months. However, those who were members of the meditation-relaxation groups reported significantly greater symptom reduction than controls. When those subjects who were still practicing their techniques at the conclusion of the study were compared with nonpracticers, the therapeutic benefits were even more pronounced despite only occasional use.

In another study conducted in the corporate offices of the Converse Rubber Company, 126 volunteers participated in a program designed to study the effects of two 15-minute relaxation breaks during the work day. One third of the group had two or three instructional sessions in the relaxation response, another third simply relaxed without focusing on anything specific or listened to music, and one third received no special instruction. The efficacy of the program was assessed by self-report of physical and mental symptoms including level of energy, improved concentration, overall efficiency, problem-solving ability, and time lost due to illness. On each of these indices, the relaxation response group showed the greatest benefits. Specific relaxation training also appeared to cause significant reductions in blood pressure. The results of such studies are encouraging since they suggest that positive benefits can result from relatively simple, inexpensive techniques that do not require highly trained personnel or specialized equipment and can be adapted to almost any work setting. However, long-term follow-up is required to demonstrate sustained improvement and such data is not readily available.

A variety of outside vendors offer stress management training programs for workers that may be delivered on site or at other locations. These programs generally provide psychologists or specially trained personnel to instruct employees in the various stress reduction techniques noted above.

One innovative approach which attempts to focus on job-related stress due to incompatibil-

ity between the individual's goals and behavior and work requirements is offered by Human Synergistics. Level 1 provides detailed information about behavior by means of a lifestyle inventory. This involves completing a questionnaire in order to reveal thinking patterns which characterize personality and lifestyle and may be productive or destructive. The results develop a profile that rates and compares concern for people and satisfaction, concern for people and security, concern for task and security, and concern for task and satisfaction. At Level 2 the same lifestyle inventory is completed by six or seven close friends or co-workers whose opinion would be respected; they describe these same aspects of the individual's behavior and attitude. The resulting composite profile helps to identify the way others perceive an individual's attitude. The similarities and differences that exist between the results of Level 1 and Level 2 evaluations provide important insights into understanding how the worker's behavior affects others. Additional levels provide further enhancements for specific groups.

The Institute for Labor and Mental Health has developed occupational stress groups that utilize trained shop stewards to conduct a highly structured 12-week course in the workplace. This is designed to increase the worker's sense of power or ability to influence working conditions and to promote a greater sense of camaraderie and trust. A major result has been a more "focused anger," directed at specific work problems, that attempts to rectify deficiencies. It is claimed that this increases productivity and reduces problems related to alcoholism and emotional outbursts or random anger at home.

RESULTS

As indicated previously, many stress reduction benefits are included in broader employee assistance programs which include exercise and counseling on alcoholism, substance abuse, marital problems, and diet. The mere establishment of an employee's assistance program may in itself have important stress reduction benefits. This provides pertinent resources for the worker as well as tangible evidence of management's interest and dedication to personal welfare. Kimberly-Clark reported a 70% reduction in on-the-job accidents as a result of their employee assistance program. At General Motors there was a 40% decrease in lost time and a 60% decrease in sickness and accident benefit payments. On-the-job accidents decreased by 50%, and so did grievances. The cost effectiveness of each dollar invested was significant, with at least a 3 to 1 return. Equitable Assurance Society estimated $5.52 and Kenecott Copper $6.00 saved for every $1.00 spent on their program. The Chief Executive Officer at Tenneco, which reports to have the "Cadillac" of corporate wellness programs, cited improved morale, better quality of life, greater inducement for recruiting, less employee turnover, and better employee-management relationships. Johnson & Johnson's "Live for Life" program far exceeded predicted cost savings and also created a greater sense of community among employees as well as between the company and its employees.

FUTURE DIRECTIONS

While some simple stress reduction techniques may provide across-the-board benefits, stress management programs ideally should be matched with the requirements of the organization and the population being served. In some instances, emphasis should be placed on specific problems such as job security or career management. For maximum effectiveness, workers should play an active role in program selection, design, and evaluation. Progress is more apt to be made by beginning with a small, focused intervention program for a specific target group that allows evaluation of efficacy and costs. This can be enlarged as results indicate the need for various modifications or greater emphasis in specific areas. This approach seems preferable to instituting a large, multifaceted smorgasbord of services. Existing facilities should be utilized whenever possible, and this usually can be accomplished with respect to exercise or fitness programs. On the other hand, it may be more efficient and economical to take advantage of existing community-based programs such as the local YMCA or established stress management facilities. These often provide exercise programs and counseling services for diet, nutrition, smoking cessation, hypertension detection, management of low back problems, etc.

Companies can best embark on such programs by learning from the experience of others, particularly organizations of similar size and demographics that have instituted successful programs. A listing of such organizations, corporations, and other resources involved in stress reduction activities may be obtained for a small fee from the American Institute of Stress.

16 BURNOUT: RENEWING THE SPIRIT

Dennis T. Jaffe, Ph.D., is director of The Center for Health Studies at Saybrook Institute in San Francisco. His book, *Healing From Within* (Simon and Schuster, 1986), received a "Medical Self-Care" book award.

Cynthia D. Scott, Ph.D., is an organizational and health promotion consultant and research associate at the University of California at San Francisco. She is the editor of *Heal Thyself: The Health of Health Care Professionals* (Brunner-Mazel, 1986).

Dr. Jaffe and Dr. Scott are co-authors of *From Burnout to Balance: A Workbook for Peak Performance and Self-Renewal* (McGraw-Hill, 1984), *StressMap* (ESSI Systems, 1985), and *Take This Job and Love It!* (1987).

The classic victim of "burnout" is a nurse or social worker who has been around the sick and dying too long without respite. In this sense, burnout is a severe manifestation of job stress. Dennis Jaffe and Cynthia Scott are studying the impact of burnout on health care practitoners' ability to treat patients and possible links with medical malpractice. In this article, they describe the symptoms and suggest a method for overcoming the the discouraging effects of burnout through improved communications, self-esteem, self-awareness, and personal mission.■

THE CRISIS OF SPIRIT

Everyone has seen it happen. A colleague who has been excited, involved, and productive slowly begins to pull back, lose energy and interest, and becomes a shadow or his or her former self. Or, a person who has been a beacon of vision and idealism retreats into despair or cynicism. What happened? How does someone who is capable and committed become a person who functions minimally and does not seem to care for the job or the people that work there?

Burnout is a chronic state of depleted energy, lack of commitment and involvement, and continual frustration, often accompanied at work by physical symptoms, disability claims and performance problems. Job burnout is a crisis of spirit, when work that was once exciting and meaningful becomes deadening. An organization's most valuable resource—the energy, dedication, and creativity of its employees—is often squandered by a climate that limits or frustrates the pool of talent and energy available.

Milder forms of burnout are a problem at every level, in every type of work. The burned-out manager comes to work, but he brings a shell rather than a person. He experiences little satisfaction, and feels uninvolved, detached, and uncommitted to his work and co-workers. While he may be effective by external standards, he works far below his own level of productivity. The people around him are deeply affected by his attitude and energy level, and the whole community begins to suffer.

Burnout is a crisis of the spirit because people who burn out were once on fire. It's especially scary and consequential because it strikes some of the most talented. If they can't maintain their fire, others ask, who can? Are these people lost forever, or can the inner flame be rekindled? People often feel that burnout just comes upon them and that they are helpless victims of it. Actually, the evidence is growing that there are ways for individuals to safeguard and renew their spirit, and, more important, there are ways for organizations to change conditions that lead to burnout.

SIGNS OF BURNOUT

It's common for a person to come to work feeling drained and tired, saying, "I'm really feeling burned-out today." This is *not* what we mean by burnout; it simply represents our fluctuating personal energy reserves available for responding to work pressure. *Burnout is an end stage, a severe crisis.* A person does not wake up one morning burned out. It is a process that develops slowly, over time—several months to several years. And burnout is not the same as everyday stress and pressure. While work demands and experienced stress can go up and down—today I feel pressure, tomorrow things will get a little better—the burnout experience does not go away or fluctuate. Once a person reaches burnout, major changes are necessary to reverse it.

The burnout experience is surprisingly uniform. Psychologist Christina Maslach has interviewed hundreds of burned-out workers, and her Burnout Inventory catalogues three major qualities of burnout:

Emotional exhaustion: feelings drained, not having anything to give even *before* the day begins.

Depersonalization: feeling unconnected to other people, feeling resentful and seeing them negatively.

Reduced personal accomplishment: feeling ineffective, that the results achieved are not meaningful.

This inner experience has clear negative effects on work relationships and performance. A burned-out worker affects the working climate for others. The organizational consequences of burnout include absenteeism, turnover, poor performance, and dissatisfaction. Burnout is everyone's concern. If more than a few employees within an organization exhibit signs of burnout, it represents an organizational challenge, not a personal problem.

BURNOUT RESEARCH: SITUATIONS, NOT PEOPLE

Burnout came to popular attention in the late 1970s when Herbert Freudenberger wrote an article about his own burnout. During the day he worked in his own psychotherapy practice, and at nights he worked as a consultant to a community service, Free Clinic in New York. The whole staff was deeply dedicated to their work and willing to work long hours at low pay. Freudenberger would often work late into the night. Then, one day he just couldn't continue. During a vacation, he slept for almost a week. He felt he had nothing more to give and had to stop work for a few months.

Human service workers—teachers, social workers, public service employees, police, nurses, and physicians—seem unusually prone to burnout. Much of the early research was concerned how burnout quickly took root among idealistic young professionals. Cary Cherniss studied the first work year of teachers, lawyers, and psychologists just out of graduate school, and he found that the signs of burnout set in very quickly. Their dedication soon began to flag. They became frustrated and experienced a crisis of purpose and meaning.

For example, social workers began work with a hope of making a difference in clients' lives, but they soon found that limits of bureaucratic regulations and difficulties in relating to clients made it hard to be helpful. The continual emotion-tinged interactions with people in need, in crisis, and in pain were difficult. The fledgling social workers felt that what they had learned in graduate school had little relation to realities of their professions. They were thrown back on their own devices and often had nobody to talk to about their struggle, as they had in grad school. These factors—the pressures of continual emotional involvement with people, not being sure what "competence" meant, the lack of colleague support and exchange, and bureaucratic limits to helpfulness—worked together to create burnout.

These people shared certain qualities. They cared deeply for their work in the beginning. They wanted to make a difference and had an inner sense of mission about what they wanted to accomplish. They were also high achievers and expected a lot of themselves. This high-octane mixture came into contact with a demanding but unreceptive or frustrating working environment. The conditions of work—such as an unresponsive bureaucracy, rejection of innovative ideas,

and difficult if not impossible problems to solve for clients—seemed designed to dampen and frustrate the fledgling professionals or managers. They took their failures personally, and, in effect, began to lose heart.

The research on burnout supports one primary principle: that it is work situations and qualities of work itself, rather than individual personality factors, that create burnout. In other words, burnout is not due to defective people, but to difficult and demanding work environments. For example, Robert Golumbiewski found that if one member of a work group is burned out, then chances are high that the rest of the group is as well. The evidence is growing that certain qualities and norms within work *environments* promote burnout.

WHO'S AT RISK?

The burnout problem does not just affect service workers—many types of managers have also come to experience it. Certain types of jobs are more likely to lead to burnout. Burnout tends to cluster in the middle and supervisory levels of an organization, in job roles that bring a person into regular and stressful contact with other people. It affects employees on boundaries between the organization and the public and people who are mediators between different levels and demands, like supervisors. These people have to balance demands from many people. And often there are real limits on their control over situations and their ability to respond. Their hands are tied, and they often have to carry bad news back and forth. They feel that no one values them.

Another factor related to burnout is receiving feedback on how well you are doing. When people operate without a clear sense of where they stand or how effective they are, they are vulnerable to the crisis of confidence that can lead to burnout. In technical tasks or in physical or routine tasks, the numbers tell the story. One achieves tangible results, meets a quota, or succeeds at a task. In human relations, results are less clear. Feedback from others lets people know if they are making a difference. For example, a supervisor who does not give any personal support or positive feedback, and whose demands are unrealistic or inconsistent, can promote burnout in a whole group.

Certain types of interaction are inherently draining and promote burnout over time. Imagine having to receive customer complaints or problems all the time. People in these positions are in toxic interactions, exchanges that are stressful for both parties. Dealing with people who are in pain or angry or upset on an ongoing basis has a detrimental effect on the listener if he doesn't take good care of himself. Continued contact with severe emotional pain and illness, for example, in a hospice environment, where it is not clear how the nurse is expected to relate, can result in burnout. These difficult environments demand special measures to prevent staff from burning out. Otherwise turnover, illness, and low morale can destroy a whole system.

SELF-RENEWAL AND MAJOR LIFE CHANGES

What does it mean when we burn out? When this happens, it should be taken as a signal to begin reassessing one's life choices and work. Burnout might be a sign that a person is beginning a major life transition, or needs to. Life has many transition points—job changes, forced shifts, choices. A person entering the job market today, even at a professional level, can expect at least five major job shifts in the course of a career. While upheaval can come from external shifts and crises (a failing company, for example), often the need for change comes from inner signals, such as restlessness or boredom.

For example, we conducted a study of physicians who had started to define their work in a new way. They had shifted from traditional medicine to what they termed a holistic perspective and style of practice. The majority reported that the shift had come when they felt burned out in their practice, when they sensed that something was wrong with the way they were practicing medicine. The burnout and dissatisfaction triggered a search for new ways.

When a person comes to such a shift point, he cannot simply change his work or life situation. Bill Bridges notes that change is followed by a transition. The transition demands major self-renewal and restructuring. Research has shown that the personal stress of change affects one's health. In addition, allowing time and space for the emotional shifts is important because one's emotional reserves are often exhausted by a change. Many people do not allow themselves time to recover from a layoff, a personal loss, or a crisis. Then they wonder why they can't sleep or be fully effective at work. For example, in our work with a company undergoing a major downsizing, the effects of the layoffs were evident for months in the surviving workers. When supervisors and managers were given a model and told to expect these signs, they were better able to help their workers manage the transition.

When burnout occurs at the personal level, it can be the signal for a major life transition. The person who is burned out may be the last one to realize it. Often family members or work colleagues see that the spark of excitement is gone and that performance has gone flat. Making adjustments of an environmental nature, such as rearranging your office or taking a vacation, will not provide sufficient excitement. Completing the renewal process usually involves shifts in attitude as well as activity.

Burnout can be turned into a positive signal to initiate a transition from one endeavor to another. This is often the case with individuals who have lost sight of the original reason for going into a particular field. For example, a human resources executive had been a fighter pilot in the Navy for a number of years before entering his present field. He took great pleasure in the freedom of flying and missed the excitement very much. After a particularly challenging job as a director of human resources, he went into a slump, feeling that his work wasn't fulfilling and that he just couldn't do one more task. He applied for a disability leave and at the same time began to have numerous physical complaints. Both his body and his spirit were burned out.

His renewal process led him to explore his

original mission in entering the human resources field and the satisfactions that he drew from it. Taking time to revisit his original dreams and seeing how he was failing to nurture them was an important part of his recovery.

He also took time to reconnect with friends whom he had become "too busy" to contact, and he recognized the importance of his relationships at work. The third step of his renewal process involved considering his needs. It became clear to him that he yearned to "fly free" unencumbered by a large corporate structure and that it wasn't the human resources activities but the environmental setting that was wrong. This understanding encouraged him to leave his position and move into a setting that allowed him much more independent judgment and initiative.

The process of renewal is not instant; it requires self-examination and the willingness to make changes. Just as burnout does not suddenly appear, neither does the renewal process manifest itself overnight. There are many paths to renewal. The most important factor is knowing how to spot burnout before the flames have consumed the spirit. There are many opportunities to prevent burnout before it takes hold.

LEVELS AND RHYTHMS
OF PERFORMANCE

Burnout is only one side of the story. At the other extreme, companies have discovered the *inspired* performer. This type of employee is excited about work, and sees his job as an opportunity to expand his capabilities. His vision and energy are contagious, and he is a great natural resource to a company, for he inspires others and continually exceeds expectations. The challenge facing the leadership of the organization or the work group is to create a climate that leads a critical mass of employees toward inspired performance and away from burnout.

It is helpful to see performance as a rhythm, moving through different levels like a wave. Because one's work energy and involvement are ever changing, describing it as a flow fits people's experience of the fluctuation. Individual

and group performance can be seen as flowing through four Performance Zones. *Optimal* performance is the very best the individual or organization is able to accomplish. There is a keen sense of accomplishment and an experience of peak performance. *Balanced* performance is steady and strong, resulting in a solid sense of accomplishment. *Strained* performance represents approximation and minimal accomplishment. The individual or organization is striving for results but not achieving them. There is a sense of futility and exasperation about not being able to do the task well. Performance in the *burnout* zone is minimal, results are negligible, and the individual or organization has a sense of flatness about the outcome. There is very little interest in quality, and people feel like they've just put in their time.

What's most interesting about the performance zones is how high performance and satisfaction are the opposites of burnout. Examining the elements of optimal performance, both organizationally and individually, can help us to avoid burnout.

COPING STYLES AND STRESS RESISTANT PERSONALITY

Although it has been found that no specific personality type is more susceptible than others to burnout, we still must explain why some people burn out while others are inspired performers, even when they work in the same environment. Researchers have explored the ways in which people respond to pressure, and they have begun to define factors that enhance effective coping or lead a person into burnout. These factors include styles of behavior, ways of relating to others, and internal cognitive and emotional ways of defining and experiencing situations.

Our own work has defined 12 coping responses that research and personal experience have linked with optimal performance or burnout. These 12 factors each have a positive and a negative pole:

These factors are described and assessed in our performance tool *StressMap*,[SM] which is designed to help managers assess their performance level in each of these dimensions.▪

OPTIMAL ZONE	BURNOUT ZONE
Key Coping Responses	
Self-Care Practices	Neglect
Direct Action	Avoidance
Support Seeking	Withdrawal
Situation Mastery	Ceaseless Striving/ Type A
Adaptability/Flexibility	Rigidity
Time Management	Disorganization
Key Cognitive/Emotional Styles	
Self-Esteem	Self-Criticism
Positive Outlook	Pessimism
Personal Power	Helplessness
Connection	Alienation
Emotional Expression	Internalizing Feelings
Compassion	Anger/Resentment

Consider the ways that optimal performers approach challenges, and compare them to the responses of burned-out co-workers. The key skills of the inspired performer include maintaining their physical health, responding directly to difficulties and demands rather than avoiding them, utilizing the help and support of others, focusing energy on mastering some part of a challenge rather than trying to do it all, taking time to rethink one's approach when things aren't working out, and effective management of time. Each of these six basic skills can be cultivated, and a person can become more effective at bringing this skill into play.

The way a person sets his own standards and looks at situations is also important in avoiding burnout. The burned-out worker tends to be highly self-critical, always saying he is not doing enough. He expects the worst and has little sense of personal capacity to effect changes. The optimal performer has a positive view of himself and

of the future, and he knows that he can use his energy to make a difference and achieve some success. Emotionally, the optimal performer's style is characterized by a sense of connection to other people, feeling comfortable expressing and sharing feelings, and having a sense of compassion.

The research that defines positive personal styles seems to indicate that there are *generic human and self-management skills* that are critical to managers today. Curiously, the same styles and attitudes that lead to effective performance also seem to promote physical health. Psychologist Suzanne Kobasa compared groups of healthy and unhealthy managers in a high-stress work environment. The healthy managers, who seemingly thrived under stress, differed from the unhealthy managers in that they were more *involved* in their work, *welcomed change* as an opportunity to learn, and felt a greater sense of *personal power*. Other studies of healthy personal styles add two more factors to this list of qualities seen in stress resistant people: drawing on other people for help and support, and having a personal sense that what one is doing is important and meaningful.

The same personal qualities that promote health also seem to promote productivity. Inspired performers combine high productivity, personal satisfaction, health, and well-being. Burnout represents the opposite extreme. Burned-out managers experience all manner of stress-related ailments—physical and emotional—and their performance is impaired as well.

An inspired performer can be put into a work setting that burns him out, and a person prone to burnout can be inspired to perform. For this reason, more and more employers are seeking to create a climate for inspired performance.

When managers are asked to think back to a project, or a situation where they felt they were an "inspired performer", and then to define the key elements of this state of performance, their reports are surprisingly similar. They felt valued as individuals within their work group, were given a clear project or task that was meaningful to them, had the autonomy to pursue the project to its conclusion, had clear and open communication with other team members and with other parts of the organization, felt they were using their creative resources within the project, and they received rewards appropriate to their success. Burned-out executives report that their work seems insignificant, that they do not feel valued or supported in their jobs, that they can't get things done, they don't know what is expected of them, and that they don't feel that their skills are being utilized.

What Can You Do To Overcome or Prevent Burnout?

In our work with burned-out managers and companies, we focus on four key areas that seem most critical to helping people overcome or prevent burnout:

Create Support Nets: People need people. As the current campaign of the California Department of Health suggests, "Friends Can Be Good Medicine." When a person begins to burn out, the best resource is to talk about pressure with others and begin to share the burdens. Even talking to another person is helpful; the other person does not have to resolve the dilemma or change it. People at work need an environment where they can ask for help and feel that their needs are taken into account. When people sue, when workers strike, when managers quit, the most cited reason is that they didn't feel respected. Work teams can rise to heights of inspired performance when they feel they are working for each other. Developing positive work relationships, having mechanisms to respond constructively to conflicts and differences, and learning the skills to share your personal needs and feelings with others—these are all aspects of creating support nets.

Enhance Personal Power: Personal power is not unlimited authority over others but the power to get what you need. Burned-out people feel they cannot get what they want or need from their work or personal lives, or they feel they are putting out vast amounts of energy, depleting themselves, without making any difference. Developing a sense of personal power includes

deciding whether you are using your energy in ways that fit your personal priorities and goals and in ways in which you can make a difference. Type A behavior has been linked with heart disease. We call it ceaseless striving. This consists of trying to get the whole world under your control, and feeling frustrated when you don't succeed. Personal power requires positive beliefs about your own abilities and those of others, which lead you to see yourself and others as resources. To avoid burnout you need to define what you want to accomplish and to direct your energy into areas where you can make a difference.

There are many ways that workplaces can be adapted to fit one's inner needs and styles and to enhance the personal power of all employees. Today we see many alternate work arrangements—flex time, job sharing, quality circles, job redesign, cross-training, parallel organization structures, project task forces—that respond directly to workers' needs to experience power and challenge in their work. These organizational interventions directly impact on the burnout level of people.

Listen to Your Inner Self: The first signals of distress are often ignored. They come in the form of vague feelings or physical symptoms that we often ignore, neglect, or mask. Discomfort is not something to avoid—it must be faced. People who become burned-out have not asked themselves questions about what they want or how they really feel. If they have, they do not do anything about their answers. Listening to oneself means taking inner feelings and needs into account, then findings ways to negotiate with others to meet those needs. It also means respecting yourself.

Recreate Your Mission: People need to find meaning in what they do. Each of us has a set of core values that we stand for and goals we want to accomplish. Often burnout means that someone has lost his original commitment to his profession. Overcoming burnout involves looking for your personal values and aligning your current work and organization with these values. Unless this connection is made between what you do and what you feel really matters, you are an empty shell. This emptiness causes people to burn out, and they need to undergo a personal renewal process to reconnect with this vital inner core.

The exploration of burnout has led from the symptoms of deep distress to ways in which the meaning of this crisis touches on some of the deepest aspects of life. Burnout is not something that can be cured by a quick fix. For individuals experiencing burnout, and for companies that find many of their employees are in that end state, a major renewal and re-examination is needed. When a person finds that something in his life has been lost, he must take steps to restore it.

PART V NUTRITION AND DIET

17 **What Is a Balanced Diet, Anyway?**
Sheldon Margen, M.D. and Michael Schwab

18 **What Do You Need to Know about Some Dietary Supplements?**
Kathryn Kolasa, Ph.D., R.D.

19 **Is Natural Better? And Other Questions about Health Foods**
Joan Dye Gussow, Ph.D.

20 **Controlling the Chemical Feast: How To Survive the Expanding Crisis in Food Safety**
James Turner, Esq.

21 **Diet, Nutrition, and Weight Control**
Anne M. Fletcher, M.S., R.D.

17 WHAT IS A BALANCED DIET, ANYWAY?

Sheldon Margen, M.D., has published 150 articles on the subject of nutrition and is editor of the Progress in Human Nutrition Series. He is chairman of the Editorial Board of Advisors of the University of California, Berkeley, *Wellness Newsletter*. He also co-authors a weekly health column for the *San Francisco Chronicle*. Dr. Margen has chaired the Department of Nutritional Sciences and the Public Health Nutrition Program at Berkeley.

Michael Schwab was associated for many years with R.D. Laing's Philadelphia Association in London, where he explored the complex web of relationships connecting nutrition, psychology, and health. He has worked as a nutritionist for the World Food Program in Haiti and the League of Red Cross Societies in West Africa. He also administered the United Nations Development Program in Malawi for 3 years. He is now pursuing a doctoral degree in nutrition, working with Dr. Margen at Berkeley.

One of the most frightening phenomena the health scene today is the gullibility of the American public on the subject of diet and nutrition. One best seller after another lands in book stores, each with a variation on the basic theme and promising dramatic results in terms of weight loss and vitality. This is troubling to those who believe the health field should be enriched with new ideas. What is known today about nutrition is quite basic. And if this basic information is appreciated, much of the hyperbole—and downright distortion—of many fad diet books will become obvious. Sheldon Margen and Michael Schwab give the thoughtful reader some simple guidelines for developing a healthy diet.■

THE DREADFUL QUESTION

What *is* a balanced diet anyway? Ask a mother of three children, ask the doctor, ask a dietitian or nutritionist, a farmer or a chef. Listen to the television or your Sunday columnist. There are many answers in the air. And perhaps this is how it should be, for, as the French nutritionist Jean Tremolieres has pointed out:

Ideas on nutrition and dietetics have never been the monopoly of any particular class. The experience of feeding is common to all, and each according to his personal experience has developed his own ideas and principles on the subject.

The trouble is that we have come to expect straightforward answers to nutritional questions. We want facts (or at least what we can accept as facts), a no-nonsense explanation of why things are the way they are, clear statements of how they ought to be. One of the themes of this chapter is that expecting straightforward answers, though it may be appropriate when dealing with machines, is usually mistaken when we deal with living organisms.

Nutrition, as a science, was built on the eighteenth century concept of "man as machine," dealing with people as if we were products off a conveyer belt, rather than unique individuals with neighbors, lovers, bills to pay. This mechanistic view still holds the high ground.

In recent years, however, a broader point of view has been emerging. There are now numerous nutritionists for whom the question "What is a balanced diet?" has become dreadfully complex. Many now admit, without apology, that there is no simple answer for the wide variety of individuals in their various situations, nor even for the same person at different times.

For those who subscribe to this complex view, the dreadful question can only be explored by asking counter questions. What are you used to eating? What kind of work do you do? How much have you got to spend on food this week? What foods are available? What do you *feel* like eating? All these (and many more) factors influence what is probably best for us to eat at any particular time. The foods we are used to eating form the foundation on which our diet is based. The kind of work we do calls for differing nutrient requirements.

Questions of finance and availability are important because our balanced diet can have no real significance outside what is affordable and available. As for what we feel like eating, this is perhaps the major (if largely unacknowledged) determinant of what we eat.

Some nutritionists have nightmares about this complex state of affairs, but the truth of the matter seems to be, as they say in Haiti, *Deye mon ge mon*: beyond the mountain, more mountains. In living systems every problem can be considered a symptom of at least one other problem. We are not machines at all but complex, interrelated organisms. A balanced diet depends on who, where, with whom, and in what state of health we are. It is influenced by an interplay of genetics, past experience, age, personality, and occupation, as well as of climate, culture and season. It certainly appears to be a dynamic thing, a state of constantly changing balance between us and our environment, not fixed at all.

Recognition of this state of affairs is nothing new, as the fifth century Greek physician Hippocrates testified:

Every doctor must learn about nature and seek to find, if he wishes to fulfill his obligations, the relationships of man to his food, his drink, and his whole way of life, and the influences exercised by each thing over each individual.

If this seems to be a tall order to the modern diagnostician, it can at least serve as a guiding principle. For diet reflects our whole way of life. A balanced diet can exist only within some system of balance among the many prevailing forces, external and internal, that make up our day-to-day lives.

FROM INTEGRATED FOLKLORE
TO FRAGMENTED SCIENCE

In traditional cultures throughout the world, food and its relationship to health are part of the overall beliefs and habits of the people. Nutritional information is based on physical experience developed through trial and error and transmitted in culinary folklore as a matter of course. In the rural areas of the Third World, folklore continues to hold a place of sorts, despite its gradual erosion over the last 200 years (and especially in the last 20) by the influx of some of the worst European and American values.

The nomadic peoples of the southern Sahara, for example, have lived for generations on the milk, blood, and meat of their herds. They live with and upon the goats and camels that comprise their wealth, that inspire their songs, that serve as the matrix for their culture. Traders in grain and salt (a trade now taken over by transcontinental trucking companies), they traditionally eat some rice and millet, and small quantities of desert dates, but their diet is based on their animals.

To the desert peoples, eating the meat of young goats—and with their rigorous sense of hospitality, offering it to their guests—is an integral part of life. Goats and rice are part of their social ecology, their traditional system of values and beliefs, their relationship with the world. Young men who leave for the city change this traditional relationship in many ways, in the matter of food by turning to dried milk, white bread, and Pepsi-Cola. What is available, what they can afford, what their peers are buying—these are just a few of the factors at play.

In the industrialized world, dietary folklore itself is all but swept away before the brooms of the newer sciences—biochemistry, physiology, and statistics. They assemble for us, in a piecemeal way, an entirely new, homogenized epistemology of food and a new kind of nutrition, approached through the intellect rather than through physical experience. This can be unnerving, as sociologist Hilary Homans points out in her comparison of Indian and Anglo-Saxon British women living in England:

Indian women conceptualize food and its relationship with health maintenance according to the Ayurvedic philosophy. British women, on the other hand, do not possess knowledge of such a coordinated belief system relating to diet; rather, their knowledge is more fragmented and derived from changing theories in nutritional science. . . .

We sometimes forget that the body of information we call nutritional sciences is young, only gradually finding its feet, only slowly building up a picture of how diet fits into the life of mod-

ern mankind. In this chapter, we review some of the steps in this growing process, and some of the dietary trends which have preoccupied nutritionists, such as the tendency for us—as we get richer—to eat more fat, more sugar, and less grain than in our traditional diets.

Like wealthy peoples before us, we eat the "fat of the land," and though we know now that eating a lot of it may bring on heart disease and perhaps cancer, fat still constitutes over 40% of Americans' national food energy intake. As we get richer, we also enjoy an astonishingly sweet life, getting through an average of a kilogram each of sugar and corn sweeteners per week, apparently despite the knowledge that it does us very little good. Other aspects of our modern highly processed diet—lots of salt and very little fiber, for example—also seem to contribute to the development of the diseases of the rich.

This dietary pattern represents a major obstacle to well-being in the modern world and a particular kind of challenge to the nutritionist. By what standards should we assess whether a diet is balanced or not? Desert nomads and other peoples throughout the world have developed their own standards in the past, but in the homogenized cultures of the modern world, these tend to lose their special validity. In the emerging science of nutrition, we have two kinds of standard: the so-called recommended daily allowances and the dietary guidelines. Where do they come from? What are their strengths and weaknesses? And how useful are they to us as individuals? And there is a third approach to the question, "What is a balanced diet?"—the way of personal experience and intuition.

RECOMMENDED DAILY ALLOWANCES: ARE THEY ANY USE?

Nutrition is a young science and, despite the millions of research papers, surveys, books, magazines and television programs devoted to the subject, we still understand relatively little.

Of course, we have identified and labelled the different kinds of biochemical matter that our bodies, and our food, are made of. In nutrition, the classifications are now common knowledge:

proteins, fats and carbohydrates, vitamins, minerals, and fiber. We know that some nutrients are crucial: the essential amino and fatty acids have probably all been identified, as have most of the vitamins and essential minerals.

We also know something about the properties of these compounds and their variable forms, but our understanding of their complex physiochemical interactions—in the cooking pot and in our bodies, with each other and with the increasing amounts of food additives that we eat—is far from complete.

Even what might seem to be a fundamental question—how much of each nutrient do we need?—remains something of a mystery. Not that nutritionists haven't tried to answer it. Nearly a century of research has given us two broad kinds of data on which to build our estimates. The first, and historically the earliest, has been the study of individual animals and humans in the laboratory. The second has been the surveying of groups or "populations" in the community. And this data has been useful. From the laboratory study of individuals we know quite a bit about how nutrients behave in the body and how deficiency and excess occur, which has helped in the recognition and treatment of classical deficiency diseases like scurvy, iron-deficiency anemia and rickets.

But studies of individuals only tell us about *those* individuals at that time. They cannot tell us how low vitamin intakes may safely fall in *others* before classical deficiency symptoms occur. For this, we need to have broader knowledge, with information about *variation* between people, and this is where the population studies have been helpful. They tell us, more or less, how much of any given nutrient is actually eaten by apparently healthy (or at least disease-free) people in a community, so that by implication we can estimate the range of their individual requirements.

A combination of these two kinds of research forms the basis of the closest thing we have to quantification of our biochemical requirements—the RDAs (Recommended Daily Allowances) as they are called in the United States, and similar national recommendations in other countries. And yet these recommendations are not require-

ments at all. For energy (calories), for example, there is a fixed RDA for each age group, by sex, with special additional recommendations for pregnancy and lactation, but the RDAs for energy are actually *average intakes* for apparently healthy persons in each group.

This is demonstrated in Figure 17-1 which shows a distribution curve for the range of energy intakes over 24 hours by a hypothetical population. The area under the curve represents the sample population. As you can see, half the population is below the RDA, even if they are getting enough to eat, while the other half is above the RDA, even if they are not getting enough. The interpretation often given to intake data—that eating less than the RDA is a sign of deficiency, or that eating more than the RDA indicates excess—is therefore obviously ridiculous.

For individual nutrients, the RDA is generally set not at the average intake but at two standard deviations above the average (Figure 17-2). This statistical device brings the RDA to the top end of the distribution curve, and it results in the setting of very high standards with a large safety margin for most people. Here, eating less than the RDA is even less likely to be associated with any manifestations of deficiency than with energy.

The RDAs are useful whenever populations are being considered in planning food supplies for

FIGURE 17-1.

DISTRIBUTION OF ENERGY INTAKES FOR A HYPOTHETICAL POPULATION

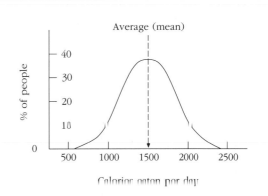

FIGURE 17-2.

DISTRIBUTION OF INTAKES OF A NUTRIENT (X)
FOR A HYPOTHETICAL POPULATION

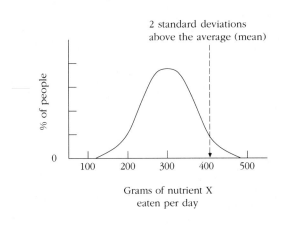

Grams of nutrient X
eaten per day

large groups; for example, they were first developed for this purpose during World War II, and they remain a humane guide to requirements in the planning of food stamp and other welfare meal programs.

But they are not a valid measure for assessing individual diets, even though they are very often used for this purpose. Elsi Widdowson, a doyenne of the Western nutrition establishment, pointed this out more than 40 years ago in the conclusion to her study of the diets of school children:

The one outstanding fact, which has been brought out again and again by this investigation, is that similar individuals may differ enormously and unpredictably in their food habits. This applies with great force to the energy value of the diets, but it is equally true of the approximate principles, minerals and vitamins, and still more of the foods themselves. Extraordinary departures from the average are compatible with normal physical development. These findings indicate that individual requirements must differ as much as individual intakes, and that an average intake, however valuable statistically, should never be used to assess an individual's requirement.

The RDAs can only serve as very crude yardsticks, and for individuals we must learn to use them in a much less absolute, more probabilistic

way. The best we can say is that the more frequently an individual does not meet or exceed the RDA, the greater the probability of deficiency; the more frequently an individual's intake exceeds the RDA, the greater the chance that it is excessive.

REQUIREMENTS AND TIME

An even more critical problem with the RDAs, and with the dicta of nutrition in general, is that they take little account of the way we and our individual requirements change over time. Granted, there are different RDAs for various age groups and time-related physiological states like pregnancy, but we know as a matter of everyday experience that our appetites vary over time for many reasons, both external and internal. And there is evidence that some of these influences on appetite— for example the season of the year, the amount of exercise we take, and the number of cigarettes we smoke—also affect our nutritional requirements. But by *how much* these requirements change, as time and our lives unfold, and the way these influences interact, we have little idea.

This is perplexing, even maddening, for those who expect science to come up with straightforward answers. The closer we look at requirements, the greater looms the possibility of variation—not only between individuals but also within each individual over time. How then shall nutritionists estimate the requirements of real people, living in their unique situations at one particular time? In our view, we may never be capable of doing this unless we are prepared to adopt a more flexible approach, less fixed in a mechanistic mold, which at least takes account of two fundamental time-related principles of biology that have only recently surfaced into modern nutrition, namely homeostasis and adaptation.

Homeostasis: The Basis for Fluctuating Requirements?

How many calories a day does a 55-year-old American woman need to maintain a healthy weight? How many calories does a 4-year-old African need? These are both important questions in the 1980s, when more than half of the world's population is said to be starving and a good many of the rest are trying to lose weight. Yet we do not have straightforward answers, for nature fluctuates. All living systems constantly adjust themselves to maintain stability. In human biology this process is known as homeostasis. Homeostasis almost certainly implies that our individual requirements also fluctuate.

Take the example of energy. Nineteenth century physiology was dominated by the study of the transformations of food energy into body mass and activity. And the models designed to explain these transformations were, like most medical research at that time, based on principles borrowed from the engineering innovations of the industrial revolution and on the world view of the body as a machine.

The mechanistic model of energy flow was developed on this basis (Figure 17-3). The remarkable ability of humans to maintain their body mass—sometimes varying by only a few pounds over half a lifetime—was believed to be due to a physiological correcting mechanism in the body

that regulated either food intake or energy output, or both. In this sense, we saw ourselves like the early steam engines designed by James Watt, which were regulated by the use of mechanical "governors." Energy requirements were believed to depend on energy output (i.e., activity), provided that body weight stayed constant. Too much food for the activity was assumed to result in increased weight; too little was assumed to lead to weight loss. And, to put a lid on the matter, this hypothetically fixed relationship between energy intake and output was assumed to be a genetically determined fact of life.

As anyone who has tried to lose weight will know, this assumption of fixed requirements was incorrect. Simply reducing food intake while maintaining the same level of activity does not necessarily result in weight loss. Despite the more recent refinement of the model—to include the energy used to maintain metabolism and the energy released as heat—mechanistic models have repeatedly shown a discrepancy between

FIGURE 17-3.

ENERGY REGULATION: THE MECHANISTIC MODEL

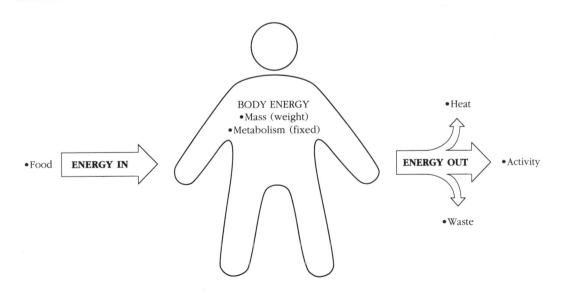

As long as body weight remains constant, energy requirements are determined primarily by activity levels. Like a machine, the body is believed to function at a fixed level of efficiency. Attempts to demonstrate this model have repeatedly failed.

els have repeatedly shown a discrepancy between energy intake and output that could not be accounted for by changes in body weight. In other words, something else goes on for which the theory of fixed requirements cannot account.

What the mechanical model failed to acknowledge was the possibility of changes in the efficiency with which the body uses energy— its "metabolic efficiency." Today we know that metabolism is a dynamic thing, constantly changing, an integrated system of chemical reactions, more than a million per minute in the human body. It regulates its own stability, or balance, within a certain range by continuous internal feedback. It is this dynamic stability we call homeostasis, a concept intuited by Claude Bernard

over a century ago and clearly formulated by the American Walter Cannon and others in the 1930s.

A somewhat similar phenomenon is known in mechanics as the "steady state," and in biochemistry as "dynamic equilibrium." But for some reason, this dynamic quality has been slow to catch on in nutritional theories. Even today, you will find little or no reference to homeostasis in any standard nutrition text.

This situation is beginning to change as researchers slowly turn their attention to the vexing question of how metabolism, and therefore requirements, change over time. Recent studies by Indian statistician P. V. Sukhatme and one of the authors, Sheldon Margen, have already demonstrated how energy and protein balance appear to

FIGURE 17-4.

ENERGY REGULATION: THE HOMEOSTATIC MODEL

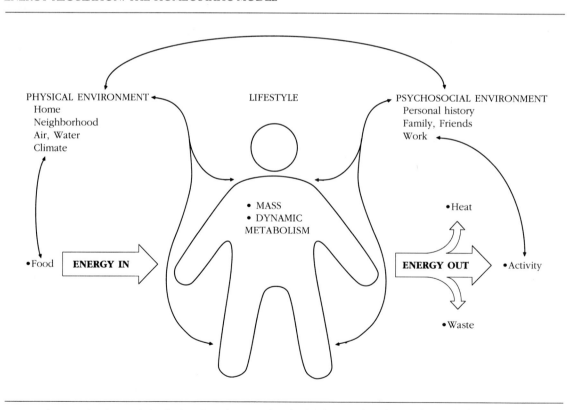

Body weight is regulated not only by food intake and activity, but also by the interplay of metabolism with the environment. Weight, energy requirements, and the balance of energy in and out of the body all fluctuate within a healthy range.

fluctuate in the manner of a homeostatic system. A new homeostatic theory of requirements has been proposed (Figure 17-4). The mechanical man in Figure 17-3 has now become a self-regulation system with food intake, body weight, metabolic efficiency, and energy output all interacting, not only with each other but with other aspects of the individual's life. Falling in love, for example, can have an immediate effect on metabolic rate and thereby on metabolic efficiency and body weight!

This realization is important for those engaged in losing weight. In slimming clinics, it has long been observed that weight gains and losses seem to be associated with changes in metabolic efficiency, even over relatively short periods of time. Popular nutrition writers have been saying for years that eating less triggers greater metabolic efficiency, so that the body can made better use of the food that is eaten; weight is maintained at a level little or no lower than before. Even when accompanied by more exercise, dieting is often ineffective in reducing weight. According to the homeostatic model of energy regulation, this is because, within a range of food intakes, body weight is maintained by homeostatic variation in the body's energy utilization. The first experimental evidence to support this view is only beginning to emerge.

Adaptation: How Far Does It Go?

The potential for changing metabolic efficiency implies that our body weight is maintained by homeostasis although, in the face of reduced food intake, we shed a few pounds before stabilizing at a new homeostatic level. This is a process of adaptation as the body adjusts to eating less food.

Now, what happens if we apply this model to malnourished children in Africa or in the United States? In the past, we have assessed the prevalence of malnutrition largely on the basis of the malnourished children's diet and growth, as compared with RDAs and average growth patterns for Western children. By this process, we find a vast population of kids who eat less and are smaller than the Western average. The question then arises: to what extent are these children adapted, without impairment, to a lower food intake? This is a deeply controversial issue. The homeostatic model suggests that some of the children in this group have adapted and that our Western estimates of world malnutrition may be exaggerated. But we do not yet understand how to tell which children can adapt in this way nor what the long-term effects of such adaptation may be. This question should not distract us, however, from the reality that millions of children die from starvation each year and that hunger afflicts millions more. These are nutritional issues of great concern. Yet the probability remains that we may be able to adapt without impairment to lower food intakes than is generally considered possible.

This is the case not only in the face of changes in food intake but also in response to or as a part of inner, physiological changes, such as those that occur in pregnancy. Though a good deal is known about the adaptations of pregnancy, relatively little has been acknowledged thus far in nutrition. Within hours of conception, a pregnant woman's body begins to change as her metabolism adapts to the presence of the blastocyte settling into the lining of her uterus; over the ensuing weeks, her heart enlarges, her blood volume increases, digestion slows down and her appetite becomes more sensitive, all of which may be seen as serving the purpose of maximizing her nutritional status. The retention of iron, for example, is enhanced by the cessation of menstruation and increased absorption from the gut. For women who usually eat iron-rich foods like meat, fish, seeds, legumes, nuts, dried fruit, and whole grains, these adaptations are generally sufficient to satisfy the additional iron requirements of pregnancy. For those whose iron stores are low—between 10 and 15% of pregnant women in the U.S., according to recent estimates—additional iron in the form of supplements is advisable.

Yet little of this remarkable adaptive process is acknowledged by nutritionists, who continue to recommend (and even insist) that pregnant women ingest vast quantities of extra iron. In the United States, this kind of guidance is justified by reference to the RDA for iron in pregnancy, which is 18 mg—more, as the RDA authors point out, than can possibly be obtained from a normal diet.

Even a quarter pound of liver contains only about 5 mg of absorbable iron! So the RDAs include the caution that *all* pregnant women should take 30–60 mgs. of supplemental iron per day (the excess being to allow for the low absorption of dietary iron) during their third trimester.

Perhaps this very high intake would be justified if it were of demonstrable benefit. But there is no evidence that it is. A recent review by American epidemiologists Hemminki and Starfield of all the controlled trials of iron supplements reported in the scientific literature of four languages showed no evidence of benefit to either mother or baby. As many women develop constipation when they take iron supplements, and some seem to develop abnormally large, fragile red blood cells, there is clearly some reason for this RDA to be reviewed.

The adaptations of pregnancy illustrate the marvelous, unfathomable complexity of all biological adaptations pervading the biosphere. We hardly begin to understand their physical nature as it has evolved. Before relying too enthusiastically on the RDAs as a guide to balanced nutrition in pregnancy (or at any other time), we should perhaps pause to consider how women ever managed to bear children over the millions of years before iron, or the RDAs, were ever thought of.

DIETARY GUIDELINES: CLOSER TO SOCIAL REALITY?

Another set of standards by which to answer our dreadful question arises from the field of public health epidemiology, which is concerned with the distribution of diseases in the community. This would include, for example, the characteristics of those who develop heart disease–their age and sex, ethnic and social origins, their jobs, their diet, and so on. Using the survey methods of the social sciences, rather than the laboratory methods of the biochemist, epidemiology places nutrition into a broader context, something more closely resembling social reality. In the 1950s and 1960s, it was through epidemiological surveys, supported by laboratory studies and the data-crunching capacities of computers, that we had the first quantified demonstration of a relationship between diet and heart disease. And from such studies emerged the now well-known phenomenon of "relative risk," which gives us the relative probabilities of developing a given disease for different categories of individuals.

This opened up new possibilities for nutrition education as a public service. By the early 1970s, there was a large enough body of epidemiological data on diet and disease to form the basis for a new kind of balanced diet standard. Though the information available was incomplete and sometimes self-contradictory, several Western nations published their own national dietary guidelines during the 1970s. Sweden was the first, closely followed by Holland, Norway, Canada, and the U.S. All followed a similar pattern: less fat (especially saturated fats and cholesterol), less sugar and salt, and less food altogether. All implied that we should eat more whole grains, vegetables, and fruit. In a rather piecemeal but nevertheless practical way, governments were—for the first time—assuming a responsibility to guide their citizens towards a balanced diet.

Immense controversy surrounded these various recommendations. Objections and counter-proposals came especially from those who had the most to lose by the recommended changes. The meat, dairy, egg, and sugar industries, with their powerful agricultural and manufacturing interests, lobbied strongly against recommendations not based, as they saw it, on established evidence. Food processing corporations using these commodities argued that alternative products would be expensive to develop and that the cost would fall on the consumer.

The Dietary Guidelines for Americans, published jointly in 1979 by the U. S. Department of Agriculture and the Department of Health and Human Services, and revised in 1985, is typical of what emerged from this controversial process. Apart from the ticklish problems of saying just how much fat or sugar or salt is "too much," or what exactly "desirable" weight means—and perhaps more importantly, who is to decide these things—they offered us a framework within which to work. At last nutritionists had something more to offer up than the RDAs and vague references to a balanced diet.

The effect seems, in some ways, to have been dramatic. The American diet *is* gradually changing in what most nutritionists would consider to be the right direction. Though we cannot say how much of this is due to the *Guidelines*, we are—according to the U.S. Food and Drug Administration— steadily reducing our intake of fat, cholesterol, and salt, while increasing the amount of fiber in our diet. Consumption of animal foods has remained fairly constant, but within this group there has been a substantial decrease in whole milk and egg consumption and a moderate decrease in red meat intake in favor of low-fat and skim milk, poultry and, to a lesser degree, fish. Vegetable and fruit consumption are also up— to their levels of thirty years ago—although potatoes, once a staple and a major source of the nation's vitamin C, continue to lose popularity, except in the form of potato chips and french fries.

An unwelcome trend is the continuing increase in the amount of sweet foods we eat. Sugar consumption is down, but its place is more than taken over by corn sweeteners. Americans now eat some 2½ pounds each per week of these two calorie rich, nutrient poor foods, with another 5 ounces equivalent of sugar in saccharine and aspartame, the so-called noncaloric sweeteners. Much of this is consumed in soft drinks, which have now overtaken milk and beer to become the nation's most popular type of beverage.

While our consumption of corn sweeteners (and of another popular carbohydrate, alcohol) goes up, the amount of grains we eat *as such* continues to decline. Nevertheless, whole grains can provide versatile, nutritious, and delicious staples at a relatively low cost. Wholewheat breads, brown rice, oats, and barley are excellent sources of most nutrients, including protein when they are eaten with beans, peas, nuts or even small quantitites of an animal food. The *Dietary Guidelines* imply that our national "dinner plate" (if we could make one up from everything we eat in a day) should contain a good deal more grains, less animal foods,

FIGURE 17-5.

THE AMERICAN DINNER PLATE: TODAY AND TOMORROW

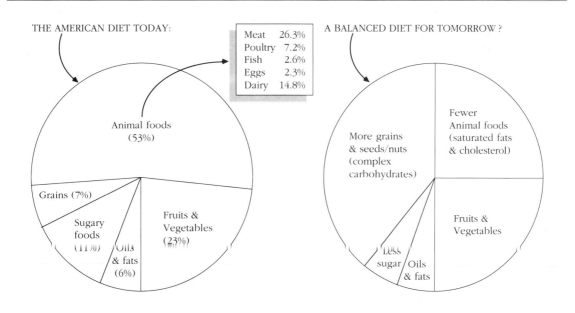

Today most of our grains go for animal feed. If we ate less meat, there would be enough grain for us and much of the hungry world.

and less of the sweet stuff. In this respect, we still have a long way to go.

If this is frustrating to those who look for rapid change, there may be some consolation in considering how long the recommendations in the *Guidelines* took to become a part of public policy at all, given that similar advice has been in limited circulation since at least the turn of the century. The pioneering American nutritionist Wilbur O. Atwater wrote in 1894 that

our diet is onesided . . . with relatively too little protein and too much fat, starch and sugar. In other words it is relatively deficient in the materials that make muscle and bone and contains a relative excess of the fuel ingredients. This is due partly to our large consumption of sugar and partly to our use of such large quantities of fat meats.

Mid-twentieth century studies, comparing the diet and health of traditional communities with the diet and health of those who had made the transition into urban civilization, pointed in the same direction: that Western civilization brings with it a more refined, fattier, saltier, sweeter diet, and that its introduction is soon followed by the so-called diseases of modern civilization— heart disease, cancer, and diabetes. Going back even further, the Reverend Graham Sylvester was preaching a gospel of whole grains and legumes in 1830, albeit as part of a larger moralistic package that included vegetarianism and sexual abstinence. Perhaps our newfound national guidelines are simply the arrival at a societal level of dietary principles that have been around for many years.

The epidemiological approach is highly computerized and produces the kind of information that impresses in the modern world—simple (if at times simplistic), statistical, and useful. With succeeding generations of computers, it becomes possible to measure more variables, which enables us to piece together more of the complexity of health and disease.

This has drawn nutrition into a broader scheme of things, showing how diet is integrally related to other aspects of our lives. For example, Ancel Keys' hypothesis about fat as the cause of heart dis-

ease, which was famous 20 years ago, has now dissolved into a broader understanding of the many physical and social risk factors involved. Age, sex, smoking habits, exercise, and diet all play a part in the etiology of heart disease, and a number of studies have now shown that stress is also implicated.

The major drawback to the epidemiological approach is that, in seeking always to know more about the world, it tends to draw us away from knowing it directly. Striving for knowledge, we detach ourselves from experience. At a personal level, the more we rely on epidemiological maps of reality, the less attention we pay to our own experience of reality. Intuition and other processes of self-knowledge are neglected. Yet it is these very processes that can provide a third way to answer the dreadful question.

INTUITIVE BALANCE

There is now a mass of public information on healthy eating. Indeed, in every realm, we are flooded with information and advice on how to lead a better life. And yet, in the last resort, we have to make our own decisions. From early childhood, we submit to an apparently endless stream of expert advice from parents, caretakers, teachers, television, doctors, and dentists, all intent on showing us the way. Yet the way is not a rigid thing. It differs for each of us and it differs for any one of us over time. If, as individuals or as families, we are to find the diet that suits us best, we need more than nutritional research, enlightened public policy with regard to nutrition, and education. We also need to draw on our own resources, our own and our culture's experience and intuition.

We are, after all, sentient creatures, with a vast capacity to feel. Few would deny it, even if scientists are supposed to ignore their own feelings when studying other people! In relation to food alone, we have an array of interacting faculties that serve to help us find the way: hunger and appetite, smell, sight and taste, as well as those intuitive processes that make us aware, in sometimes inexplicable ways, what it is we need to do in a given situation. In the real world, these personal, subjective feelings may be no less important indicators of a balanced diet than those many factors studied by the apparently objective measures of science. Unfortunately, we often tend to mistrust these feelings because we are led to believe that only the so-called experts know what is true.

Hunger, for example, is usually an indicator of a need for food, and satiety is a sign that hunger has been satisfied. Though there are many who become hungry in the face of frustration, boredom, and anger, everyday experience tells us that hunger, and its absence, *can* serve as a guide in the matter of when and how much to eat.

Perhaps more controversially, appetite also seems to serve a physiological function. As a refinement of hunger, appetite reaches out into the world from within us toward particular foods. Most people know the feelings of having had enough pasta but still having an appetite for dessert. To what extent the appetite of healthy individuals is an indicator of what foods their bodies *need* is a fascinating subject. The idea of the "nutritional wisdom" of the body has fascinated psychobiologists for more than 50 years and there is some evidence—at least in animals and children—that intuitive appetite can be a reliable guide to a balanced diet. Clara Davis' study of the self-selection of diets among young children remains as provocative now as it did them. Despite some novel meal combinations that would make most nutritionists' hair stand on end (one child ate 11 bananas in a day), all her subjects selected a balanced diet over a period of weeks. Davis found, however, that the kids' intuitive choice only worked if unrefined and unprocessed foods were offered; with the introduction of sugary foods, their balanced choices broke down.

The idea of nutritional wisdom posits that we are all endowed with potential intuitive understanding of what our bodies need for good health. Walter Cannon, who first used the word *homeostasis* in biology, is sometimes credited with having also coined the expression *wisdom of the body*, though the idea has certainly been understood for centuries. The diets of older civilizations seem to have been based on nutritional wisdom with, for example, their balance of proteins

in grains and legumes, or the traditional Mexican addition of lime juice to tortilla flour which effectively protects the consumer against the vitamin deficiency disease pellagra.

Yet in the modern world, we resist feelings of the body, distrust ourselves and our prescientific traditions. From the earliest days of life, most of our babies are fed formula by the clock from a manmade bottle, rather than human milk from the woman's breast according to the intuitive wisdom and timing inherent in her relationship with her child. As kids grow, the dictates of the marketplace tend to dominate their nutritional choices rather than any wisdom of their bodies or their parents. The average American child internalizes more than 20 TV food commercials a day, most of them for products of marginal or negative nutritional value.

There are also family eating patterns to consider with their many variations on the use of food as a response to stress or as bribes and threats and rewards. All these phenomena serve to draw children, and the adults they become, away from sensing what they need to eat.

And yet we can regain ourselves by learning (or relearning) to turn our attention away from the information that floods us from outside, towards our own experience, the wisdom of the body, through observation and reflection—in meditation, art, psychotherapy, or some other regular practice that reminds us who we are and what it is we feel. Experts—be they parents, teachers, health professionals, neighbors, or friends—cannot know more about our bodies than our bodies already know.

CONCLUSION

For those in search of a personal answer to the dreadful question, there is the need to seek a balance. The RDAs are best left to those who deal with populations, and even then they should be used with caution, but the government's dietary guidelines do provide a useful framework on which individuals may build. By simply keeping a record of everything you eat over a week, you can check how your "dinner plate" corresponds with the recommended guidelines. If you see a need to change, the next step is up to you. Some opt for dramatic alteration, by completing cutting out, say, sugar or red meat. Others prefer to change more slowly, establishing a new balance by trial and error.

Either way, more than a change of diet tends to result. New diets go hand in hand with new lifestyles; patterns of social interaction, work and leisure tend to change, too. This is where intuition becomes invaluable, for nobody knows our individual needs and capacities to change better than we do. By all means, let's listen to the experts and bear in mind their guidelines, but we should also remember to listen to ourselves.

18 WHAT DO YOU NEED TO KNOW ABOUT SOME DIETARY SUPPLEMENTS?

Kathryn Kolasa, Ph.D., R.D., is professor and section head of Nutrition Education and Services at East Carolina University. She is a registered dietitian and she specializes in providing nutrition information to consumers so they can make informed choices. Dr. Kolasa is past president of the Society for Nutrition Education.

The field of dietary supplements has become a battleground. On one side are the health food purists, who believe and argue that only fruits and vegetables grown on ground untainted by chemicals and unadorned by anything the food distributor might add are to be considered healthy. They are opposed by the major food distributors who are driven by economical and technological considerations to sprinkle, spray, and otherwise infuse our food with chemicals. As with so many subjects, the truth must lie somewhere between these two extremes. Kathryn Kolasa explains her view of this chemical warfare and reminds us of the importance of using common sense. ▪

"Please pass the red, blue and yellow food packages." Many writers of the late 1970s described a growing trend in the United States toward the consumption of a synthetic diet. Some writers warned that real food would become an endangered species. We would eat food packages, similar to those developed in the space program, and eat pills to take care of our hunger and nutrient needs, with no fuss or muss.

But people worldwide find that food is more than just a mix of chemicals, more than a biological necessity. Food is a major ingredient in the pleasures we find in eating. We now have the capability to manufacture food by chemical synthesis, but consumers want real food. At the same time, however, when we feel our selections are not good enough to nourish us, many of us turn to manufactured nutrient supplemental powders, tablets, liquids, and pills.

Americans have received a flood of dietary recommendations to help reduce the risks of chronic and degenerative diseases such as cancer, osteoporosis, hypertension, and heart disease. We have responded by being more concerned about our health and fitness. Even so, many of us do not want to change the way we eat. Many of us look for easy answers. And in the face of much of this conflicting dietary advice, we have begun supplementing our diets with vitamins, minerals, fiber, fatty acids, amino acids, and more. The commonly asked questions are which supplements, what form, whose brand and how much.

Supplements and information about supplements are big business. Quack advice and good advice are often difficult to separate. So, in this chapter, we will review the advice that qualified health professionals have given the public about dietary supplementation. Some of the popular concerns of food versus supplements as the source of nutrients will be highlighted.

Note that research about and practice of supplementation covers a wide variety of nutrients in both the prevention and the treatment of diseases. For example, since 1924, salt has been fortified with iodine to supplement the low levels of iodine in some of our diets. This was done as a public health measure to prevent the incidence of goiter,

a disease characterized by swelling in the neck as a result of the enlargement of the thyroid gland. Since the 1940s, enrichment of cereals with B vitamins has been practiced to reduce the incidence of beriberi, a disease in which the nerves and muscles degenerate, ultimately leading to paralysis. Today, health professionals are studying the possibilities of supplementing the diet with different types of fiber, with beta carotene to delay or prevent the onset of cancers, and with calcium to prevent or minimize the debilitating effects of osteoporosis, a disease of reduced bone density in old age, which makes bones fragile. These are examples of supplementation to prevent diseases.

Scientists, too, are studying the use of supplements in treating and curing diseases. For example, researchers are using selenium to treat skin cancer and dietary fibers to control blood glucose levels in diabetics. But using supplements to cure disease is beyond the scope of this chapter.

THE TRADITIONAL NUTRITION WISDOM: EAT A BALANCED DIET

Get your nutrients from foods. Nutritionists have been advising Americans about their dietary practices for approximately a century. This advice has evolved from knowledge of human nutritional needs and of the relationship of diet to health and disease. The advice may change from time to time because it is based on imperfect and incomplete knowledge. A variety of eating guides have been developed over the years. These eating patterns translate what is known about nutrient requirements into a plan that will help consumers select the kinds and amounts of foods for a nutritionally sound diet. The best known plan is called the Basic Four Food Groups. The traditional nutrition wisdom was that an individual could obtain *all* his nutrients from eating a balanced diet and therefore supplementation with vitamin or mineral pills was neither necessary nor desirable. "Get your nutrients from food, not pills" was a common piece of dietary advice. Recently, the Food and Drug Administration (FDA), many nutrition scientists, and the American Dietetic Association (ADA) have reiterated that advice.

Until the late 1970s, all food guides were

devised to ensure that the nutrient and caloric needs of individuals, as described in the Recommended Dietary Allowances, were met. The Recommended Dietary Allowances (RDAs) are suggested amounts of energy, protein, and key minerals and vitamins for an adequate diet for practically all healthy persons. The RDAs have been revised at regular intervals to incorporate new knowledge of nutrient requirements for people of various ages. In terms of diet and health concerns such as fat, cholesterol, sugar and fiber are not addressed in the RDAs or in the Basic 4. As a result, some other types of dietary advice have been promoted since 1979.

MORE RECENT WISDOM:
AVOID AND ABSTAIN

Dietary goals for the nation were announced in 1977 emphasizing prevention of killer diseases. These goals were the first to suggest that Americans should avoid high fat and high sodium intakes. No advice was given about dietary supplementation.

Soon after these goals were promoted by the Senate Select Committee on Nutrition, the U.S. Department of Agriculture (USDA) and the U.S. Department of Health and Human Services (HHS) jointly issued *Nutrition and Your Health: Dietary Guidelines for Americans* in 1980. The healthy population was advised to:

1. Eat a variety of foods.
2. Maintain ideal weight.
3. Avoid too much fat, saturated fat, and cholesterol.
4. Eat foods with adequate starch and fiber.
5. Avoid too much sugar.
6. Avoid too much sodium.
7. If you drink alcohol, do so in moderation.

Americans were advised that they did not need to supplement their diets:

There are no known advantages to consuming excess amounts of any nutrient. You will rarely need to take a vitamin or mineral supplement if you eat a wide variety of foods. There are some exceptions to this general statement: women in their childbearing years may need to take iron supplements to replace the iron they lose with menstrual bleeding. Women

who are no longer menstruating should not take iron supplements routinely. Women who are pregnant or who are breastfeeding need more of many nutrients, especially iron, folic acid, vitamin A, calcium and sources of energy.

To make sure you get enough fiber in your diet, you should eat fruits and vegetables, whole grain breads and cereals. There is no reason to add fiber to foods that do not already contain it.

The second edition of these guidelines, with few modifications, was issued in 1985. The statements and philsophy of dietary supplementation remain basically unchanged. The revised guidelines tells us:

In chronic conditions where diet may be important—heart disease, high blood pressure, strokes, tooth decay, diabetes, osteoporosis, and some forms of cancer—the role of specific dietary substances has not been defined fully.

A caution was added that there may be harm in consuming excessive amounts of a nutrient and that "large dose supplements of any nutrient should be avoided." In 1986, the Food and Drug Administration (FDA) began a campaign asking physicians to record the use of supplements by individuals who take massive doses and to monitor for any side effects.

The guidelines stated that "elderly people who eat a varied diet do not generally need vitamin and mineral supplements. However, some medications used for the treatment of disease may interact with nutrients. In such instances, a physician may prescribe supplements." The guidelines further suggested eating foods containing fiber naturally rather than adding fiber to foods.

Between the 1980 and 1985 publications of these guidelines there was a great deal of nutrition activity. Nutrition studies about diet and disease were conducted. Guidelines were issued by the American Heart Association, the American Cancer Society, and others. Food and supplement advertising and marketing campaigns were vigorously conducted. Some of these are described below.

Cancer Guidelines. In 1982, the National Academy of Sciences issued dietary guidelines to help Americans reduce the risk of diet-related cancers. Researchers warn that it is not possible and may never be possible to specify a diet that will protect everyone against all forms of cancer, but we can benefit from doing all of the following:

- Reduce intake of saturated and unsaturated fats.
- Include fruits, vegetables, and whole grain cereal products in the daily diet for dietary fiber and Vitamin A or its precursors.
- Minimize consumption of foods preserved by salt curing and smoking.
- Minimize consumption of foods with carcinogens from any source.
- Drink alcohol in moderation if at all.

These guidelines specifically noted that food and not supplement products should be the source of individual nutrients. In spite of these statements, consumer interest in taking vitamin A and fiber supplements to prevent cancer has soared.

More Cancer Guidelines. The American Cancer Society echoed the above recommendations and included a statement in 1984 that consumers should avoid taking high dosage supplements. The National Cancer Institute recommended eating a variety of foods and especially eating more vegetables and fruits rich in vitamins A and C.

Aggressive Product Promotion. Newspaper stories and magazine ads scream at consumers to take stress vitamins to replace lost vitamins or rebalance their diets, take antacids for calcium, take vitamin C to prevent colds, and take dietary supplements to reduce premenstrual syndrome (pms) effects. Many campaigns target the generalized feelings that none of use eat the way we should. We are told that taking a supplement is getting insurance for yourself. In some states, the product promotions have become so aggressive that consumer advocate groups are concerned that the public is being misled. In New York, some ads were judged misleading by the attorney general and the manufacturer was fined.

A "fiber war" is being waged on the breakfast cereal and specialty bread shelves of the grocery store. Consumers are encouraged to eat specific fiber-rich foods to prevent cancers, prevent constipation, and perhaps lower their cholesterol levels. There appears to be some impact from this pro-

motion. One national poll reports that 43% of Americans are eating more fiber, some of it as supplements.

CHANGING PROFESSIONAL ATTITUDES ABOUT RESPONSIBLE SUPPLEMENTATION

Consumers have been receiving information about supplementation from many sources and are asking professional nutritionists and physicians the types of questions mentioned earlier—Do I need a supplement? If so, what kind and how much should I take?

Official dietary guidelines downplay the need for dietary supplementation. But many health care professionals and the food industry are reevaluating these recommendations. Most health care professionals remain convinced that we should try to get all our needed nutrients and other food components from food. Yet, some health care professionals are reluctantly admitting that it is not always possible to do so within the number of calories most Americans are consuming or given the types of foods we prefer to eat. Health care professionals are cautious in their recommendations on the use of supplements, noting that we have only limited understanding of food composition, nutrition, and the human body's use of food ingredients. It is not known, for example, if a manufactured vitamin A supplement, natural or synthetic, has the same properties as beta carotene found in food. Perhaps the health benefit is from an undiscovered element in the food.

The dialogue about reasonable and rational dietary supplementation by Americans was joined in 1983 by the Council for Responsible Nutrition (CRN), a trade association of manufacturers and distributors of nutrient supplements. CRN reported that about 40% of the American population relied on nutrition supplements and predicted use to double by 1988. The Council issued a position paper that "outlined the role nutrient supplementation can and should play in an overall nutrition and health plan." CRN suggested that there are many people whose diets fall short in nutrients: people who do not eat enough food, whose eating habits are poor, who have lifestyles that compromise nutritional status, who have disease or surgery, and who are passing through special life periods. These people must rely on dietary supplementation to obtain needed nutrients.

The less food you eat the harder it is to get all the needed vitamins and minerals. Diets of fewer than 1,800 calories must be very carefully planned to meet the RDAs. Many Americans, however, would not maintain their desirable weight if they routinely ate more than 1,800 calories. So, many nutritionists will recommend that we increase activity levels so we can eat more food and get nutrients in necessary amounts. If increasing activity is not possible, it probably is necessary to supplement the diet with the nutrients in the amounts that are missing from food. We will discuss how to do that below.

The food industry, too, is reviewing the market demands. Fortification of foods is regulated by the FDA, so consumers are somewhat protected from a fortification horse race. However, manufacturers note that market possibilities exist for drinks and desserts with added vitamins, breads with high fiber ingredients, and so on.

There are several books you can read for a comprehensive review of information about vitamins, minerals, and other supplements. For the rest of this chapter, some of the most frequently asked questions will be answered.

Shall We Take a Daily Multiple Vitamin Supplement?

Based on consumer polls, there is a high probability that you or a member of your family already are taking a vitamin or mineral supplement. A 1982 Gallup Poll found 37% of American adults took vitamin supplements. The 1981 National Health Interview Study found that 36% of the children under the age of 18 had taken a supplement during the 2 weeks before the interview. Almost half of the children between 3 and 6 years of age were taking vitamins. Parents report giving supplements to their children because 1) the children are picky eaters and parents fear the diet is inadequate, 2) the doctor has recommended supplements, or 3) parents hope the supplements will prevent winter colds.

The American Academy of Pediatrics says there is little need for routine use of nutrient supplements by normal children. Those children with extreme dietary limitations or preferences should follow the advice of their physician. Studies of children 3 to 9 years of age report that, overall, the diets of children supply enough water-soluble vitamins and that taking supplements offers no clear improvement in the blood and urine levels for those nutrients. These results, however, did not necessarily apply to children of parents with low incomes or limited interest in health care.

The FDA surveyed the level of adult usage in 1980 and found about 40% used some type of supplement. The usage was higher among women than men, higher among whites than nonwhites, higher in the western part of the U.S. than in other regions, and higher among those with more education.

Is this supplementation necessary? A wise consumer must do more than just swallow that vitamin or mineral supplement. First, take a careful look at your regular food intake. There are many microcomputer programs that allow you to compare your food intake with your nutrient needs. Of course, you can do it the old-fashioned way and compute your nutrient intake by hand, using the food composition tables found in most nutrition books. Look up the nutrients for the foods you eat throughout an entire day, add up the figures, and then compare them with the RDA.

If you find a nutrient shortfall, change your eating habits and include foods high in the nutrients you are lacking. If you do not choose to change your food intake, then perhaps taking a multiple vitamin supplement is appropriate. Don't take a supplement without carefully analyzing what nutrients you are already getting. It's best to check with a registered dietitian, nutritionist, or other health care professional first. Remember that accidental poisonings do occur due to the accessibility of supplements in the home. Also, some health experts believe that we should avoid teaching children at an early age to depend upon pills.

If you are using supplements, read the label of the supplement to select the one best for you and your family. Remember, that *more* is not necessarily *better*. Select the supplement of vitamins or minerals in the dose that covers only your nutrient shortfall.

Many people are getting far more nutrients in their supplements than they are missing from food. An FDA survey of adult vitamin use found many adults were getting between 100% and 200% of the RDA from supplements alone. For eight nutrients (thiamine, riboflavin, vitamin C, pantothenic acid, vitamin E, vitamin B_{12}, niacin and vitamin B_6), the median intake was greater than 200% of the RDA. These high intakes are alarming. Remember, some of the old and easy nutrition rules don't necessarily work anymore. For instance, you may have learned in the past that fat-soluble vitamins are potentially harmful if taken in excess because they are stored in the liver. We continue to be concerned about high levels of intake of fat-soluble vitamins and their potential toxicity. But we have new toxicity concerns.

The old nutrition rule for water-soluble vitamins was that if you took too many water-soluble vitamins you probably would not do any harm, because excess water-soluble vitamins were excreted in urine or sweat. But toxicities from overconsumption of some water-soluble vitamins have been reported. Vitamin B_6 is of special concern, because it is being used to treat the symptoms of PMS and to relieve nausea during pregnancy. Ill effects have been reported in medical journals. Burning, shooting, and tingling pains in the limbs as well as clumsiness and numbness have been observed in women taking between 500 and 3000 mg per day. These are large doses considering that RDA is 2 to 4 mg/day. Toxic effects of niacin, vitamin C, thiamin, folic acid, and panthothenic acid have also been reported. Reports from hospitals of acute overdoses of children's multiple vitamins, particularly sweetened preparations, have increased in recent years.

Water-miscible preparations of fat-soluble vitamins are also more available. Remember, a water-miscible preparation of vitamin A is really designed for patients who have trouble absorbing fat-soluble vitamins because of a disease. For the normal individual, water-miscible fat-soluble vita-

mins should be taken with the same care as fat-soluble preparations, because the same ill effects can occur with overuse. (See tables 8-1 to 8-8 on pages 141-148).

Will Supplements Improve My Athletic Performance?

The use of vitamin and/or mineral and protein or amino acid supplements by athletes and those involved in physical fitness is commonplace. Each person has his or her own reason for using supplements, but most believe that the supplement will enhance performance and endurance. It's difficult to provide recommendations based on scientific information at this time, because the scientific reports are still inconclusive. The following is typical:

Well trained male runners from a club were given a vitamin/mineral supplement with amino acids and essential fatty acids to see if it would improve their athletic performance and endurance. There were no effects on any of the indicators of improved performance or endurance, including no difference in maximum oxygen consumption, no change in submaximal endurance run, no difference in muscle glycogen, no difference in glucose concentration, and no change in free fatty acid levels or lactate. It would seem from this report that the supplement has no physiological value to an athlete who is already consuming a nutritionally balanced diet.

Will Taking a Calcium Supplement Prevent Osteoporosis or Reduce My Hypertension?

All consumption studies show that most American women do not meet their dietary need for calcium. Most consume 450 to 550 of the 800 mg necessary according to the 1980 RDAs. Many health care professionals believe that even 800 mg is below the needed daily calcium intake to prevent osteoporosis in women. The NIH Consensus Conference called for 1000 mg for premenopausal and estrogen-treated women. Postmenopausal women who are not treated with estrogen require about 1500 mg/day for calcium balance.

TABLE 18-1. RECOMMENDED DAILY DIETARY ALLOWANCES, revised 1980.[a] DESIGNED FOR THE MAINTENANCE OF GOOD NUTRITION OF PRACTICALLY ALL HEALTHY PEOPLE IN THE U.S.A.

Group	Age (years)	Weight (kg)	Weight (lbs)	Height (cm)	Height (in)	Protein (g)	Vitamin A (μg R.E.)[b]	Vitamin D (μg)[c]	Vitamin E (mg T.E.)[d]	Vitamin C (mg)	Thiamin (mg)	Riboflavin (mg)	Niacin (mg N.E.)[e]	Vitamin B6 (mg)	Folacin (μg)[f]	Vitamin B12 (μg)	Calcium (mg)	Phosphorus (mg)	Magnesium (mg)	Iron (mg)	Zinc (mg)	Iodine (μg)
Infants	0.0-0.5	6	13	60	24	kg x 2.2	420	10	3	35	0.3	0.4	6	0.3	30	0.5[g]	360	240	50	10	3	40
Infants	0.0-1.0	9	20	71	28	kg x 2.0	400	10	4	35	0.5	0.6	8	0.6	45	1.5	540	360	70	15	5	50
Children	1-3	13	29	90	35	23	400	10	5	45	0.7	0.8	9	0.9	100	2.0	800	800	150	15	10	70
Children	4-6	20	44	112	44	30	500	10	6	45	0.9	1.0	11	1.3	200	2.5	800	800	200	10	10	90
Children	7-10	28	62	132	52	34	700	10	7	45	1.2	1.4	16	1.6	300	3.0	800	800	250	10	10	120
Males	11-14	45	99	157	62	45	1000	10	8	50	1.4	1.6	18	1.8	400	3.0	1200	1200	350	18	15	150
Males	15-18	66	145	176	69	56	1000	10	10	60	1.4	1.7	18	2.0	400	3.0	1200	1200	400	18	15	150
Males	19-22	70	154	177	70	56	1000	7.5	10	60	1.5	1.7	19	2.2	400	3.0	800	800	350	10	15	150
Males	23-50	70	154	178	70	56	1000	5	10	60	1.4	1.6	18	2.2	400	3.0	800	800	350	10	15	150
Males	51+	70	154	178	70	56	1000	5	10	60	1.2	1.4	16	2.2	400	3.0	800	800	350	10	15	150
Females	11-14	46	101	157	62	46	800	10	8	50	1.1	1.3	15	1.8	400	3.0	1200	1200	300	18	15	150
Females	15-18	55	120	163	64	46	800	10	8	60	1.1	1.3	14	2.0	400	3.0	1200	1200	300	18	15	150
Females	19-22	55	120	163	64	44	800	7.5	8	60	1.1	1.3	14	2.0	400	3.0	800	800	300	18	15	150
Females	23-50	55	120	163	64	44	800	5	8	60	1.0	1.2	13	2.0	400	3.0	800	800	300	18	15	150
Females	51+	55	120	163	64	44	800	5	8	60	1.0	1.2	13	2.0	400	3.0	800	800	300	10	15	150
Pregnant						+30	+200	+5	+2	+20	+0.4	+0.3	+2	+0.6	+400	+1.0	+400	+400	+150	h	+5	+25
Lactating						+20	+400	+5	+3	+40	+0.5	+0.5	+5	+0.5	+100	+1.0	+400	+400	+150	h	+10	+50

[a] The allowances are intended to provide for individual variations among most normal persons as they live in the United States under usual environmental stresses. Diets should be based on a variety of common foods in order to provide other nutrients for which human requirements have been less well defined. See table 18-3 for heights, weights and recommended intake.

[b] Retinol equivalents. 1 Retinol equivalent = 1 g retinol or 6 g B carotene. See text for calculation of vitamin A activity of diets as retinol equivalents.

[c] As cholecalciferol. 10 g cholecalciferol = 400 I.U. vitamin D.

[d] a-tocopherol equivalents. 1 mg d-a-tocopherol = 1 a T.E. See text for variation in allowances and calculation of vitamin E activity of the diet as a-tocopherol equivalents.

[e] 1 N.E. (niacin equivalent) is equal to 1 mg of niacin or 60 mg of dietary tryptophan.

[f] The folacin allowances refer to dietary sources as determined by $Lactobacillus\ casei$ assay after treatment with enzymes ("conjugases") to make polyglutamyl forms of the vitamin available to the test organism.

[g] The RDA for vitamin B_{12} in infants is based on average concentration of the vitamin in human milk. The allowances after weaning are based on energy intake (as recommended by the American Academy of Pediatrics) and consideration of other factors such as intestinal absorption; see text.

[h] The increased requirement during pregnancy cannot be met by the iron content of habitual American diets nor by the existing iron stores of many women; therefore the use of 30-60 mg of supplemental iron is recommended. Iron needs during lactation are not substantially different from those of non-pregnant women, but continued supplementation of the mother for 2-3 months after parturition is advisable in order to replenish stores depleted by pregnancy.

TABLE 18-2. Recommended daily dietary allowances, revised 1980.[a]

	Age (years)	VITAMINS			TRACE ELEMENTS[b]						ELECTROLYTES		
		Vitamin K (g)	Biotin (g)	Pantothenic Acid (mg)	Copper (mg)	Manganese (mg)	Fluoride (mg)	Chromium (mg)	Selenium (mg)	Molybdenum (mg)	Sodium (mg)	Potassium (mg)	Chloride (mg)
INFANTS	0-0.5	12	35	2	0.5-0.7	0.5-0.7	0.1-0.5	0.01-0.04	0.01-0.04	0.03-0.06	115-350	350-925	274-700
	0.5-1	10-20	50	3	0.7-1.0	0.7-1.0	0.2-1.0	0.02-0.06	0.02-0.06	0.04-0.08	250-750	425-1275	400-1200
CHILDREN	1-3	15-30	65	3	1.0-1.5	1.0-1.5	0.5-1.5	0.02-0.08	0.02-0.08	0.05-0.1	325-975	550-1650	500-1500
AND	4-6	20-40	85	3-4	1.5-2.0	1.5-2.0	1.0-2.5	0.03-0.12	0.03-0.12	0.06-0.15	450-1350	775-2325	700-2100
ADOLESCENTS	7-10	30-60	120	4-5	2.0-2.5	2.0-3.0	1.5-2.5	0.05-0.2	0.05-0.2	0.1-0.3	600-1800	1000-3000	925-2775
	11+	50-100	100-200	4-7	2.0-3.0	2.5-5.0	1.5-2.5	0.05-0.2	0.05-0.2	0.15-0.5	900-2700	1525-4575	1400-4200
ADULTS		70-140	100-200	4-7	2.0-3.0	2.5-5.0	1.5-4.0	0.05-0.2	0.05-0.2	0.15-0.5	1100-3300	1875-5625	1700-5100

Estimated Safe And Adequate Dietary Intakes Of Selected Vitamins And Minerals.

[a]Because there is less information on which to base allowances, these figures are not given in the main table of the RDA and are provided here in the form of ranges of recommended intakes.

[b]Since the toxic levels for many trace elements may be only several times usual intakes, the upper levels for the trace elements given in this table should not be habitually exceeded.

TABLE 18-3. MEAN HEIGHTS AND WEIGHTS AND RECOMMENDED ENERGY INTAKE.[a]
Recommended dietary allowances, revised 1980

Category	Age (years)	Weight (kg)	Weight (lb)	Height (cm)	Height (in)	Energy needs (with range) (kcal)	Energy needs (with range) (MJ)
Infants	0.0-0.5	6	13	60	24	kg x 115 (95-145)	kg x 48
	0.5-1.0	9	20	71	28	kg x 105 (80-135)	kg x 44
Children	1-3	13	29	90	35	1300 (900-1800)	5.5
	4-6	20	44	112	44	1700 (1300-2300)	7.1
	7-10	28	62	132	52	2400 (1650-3300)	10.1
Males	11-14	45	99	157	62	2700 (2000-3700)	11.3
	15-18	66	145	176	69	2800 (2100-3900)	11.8
	19-22	70	154	177	70	2900 (2500-3300)	12.2
	23-50	70	154	178	70	2700 (2300-3100)	11.3
	51-75	70	154	178	70	2400 (2000-2800)	10.1
	76+	70	154	178	70	2050 (1650-2450)	8.6
Females	11-14	46	101	157	62	2200 (1500-3000)	9.2
	15-18	55	120	163	64	2100 (1200-3000)	8.8
	19-22	55	120	163	64	2100 (1700-2500)	8.8
	23-50	55	120	163	64	2000 (1600-2400)	8.4
	51-75	55	120	163	64	1800 (1400-2200)	7.6
	76+	55	120	163	64	1600 (1200-2000)	6.7
Pregnancy						+300	
Lactation						+500	

[a] The data in this table have been assembled from the observed median heights and weights of children shown in Table 18-1, together with desirable weights for adults given in Table 18-2 for the mean heights of men (70 inches) and women (64 inches) between the ages of 18 and 34 years as surveyed in the U.S. population (HEW/NCHS data).

The energy allowances for the young adults are for men and women doing light work.

The allowances for the two older groups represent mean energy needs over these age spans, allowing for a 2% decrease in basal (resting) metabolic rate per decade and a reduction in activity of 200 kcal/day for men and women between 51 and 75 years, 500 kcal for men over 75 (see text). The customary range of daily energy output is shown for adults in parentheses, and is based on a variation in energy needs of 400 kcal at any one age (see

text and Garrow, 1978), emphasizing the wide range of energy intakes appropriate for any group of people.

Energy allowances for children through age 18 are based on median energy intakes of children of these ages followed in longitudinal growth studies. The values in parentheses are 10th and 90th percentiles of energy intake, to indicate the range of energy consumption among children of these ages (see text).

TABLE 18-4. AICR GUIDE TO VITAMINS

Vitamins (U.S. RDA)	Best Sources	Functions	Deficiency symptoms
A CAROTENE (5,000 IU)	Liver, eggs, yellow and green fruits and vegetables, milk and dairy products, fish liver oil	Growth and repair of body tissues (resist infection), bone and tooth formation, visual purple production (necessary for night vision)	Night blindness, dry scaly skin, loss of smell and appetite, susceptibility to infection, frequent fatigue, tooth decay
B_1 THIAMIN (1.5 MG)	Wheat germ, yeast, liver, whole grains, nuts, fish, poultry, beans, meat	Carbohydrate metabolism, appetite maintenance, hence function, growth and muscle tone	Heart irregularity, nerve disorders, fatigue, loss of appetite, forgetfulness
B_2 RIBOFLAVIN (1.7 MG)	Whole grains, green leafy vegetables, organ meats	Necessary for fat, carbohydrate, and protein metabolism, cell respiration, formation of antibodies and red blood cells	Eye problems, cracks in corner of mouth, digestive disturbances
B_6 PYRIDOXINE (2.0 MG)	Fish, poultry, lean meats	Necessary for fat, carbohydrate and protein metabolism, formation of antibodies, maintains sodium/potassium balance (nerves)	Nervousness, dermatitis, blood disorders, muscular weakness, insulin sensitivity, skin cracks, anemia
B_{12} COBALAMIN (6 MCG)	Organ meats, eggs, milk, fish, cheese	Carbohydrate, fat, protein metabolism, maintains healthy nervous system, blood cell formation	Pernicious anemia, nervousness, neuritis, fatigue, brain degeneration
Biotin (300 MCG)	Yeast, organ meats, legumes, eggs	Carbohydrate, fat, and protein metabolism, formation of fatty acids, helps utilize B vitamins	Dry, grayish skin, depression, muscle pain, fatigue, poor appetite
CHOLINE (NO RDA)	Organ meats, soybeans, fish, wheat germ, egg yolk	Nerve transmission, metabolism of fats and cholesterol, regulates liver and gall bladder	High blood pressure, bleeding stomach ulcers, liver and kidney problems
Folic acid FOLACIN (400 MG)	Green leafy vegetables, organ meats, milk products	Red blood cell formation, protein metabolism, growth and cell division	Anemia gastrointestinal troubles, poor growth
Niacin (20 MG)	Meat, poultry, fish, milk products, peanuts, brewer's yeast	Fat, carbohydrate and protein metabolism, health of skin, tongue and digestive system, blood circulation	General fatigue, indigestion, irritability, loss of appetite, skin disorders
Pantothenic acid (10 MG)	Lean meats, whole grains, legumes	Converts nutrients into energy, formation of some fats, vitamin utilization	Vomiting, stomach stress, restlessness, infections, muscle cramps
C ASCORBIC ACID (60 MG)	Citrus fruits, vegetables, tomatoes, potatoes	Helps heal wounds, strength to blood vessels, collagen maintenance, resistance to infection	Bleeding gums, slow healing wounds, bruising, aching joints, nosebleeds, poor digestion
D (400 IU)	Fish-liver oils, egg yolks, organ meats, fish, fortified milk	Calcium and phosphorus metabolism (bone formation), heart action, nervous system maintenance	Rickets, poor bone growth, nervous system irritability
E (30 IU)	Vegetable oils, green vegetables, wheat germ, organ meats, eggs	Protects red blood cells, inhibits coagulation of blood, protects fat soluble vitamins, cellular respiration	Muscular wasting, abnormal fat deposits in muscles, gastrointestinal disease, heart disease
K (NO RDA)	Green leafy vegetables, fruit, cereal, dairy products	Important in formation of blood clotting agents	Tendency to hemorrhage

TABLE 18-5. AICR GUIDE TO MINERALS

Mineral (U.S. RDA)	Best sources	Function	Deficiency symptoms
Calcium (1000 MG)	Milk and milk products	Strong bones, teeth, muscle tissue, regulates heart beat, muscle action and nerve function, blood clotting	Soft brittle bones, back and leg pains, heart palpitations, tetany
Chromium (NO RDA)	Corn oil, clams, whole grain cereals, brewer's yeast	Glucose metabolism (energy), increases effectiveness of insulin	Atherosclerosis, glucose intolerance in diabetics
Copper (2 MG)	Oysters, nuts, organ meats, legumes	Formation of red blood cells, bone growth and health, works with vitamin C to form elastin	General weakness, impaired respiration, skin sores
Iodine (150 MCG)	Seafood, iodized salt	Component of hormone thyroxine which controls metabolism	Goiter, dry skin and hair, nervousness, obesity
Iron (19 MG)	Meats and organ meats, fish, leafy green vegetables	Hemoglobin formation, improves blood quality, increases resistance to stress and disease	Anemia (pale skin, fatigue), constipation, breathing difficulties
Magnesium (400 MG)	Nuts, green vegetables, whole grains	Acid/alkaline balance, important in metabolism of carbohydrates, minerals and sugar	Nervousness, tremors, easily aroused anger, disorientation, blood clots
Manganese (NO RDA)	Nuts, whole grains, vegetables, fruits	Enzyme activation, carbohydrate and fat production, sex hormone production, skeletal development	Dizziness, poor muscle coordination, ear noises
Phosphorus (1000 MG)	Fish, meat, poultry, eggs, grains	Bone development, important in protein, fat and carbohydrate utilization	Poor bones and teeth, arthritis, rickets, appetite loss, irregular breathing
Potassium (NO RDA)	Lean meat, vegetables, fruits	Fluid balance, controls activity of heart muscle, nervous system, kidneys	Poor reflexes, irregular heartbeat, dry skin, general weakness
Selenium (50-200 MCG PROVISION RDA)	Seafood, organ meats, lean meats, grains	Protects body tissues against oxidative damage from radiation, pollution and normal metabolic processing	Heart muscle abnormalities
Zinc (15 MG)	Lean meats, liver, eggs seafood, whole grains	Involved in digestion and metabolism, important in development of reproductive system, aids in healing	Retarded growth, prolonged wound healing, loss of appetite

TABLE 18-6.

HOW TO READ A VITAMIN SUPPLEMENT LABEL

This is the brand name of the product. Multivitamin supplements contain more than one vitamin and are to be used to supplement the diet. Terms such as "therapeutic", "high potency", "stress" and "geriatric" are generally associated with formulations containing more than 100% of the U.S. RDA for one or more of the ingredients.

Recommended dosage by the supplement manufacturer.

This indicates how much of the U.S. RDA, for each nutrient, is contained in each tablet, capsule or liquid measure.

The source or form of each vitamin in the supplement is listed in descending order by weight. In addition to listing the vitamins, this list may also contain ingredients used to formulate the tablet or capsule.

All supplements should be stored this way in their original containers.

The product should be used before this date.

The manufacturer or distributor is required to put their name, address and zip code on the label.

**BRAND NAME
MULTIVITAMIN SUPPLEMENT
FOR ADULTS AND CHILDREN
FOUR OR MORE YEARS**

Directions : One (1) tablet daily as a dietary supplement

ONE; (1) TABLET SUPPLIES	POTENCY	% U.S. RDA
Vitamin A	5,000 IU	100
Vitamin D	400 IU	100
Vitamin E	30 IU	100
Vitamin C	60 mg	100
Folic Acid	0.4 mg	100
Thiamine	1.5 mg	100
Riboflavin	1.7 mg	100
Niacin	20 mg	100
Vitamin B6	2 mg	100
Vitamin B12	6 mg	100
Biotin	0.3 mg	100
Pantothenic Acid	10 mg	100

*Percentage of the U.S. Recommended Daily Allowance for Adults and Children four or more years of age.

Ingredients : Ascorbic Acid, Vitamin E Actate, Niacinamide, Calcium, Panthothenate, Riboflavin, Pyridoxine, Hydrochloride, Vitamin A Acetate, Thiamine, Mononitrate, Folic Acid, Biotin, Cyanocobalamin, Ergocalciferol (D).
Storage: Keep tightly closed in a dry place; do not expose to excessive heat.

KEEP OUT OF THE REACH OF CHILDREN

EXPIRATION DATE: Nov '84

Manufacturer's or distributor's name, address and zip code

100 Tablets

The U.S. Recommended Daily Allowance (U.S. RDA) is the most commonly used labeling guideline recommended by the Food and Drug Administration. The U.S. RDA's represent estimated amounts of nutrients needed every day by healthy people. By appearing on dietary supplementary labels, they provide consumers with a means to compare the vitamin content of a product to the daily needs of adults and children four or more uears of age. Minimum Daily Requirement (MDR) is a measurement that may sometimes appear on a supplement label. The MDR measurement, however, contains vitamin requirement levels that are out-of-date and do not include as many nutrients as the U.S. RDA.

International Unit is a form of measurement for fat-soluble vitamins — A, D, and E. Fat-soluble vitamins occur in different biological forms. "I.U." serves as one standard measurement which takes these variations into account.

Water-soluble vitamins—C and the B-complex—are measured in milligrams (mg) and micrograms (mcg). A milligram is equal to one thousandth of a gram; a microgram is one millionth of a gram. There are 28 grams in one ounce.

All dietary supplements should be kept out of the reach of children.

The manufacturer is required to indicate the quantity of tablets or capsules in the bottle.

TABLE 18-7. VITAMIN SAFETY INDEX

Vitamin	Recommended Adult Intake[a]	Minimum Toxic Dose (MTD)	Vitamin Safety Index (VSI)
Vitamin A	5,000 IU	25,000 to 50,000 IU	5 to 10
Vitamin D	400 IU	50,000 IU 1,000 to 2,000 IU [b]	125 2.5 to 5
Vitamin E	30 IU	1,200 IU	40
Vitamin C	60 mg	2,000 to 5,000 mg 1,000 mg [c]	33 to 83 17
Thiamin (B$_1$)	1.5 mg	300 mg	200
Riboflavin	1.7 mg	1,000 mg	588
Niacin	20 mg	1,000 mg	50
Pyridoxine (B$_6$)	2.2 mg	2,000 mg 200 mg [d]	900 90
Folacin	0.4 mg	400 mg 15 mg [e]	1,000 37
Biotin	0.3 mg	50 mg	167
Pantothenic Acid	10 mg	10,000 mg	1,000

a. The highest of the individual Recommended Dietary Allowance (RDA) — except those for pregnancy and lactation — or the U.S. Recommended Daily Allowance, whichever is higher.

Lower MTD's are identified for special circumstances:

b. For infants and also for adults with certain infections or metabolic diseases; 50,000 IU for most adults
c. To produce slightly altered mineral excretion patterns
d. For antagonism of some drugs; 2,000 mg for most adults
e. For antagonism of anticonvulsants in epileptics; 400 mg for most adults

As a result, most health professionals encourage women to incorporate more food sources of calcium in the diet but recommend supplementation with calcium to make up only the deficit. Higher doses are discouraged because some women might develop urinary tract stones. Some health care professionals also recommend that if you take a calcium supplement, you should also have a vitamin D supplement, especially if you have little exposure to sun.

The major sources of calcium in the American diet are milk and other dairy products. Each 8 ounce glass of milk contains about 300 mg of calcium. For those women concerned about fat and caloric intake, low-fat and skimmed dairy products are recommended. Other food sources include sardines and fish with cooked bones and dark green leafy vegetables.

Women who choose to supplement their diet need to determine the appropriate type of calcium supplement. Different forms of supplements are available with differing kinds and amounts of cal-

TABLE 18-8. MINERAL SAFETY INDEX

Mineral	Recommended Adult Intake[a]	Minimum Toxic Dose (MTD)	Mineral Safety Index (MSI)
Calcium	1,200 mg	12,000 mg	10
Phosphorus	1,200 mg	12,000 mg	10
Magnesium	400 mg	6,000 mg	15
Iron	18 mg	100 mg	5.5
Zinc	15 mg	500 mg	33
Copper	3 mg	100 mg	33
		<3 mg[b]	<1
Fluoride	4 mg	20 mg	5
		4 mg[c]	1
Iodine	0.15 mcg	2 mg	13
Selenium	0.2 mcg	1 mg	5

From "Quantitative Evaluation of Vitamin Safety", *Pharmacy Times*, May 1985, By John N. Hathcock, Ph. D.

a. The highest of the individual Recommended Dietary Allowance (RDA) —except those for pregancy and lactation— or the U.S. Recommended Daily Allowance, whichever is higher.

b. For people with Wilson's disease.
c. Level producing slight fluorosis of dental enamel.

cium as ingredients. Some health care professionals and television ads recommend antacids as a source of calcium. It is important to realize that some antacids, but not all, are sources of calcium. Read the label. Also, some women experience acid rebound or indigestion after using antacids as their supplements. If you have this type of reaction, use a different type of calcium supplement.

The most common ingredients in the supplements are calcium carbonate, calcium lactate, calcium gluconate, dicalcium phosphate, and oyster shell. They come in tablet, capsule, powder, or liquid. Traces of lead and other toxic heavy metals have been found in oyster shells, dolomite, and bone meal and therefore many nutritionists warn against taking these "natural" supplements.

Remember, before taking any supplement, first determine how much calcium you eat in foods daily, then only make up the deficit. Some researchers believe that the body can only use moderate amounts of calcium at any one time and therefore recommend taking the supplement at a meal with few other calcium-rich foods.

Even though calcium supplementation appears to be a reasonable practice at this time, research is still needed to determine if supplementation will prevent, reverse, or treat osteoporosis.

The value of taking calcium to reduce hypertension is being hotly debated. Preliminary research reports, national surveys, and epidemiological data have noted a relationship between high blood pressure and low intakes of dietary calcium. Clinical trials are under way to determine if supplementation with 1000 mg of calcium daily can lower blood pressure. Some researchers enthusiastically believe that patients with mild or moderate hypertension can be treated safely over an 8-week period. Other clinicians are more skeptical and believe that it is premature to make recommendations for calcium supplementation by people with hypertension. These clinicians believe that the small reductions in blood pressure that have been seen are not enough to recommend long-term supplementation, the effects of which are unknown. Many believe at this time that weight loss produces more impressive reductions in blood pressure than calcium supplementation.

All researchers, including those advocating calcium supplementation for control of blood pressure, recognize the need for further research on the efficacy and safety of long-term treatment for hypertension with calcium supplements or dietary calcium.

I Hate Liver, So Do I Need To Take an Iron Supplement?

Iron deficiency anemia is considered the most common single nutrient deficiency in the world. Consumers have heard for years about "iron-poor blood" in advertisements for supplements. Since iron is responsible for carrying oxygen in the blood, a person with too little iron may have less energy and generally feel tired. There is a problem in the United States with iron deficiency anemia. Between 4% and 6% of the infants, teenage girls, young women, and elderly men in this country suffer from iron deficiency anemia, and half of the women 19 to 50 years of age consume less than their RDA for iron. It is believed that a larger percentage of the poor suffer from iron deficiency anemia.

Since iron deficiency can have detrimental effects on behavior and learning, it is common for supplemental iron to be recommended for infants and young women. Other health problems that can result from inadequate dietary iron intake include decreased work performance, increased risk of maternal and fetal illness and death, increased risk of infection and immunological disorders, and stunted growth. Iron from animal foods such as liver and other meats, poultry, fish, and oysters tends to be better absorbed than from the plant foods like peas, beans, spinach, and other dark green leafy vegetables, whole grain and enriched breads and cereals, and dried fruits. Eating foods high in Vitamin C at the same time, seems to improve the body's use of iron.

In recent years iron-fortified milk formulas and cereals have been available for infants and, when used, have dramatically reduced the incidence of iron deficiency anemia.

A rather simple blood test can help determine whether you have iron deficiency anemia and need to take a supplement or just eat more iron-rich foods.

There Is a Dietary Goal That Says To Eat Adequate Starch and Fiber. Shall I Take a Fiber Supplement?

Many polls show that Americans have increased their fiber consumption during the last 5 years. Many believe that the adequate consumption of dietary fiber can prevent constipation, cancer, and heart disease and control diabetes. It has not been conclusively proven, however, that fiber can accomplish all these tasks. Also, all dietary fibers are not the same.

Dietary fiber is an all-inclusive name for a variety of substances. It is the plant material we eat that is resistant to digestion by the juices in the human gastrointestinal tract.

Many consumers are confused by the claims made on bread wrappers and cereal boxes, such as "Maximum Fiber" or "Ultimate Fiber." The cereals with these labels are all similar in fiber content with between 7 and 12 grams of fiber per serving. Read the label on the package to find out the amount of fiber in a serving of that food. Then, before worrying about adding fiber to your food or choosing among those cereals, look at your total daily consumption of food and all breads, cereals, fruits, and vegetables consumed.

The role of fiber in laxation or keeping regular is well-known and undisputed. Fiber softens and enlarges the stools and makes elimination easier. It appears that cereal fiber is more effective than fruit and vegetable fiber in treating constipation.

Neither bran nor pectin has been shown to have properties that prevent cancer. In fact, excess fiber can actually interfere with absorption of other nutrients in the intestine. The work of researchers in the 1970s brought to the forefront the relationship of fiber-rich diets to low incidences of cancer. There are scientists who believe there is enough epidemiological data to suggest that a diet low in fiber might increase an individual's risk of developing cancer of the colon. However, most scientists don't believe it is that simple of an issue. Therefore, studies about the composition and solubility of dietary fibers are being done to see what happens when cereal or vegetable dietary fibers pass through the gut. It is known that all fibers do not act the same.

Food manufacturers have claims that dietary fiber reduces the risk of colon cancer. Most scientists, however, believe that the role of fiber in removing carcinogens is still unproven and there is no reason to supplement the diet with extra fiber in hopes of preventing cancer. Eating foods high in fiber is still recommended, however.

Not only is fiber thought to prevent constipation and cancer, but some researchers believe some types of fiber may be helpful in controlling blood cholesterol levels. Can the dietary fiber in rolled oats, oat bran, red spring wheat bran, pectin, and guar gum fibers lower cholesterol levels? At this time we can only guess. Scientists cannot agree if there is enough evidence to recommend supplementation with some fibers to control cholesterol. Some physicians recommend that their patients at risk for heart disease use some of these types of fiber foods to see if they lower their blood cholesterol. These patients are monitored for potential benefits.

Until we know more about the role of different fibers in preventing diseases, most health care professionals recommend that rather than take a supplement, we should all select foods with natural sources of fiber—a variety of fruits and vegetables, fresh, canned and frozen; a variety of breads and cereals; and a variety of nuts, seeds, popcorn, peas, and beans.

Shall We Take Cod Liver or Other Fish Oils?

It amuses and amazes us when old folk remedies prove to have a potential benefit to health. The latest is the discovery that fish oil supplements might be beneficial to our health. This time, rather than as a preventative or treatment of rheumatism or lameness, the fish oil ingredient eicosapentaenoic acid (EPA)— also referred to as dietary omega 3 fatty acids—may provide protection against heart disease.

Scientists have noted that Eskimos eat large amounts of fish oils and have no heart disease. Now research is showing that if an individual can significantly increase his dietary omega three fatty acids, this might affect the synthesis of some prostaglandins and reduce heart disease. Studies over time in the Netherlands found that men who ate one or two fish dishes a week had a lower risk of death by coronary heart disease. Unfortunately, the researchers cannot explain how this works. Even so, they recommend that we eat one or two fish dishes a week to prevent heart disease. They stress that we should eat fish rather than take supplements, because they are not yet sure whether the EPA is the only important ingredient or if something else in the fish oil is important as well. Other tests have shown that blood triglyceride levels can be reduced by taking a large supplement of fish oil, comparable to the amount of fish oil in ½ to 1½ pounds of salmon or mackerel. Thus far, small daily consumption of high-fat fish has not produced the same kinds of results.

It appears that the EPA reduces blood thickness, making it easier for blood cells to squeeze through constricted capillaries and thereby letting oxygen travel to muscles. As exciting as these results are for persons prone to heart disease, it has not been proven that taking fish oil supplements or eating enough foods with EPA will affect illness or death from heart disease.

It is only fair to note that other researchers have not been able to find the same relationship between eating fish and reducing the risks of heart disease. The debate will continue for some time, but it seems reasonable to encourage Americans to eat fish one or twice a week to lower the risk of heart disease. It is unclear, however, if drinking fish oils as a dietary supplement will be of any benefit in treating high cholesterol or other heart disease risk factors. There is not enough evidence to make the whole family pucker up for their daily teaspoon of cod liver oil.

SUMMARY

These are only a few of the contemporary questions about dietary supplementation. Others include:

- Does vitamin C prevent colds and/or cure cancer?
- Do zinc supplements improve acne, promote healing, or affect taste disorders?
- Does vitamin B_6 reduce morning sickness?
- Does selenium have an antitumor effect?
- Will EPA relieve rheumatoid arthritis?
- Is a zinc deficiency a factor in the development of AIDS?
- Is zinc deficiency a factor in producing amenorrhoea in teens?
- Will a high intake of vitamin A reduce lung cancer?

The list is almost endless. But nutrition is a young science, and more research is needed before we encourage everyone to increase their intake of various nutrients by eating specific foods or by taking supplements to prevent or cure diseases. At this time it would be unwise for an individual to take therapeutic or huge doses of vitamins, minerals, or other food components without the advice of a physician.

Before you take any supplement, make sure you scrutinize your regular diet. Record your food and beverage intake for 3 or 4 days, then calculate the nutrients you are generally eating. If you find a regular shortfall, then examine your food habits and make appropriate changes or select an appropriate supplement. When selecting a supplement, be sure to read the labels. Select the supplement that meets your needs in the correct amounts. Remember that in the case of supplementation, the old adage "if a little is good, more is better" *is not true*. If you experience any side effects, stop taking the supplement immediately and contact your health care provider.

19

IS NATURAL BETTER? AND OTHER QUESTIONS ABOUT HEALTH FOODS

Joan Dye Gussow, Ph.D., is associate professor and former chair of the Department of Nutrition and Education at Columbia University.·Her interests center around the social and technological factors affecting long-term sustainability of the human food chain, with special emphasis on women's relationship with food. She serves on the Food and Nutrition Board of the National Academy of Sciences and the Board of Directors of the National Gardening Association. Her most recent book is *The Nutrition Debate*, (Bull Publisher, 1986).

Anyone who has visited the local A&P (or even the Mom and Pop neighborhood store) knows that much is made these days about natural foods. But some consumers wonder whether we aren't being misled by the advertisers' use of *natural*. Joan Dye Gussow notes that "*natural* has proliferated in the last decade far beyond the boundaries of any rational definition" and she examines the question of whether organic and health foods (including natural instant bouillon) are really safer and more nutritious than competing brands. After reading this article, your next shopping trip may become an intellectual adventure.▪

There are many adjectives you can use to describe foods in the United States without getting into an argument: fresh, colorful, sweet, imported, domestic, canned, salty, frozen, dehydrated, convenience, unprocessed, delicious, greasy, and so on. But there are three adjectives you can't apply to foods in front of a nutritionist without risking an argument. The contentious descriptors are *natural, organic,* and *health*. Several years ago when the Federal Trade Commission proposed banning those terms from food advertising, many otherwise sensible professionals found themselves recommending that the government should actually outlaw these common and harmless words! Such aversion requires some explaining.

While the term organic has ambiguous implications—organic agriculture sounds benign enough, but organic disease and organic hydrocarbons are less appealing—the adjective natural and the noun health seem inarguably pleasant. My dictionary says natural is an *adjective* meaning "not artificial or manmade"; but the word has such benevolent overtones that we have made it into an approving *noun*. "She's a natural," we say about someone who is spontaneously good at something. Robert Redford was "The Natural." So it seems obvious that a natural food ought to be a good thing in everyone's book, as should be a food that had the term *health* tacked onto it. All of which is designed to make the point that the controversy over organic, natural, and health foods has nothing to do with the words themselves but with the very different load of implications they carry for different groups of people.

For much of the public, it is clear the terms convey a special aura of goodness. Natural and organic foods seem on the whole *better* than foods which are unnatural and nonorganic. And health foods are—well—healthy. As far as nutritionists are concerned, this is precisely the problem. They argue that the cachet of "betterness" is undeserved, that there is nothing intrinsically better about such foods where nutrition and health are concerned. Which group is right? To some extent both of them are.

Let's begin with some definitions. Many years ago, testifying before the New York State Attorney General at a hearing on organic foods, I gave a definition of what these three provocative terms are supposed to mean. It remains as useful historically as any other.

Health foods is a term which I understand to cover that dazzling array of items ranging from special foods for those on salt- or sugar-free diets to the latest aphrodisiac import. Many so-called health food stores devote more space to vitamin and other supplements than they devote to food—a circumstance I find contradictory if their owners really believe that the foods they are selling are nutrient charged.

As I suppose my definition makes clear, I think a lot, not all by any means, but a lot of what turns up in health food stores is, in the vernacular, a "rip off" nutritionally and otherwise. (Of course, as the Food and Drug Administration regularly reminds us, much of what is sold in your corner drugstore for the cure of human unhealth or unhappiness is also of questionable value—a fact we should not lose sight of.)

Natural food stores, on the other hand, don't usually sell vitamins. They carry foods which may or may not have been grown organically but which have been minimally processed and are presumably additive free. These include various grains, whole and ground, nuts, dried fruits, beans, seeds, honey, and so forth. Some of these foods contain more nutrients than similar foods available at the supermarket—the whole grain flours and meals, for example, are more nutritious than their refined counterparts—and some of the foods, like the unsulfured dried fruits, may be less nutritious since sun-drying destroys more of the vitamins A and C in fruits which have not been sulfured.

Since virtually all foods are organic, the term organic foods is really a misnomer. It refers to food grown by the organic method. Since organically grown foods are usually natural, that is, minimally processed, they share whatever nutritional advantages natural foods have. What seems to be at issue, however, is something else—namely, whether these foods, by virtue of the manner in which they are grown, contain either more nutrients or nutrients which are in some way better than those in foods not so grown.

The question of whether organic foods are more nutritious remains an issue—one to which I will turn shortly. What must be said immediately, however, is that several things have changed in the decade and a half since I wrote that testimony. First, health, natural, and organic foods have moved out of that little run-down store in the unfashionable part of town to the fanciest supermarket boutiques. Second, the Federal Trade Commission has decided not to ban the terms health, natural and organic in food advertising, not to give them a legal definition. So anything goes. Third, the marketers have rushed in to fill the new demand for "health." So it is now possible to find, as *Consumer Reports* and others have pointed out, natural margarine, natural instant bouillon, natural onion rings made from chopped and reformed onions, natural yoghurt chips, natural dog food, natural lemon-flavored creme pie (that it's not *cream* is a clue to its naturalness!), and even natural cigarettes.

So the answer to the question "Is natural better?" is "It all depends on what you mean by 'natural.'" As my earlier definition indicates, if natural means minimally processed foods (whole foods, as the British call them), then such foods are often likely to be more nutritious and to have their nutrients better balanced than foods which are extensively processed or fabricated from a few highly refined ingredients. Using whole fresh foods moves one a long way toward naturalness, and if the foods are well chosen and simply prepared, such choices can, in turn, move one a long way toward a diet lower in added salt, sugar, and fat and higher in complex carbohydrate and fiber—just the sort of diet that has been recommended as lowering the risk of many degenerative diseases. In that sense then, natural diets, made up of natural foods can be healthier. If you want to go further than that, you're on your own.

As a quick aside, let's dispose of health foods here. As my earlier definition was intended to indicate, even those of us who urged the Federal Trade Commission to define natural and organic were hard pressed to find a reason for defending the term health food. Foods are healthy in specific contexts. Diets are healthy. (*Some* diets are healthy!) If "natural" has proliferated in the last decade far beyond the boundaries of any rational definition, health foods never had such boundaries.

As I was saying, if you want to go further than fresh and unprocessed in seeking natural foods, the terrain is tricky. Obviously you can't use labels to help you determine what's natural because there is no legal definition of what can be so labeled. Natural beef *may have* been raised without antibiotics or steroid hormones because many customers are increasingly wary of these growth promoters; not using them may allow a producer to sell his animals for a higher price. But the operative phrase here is *may have*. If you trust your butcher, ask him—perhaps he trusts his supplier. Natural eggs may come from chickens whose feet have touched the earth, but you can't be sure unless someone responsible assures you it is true. But do you even need to ask? Does if matter if your apples are unwaxed, if your maple syrup was extracted from the tree without formaldehyde, if your oil was cold-pressed from organically raised walnuts? Is it worth the trouble to read labels and hunt for such foods? This is where the real dilemma arises.

It is easiest to address this question by trying to answer it first in terms of foods called organic. The reason for this is simple. There are several legal definitions of organic foods, so there is at least broad agreement about what the term means. Although many scientists point out that all foods are organic (because all are made up of chemicals containing carbon), the term organic is recognized by many people (including most scientists) to have another popular meaning when applied to food. *Organic Gardening and Farming*, a magazine dealing with just what its title suggests, has laid out the basic definition:

Organically grown food is produced on humus rich soil whose fertility has been maintained with organic materials and natural mineral fertilizers. No pesticides, artificial fertilizers or synthetic additives are used in the production of organic foods.

A very similar definition has been written into law in the State of Oregon and related regulations are now on the books or being written in California, Maine, and several other states. Oregon also specifies the conditions under which "organically raised" animals must be produced.

Are foods produced in such a manner better? If the question refers to whether they are better for your health, the answer at the moment has to be that we simply don't know. We have no convincing evidence that they are, but on the other hand we really haven't tried to find out. The most thorough review of this question to appear in the United States was published by food scientist Deitrich Knorr in 1982. Despite his obvious interest in finding significant differences between organically grown foods and their conventionally grown counterparts, he was able to report only that there were "certain compositional differences" between these products—meaning that sometimes organic foods had higher levels of certain vitamins or minerals than conventionally grown foods or lower levels of moisture. Often organic produce has lower levels of pesticide residues (it should have since it is supposed to be produced without synthetic pesticides), but when organic food is tested for such residues (usually by someone trying to prove that such produce is a fraud), small amounts of such residues are usually found. This is a reflection of the fact that we have done a thorough job of polluting the planet; most living things contain pesticide residues.

Findings of more vitamins or minerals or less water or pesticides in organically grown foods—even if they were consistent—are not proof that those who eat the organic foods are healthier than persons consuming foods grown in more conventional ways. The difficulty in making a valid comparison starts long before the food is actually harvested. As Knorr points out, many of the studies which purport to compare the influence of organic and conventional farming practices on the nutritional qualities of foods "lack an adequate design for sufficient comparisons, the most common problem being the insufficient duration of the studies."

In order to demonstrate that there were or were not marked differences in nutritional quality related entirely to the method of growing, one would have to carry out a very carefully controlled long-term experiment, an experiment in which all variables other than management practices—site, seed, water availability, soil type, and so on—were identical to begin with. Then, since the differences between soils managed organically and conventionally may take years to emerge, the plots would have to be carried on with their different treatments over a long enough period of time to permit each of them to acquire the characteristics of their respective management techniques. (This is assuming, incorrectly, that there is a single technical package called organic and another technical package called convention, rather than a range of practices shading into each other.)

Only then would it be possible to begin an experiment in which goods were grown for the purpose of comparing their nutritive value. At this point a diet composed of identical foods grown in the one case organically and in the other case conventionally would have to be fed to someone—or something. The surrogate of choice in experiments is usually a rat, not because it is so close to humans in its biochemical reactions or temperament but because it's cheap, small, and has a fairly short life-span so that intergenerational studies can be done in a reasonable length of time. But a rat does best on lab chow, which illustrates only one of the major differences between rats and humans—namely, that you can keep rats on monotonous controlled diets over long periods of time, which is a tough thing to do with people.

So the requisite experiments have simply not been done. They would be long and expensive. The people who grow organically don't have the money to spend and the Department of Agriculture, which might have the money to spend, seems to think that organic growing is a bit of a fraud, anyway, and so is unlikely to carry out the experiments. (Also, it should be noted that there is a tendency for both sides in this dispute to think they're right, anyway, so there isn't a lot of motivation to carry out the needed studies.)

Now there *are* anecdotal accounts of slow and sickly children, brought to a farm to eat fresh organic vegetables, who have grown into healthy, brilliant teenagers, etc. There is nothing wrong with such accounts. They may well be true. But they simply are not proof of the superiority of organically grown food because there are too many other uncontrolled changes going on. Perhaps the fresh air and country life alone would have done it, even if the vegetables were not organically grown.

What we do know about organically grown crops, from a variety of interesting observations and experiments over the last half century, is that soils treated organically behave differently than soils not so treated, and that animals fed on forage crops raised on organically fertilized soils have shown certain differences in total fertility, feed efficiency, and so on. Whether the ability to sustain fertility longer or to produce more weight gain on less forage are desirable qualities in human foods is at least questionable. What is most important is that we simply don't know whether those findings mean anything in terms of human health and longevity.

Which brings us back to the question of whether natural foods are healthier. You will by now have noted that organic refers in this context to a method of production whereas natural refers to what happens to the food after it is harvested. In a rational world, a natural food would be organically produced and then "naturally" treated prior to reaching your table, since otherwise the term doesn't mean much. So the answer is really the one I gave earlier: if natural processing leaves more nutrients, then the food so processed will be more nutritious than an "unnaturally" processed food (for which you will have to supply your own example—I can thing of plenty!).

So where does all this leave us? One of the best definitions I've seen says that the task of nutrition science is:

... to formulate a diet over the lifetime of an individual that will optimize health, well-being and longevity. This calls for providing the necessary chemical components in the right proportion and avoiding or minimizing toxic substances.

The only way we know how to do this at the moment is to eat a diet made up of a variety of foods (and the operative concept here is biological variety, not the supermarket type where only a few raw food materials are transformed into hundreds of different cookies, cakes, and breakfast cereals) and to eat them in a form in which they are minimally processed except for removing or detoxifying known poisons. It is worth noting here that people concerned with the relationship between food and health—as opposed to supplementation and health—often make wiser food choices, tending to avoid most of the 1500 new food products that enter the supermarket race each year.

But there is something more to be said. From the standpoint of our fellow organisms, it would probably be a very good idea if the foods we selected were grown by methods which make minimum use of insecticides and herbicides and maximum use of fertilizers. While we cannot prove that foods grown organically and processed minimally extend human life, it is clear that our food system, like the rest of our environment, is under stress. We depend for our survival as a species on the continued functioning of a series of complex systems that maintain the flow of materials and energy through the biosphere. We do not fully understand these systems and probably never will. But we do know that many thousands of species other than our own (which ones we are not sure) are essential to keep those systems functioning.

A noted scientist recently observed in an issue of *Science 84* that DDT taught us one very big lesson: if we protect the life below us on the phylogenetic scale, we protect ourselves, but the reverse is not necessarily true. We are hardier than some other species—which does not mean we are more essential. Whatever we do that negatively affects other life forms with whom we share the planet may, in the end, negatively affect us. Organic food is the product of a method of growing that considers the health of the earth as one of its products. For that reason it may be worth buying, even if it won't help *us* live forever!

20 CONTROLLING THE CHEMICAL FEAST: HOW TO SURVIVE THE EXPANDING CRISIS IN FOOD SAFETY

James S. Turner, Esq., is the author of *The Chemical Feast* (New York, Grossman, 1970), *The FDA Report* and *Making Your Own Baby Food* (New York, Workman Publishing Co., 1972), as well as numerous food safety articles. He serves as a consultant to the Congressional Office of Technology Assessment, chairman of the Consumer Liaison Panel of the National Academy of Sciences, and board member to the Food Safety Council. He served as special counsel to the Senate Select Committee on Nutrition and Human Needs and to the Government Operations Subcommittee on Science. Mr. Turner is now writing a book concerning the safety of aspartame.

Few people are as passionate about their work as Jim Turner is. Perhaps this is because Jim, having worked with Ralph Nader, has a fundamental distrust of the producer. Perhaps it is because Jim is a lawyer. He believes that certain food additives are not as safe as the public believes. Moreover, he states in this article that some additives, known by scientists to be dangerous to human health, are accepted as tolerable risks by regulatory authorities. Jim asks his readers to judge whether our current efforts to ensure the quality of our food supply are adequate.∎

On April 18th, 1986, the FDA approved, without hearings, nuclear irradiation for produce preservation. The FDA convinced the Supreme Court to overturn a U.S. Court of Appeals decision that had blocked tolerances, set without oversight, for small amounts of several dangerous, commonly used food chemicals. For example, it allowed the use of food colors not yet proved safe, despite the 1960 Color Additive Law. A House Committee found that 90% of FDA-allowed animal drugs had not been proved safe, and that the FDA had no way to monitor 70% of permitted trace residues.

On April 21, 1986, the U.S. Supreme Court affirmed that no facts had been presented which would force the Food and Drug Administration (FDA) to hold public hearings on the safety of NutraSweet. That same day an FDA committee met behind closed doors to discuss new evidence connecting epileptic seizures in 86 patients with consumption of NutraSweet.

While these and other food safety battles rage, individual consumers must continue to make food choices. To do this, a food consumer needs a *conceptual framework, self knowledge*, a *time allocation plan*, and *information*.

A CONCEPTUAL FRAMEWORK

It is no longer possible—if it ever was—to accept items sold in food stores as unquestionably safe. Selling food is an enormous ($300 billion) economic undertaking. At every stage of decision making, economic gains and losses are traded off against health gains and losses. In the past decade, food safety has shifted in concept from social, objective, and absolute to personal, subjective, and relative.

Still, death and disability do not ride on every forkful of food. Suffering acute toxicity—falling over dead or becoming severely ill—from eating commonly available food is rare in America. Food chemical debates focus mostly on emerging areas of scientific and regulatory controversy—chronic (cancer, heart disease, and stroke), neurological (brain damage, seizures, depression), and immunological (immune deficiency, allergic) disorders about which little is known.

In this subjective balancing of subtle health risks against obvious economic costs, the food consumer is his or her own primary advocate. Each food consumer balances individual resources—time, energy, money—against potential personal risk. Those who are comfortable taking health risks expend fewer resources avoiding food chemical danger than those who are averse to taking health risks.

Zero tolerance for potential food chemical danger, firm distinctions between safe and unsafe chemicals, and absolute safety of chemicals added to food are concepts in the food chemical safety laws. Corporate and government food safety decision makers reject these concepts as unrealistic. The individual food consumer, pursuing effective self-protection, needs to know the rules of the food chemical safety game. They are *safety, data,* and *disorders.*

Safety.   Food chemical safety is personal, subjective, and relative. What one person can live with may cause another person to suffer blindness, depression, cancer, or another disability. The law bars the use of a chemical "if a fair evaluation of the data . . . fails to establish that the proposed use . . . will be safe: . . . no additive shall be deemed safe if it is found to induce cancer."

The FDA, supported by courts and Congress, allows a chemical to be added to food if "there is reasonable certainty that it will cause no harm." Compare the following two assurances: "The substance is safe." "We can be reasonably certain that the substance will cause no harm." Who is "we"? What is "reasonable certainty"? When is there "no harm"?

"We" is corporate officials proposing the chemical to make money and the FDA officials with possible, if not likely, future corporate jobs, reviewing the corporate proposal. Consumers reassured by this "we" can relax and eat with comfort.

"Reasonable certainty" means "we" have *seen* nothing to cause us to withdraw, now or in the future, the fruits of our research and development. Consumers who believe that "we" have looked everywhere can relax.

"No harm" means the absence of general, widespread, obvious harm—not of unique, subtle, personal harm such as idiosyncratic, allergic, or genetically anomalous injury. Sensibly, a chemical harmful only to some need not be banned for all. But individuals must understand this distinction.

The absolute food chemical safety set out by law is in practice relative, the result of balancing the trade off.

Data.   Food chemical owners supply the data for FDA safety assessments. NutraSweet's manufacturer sought to influence FDA reviewers by developing in them "a subconscious spirit of participation" in company safety studies. While unique because written in a company memo, this attitude captures the general tone of the food company/regulatory agency relationship.

In this atmosphere, chemical safety data presented to FDA lags behind new science. Until 1958, food safety policy focused on acute toxicity—food poisoning, caustic trauma, etc. As workplace studies connected cancer to chemical causes, food safety expanded to look for similar connections with food chemicals.

In the 1960s, after the drug thalidomide caused hundreds of grotesque birth defects, the FDA added this danger to its food chemical concerns. In the 1970s, the "genotoxin" concept expanded the cancer and birth defect concerns to include all chemically-caused general gene-related disorders. In the 1980s, brain toxicity is the new danger.

The FDA addresses new concerns slowly, often after approval of a potentially dangerous chemical. For example, on June 17, 1986, 3 years after approving NutraSweet for diet soda, the FDA asked for assistance in developing an "animal model . . . [for use] in evaluating the safety food chemicals [such as aspartame—NutraSweet] for neurochemical and neurobehavioral effects . . . relatively new aspects of food safety."

The FDA bases food safety approvals on limited data provided by chemical sponsors.

Disorders.   No one systematically monitors the relationship between food chemical consumption and cancer, birth defects, genetic damage, seizures, or mental retardation, all of which happen frequently, usually with no apparent cause. Since science connects these disorders in large

part with the environment, which includes food and its chemical additives, food must be considered a potential source of these diseases and disabilities.

Approximately 3,000 chemicals are routinely added to the food supply in thousands of combinations and variations for flavoring, coloring, texturizing, preserving, extending, and sweetening. Each has a commercial sponsor. Each has the status of FDA acceptance, if not approval. None has been shown to be absolutely safe, i.e., incapable of hurting anyone.

Scientists agree that the sweetener saccharin, a coal tar derivative used primarily for industrial photoplating, causes animal cancers. Estimates of annual saccharin-caused human cancers range from 1 to 100 per million. In 1977, Congress blocked an FDA-proposed saccharin ban, but required label and store safety warnings.

Sulfite is allowed in some processed foods, though banned from salad and produce. Fifteen sulfite deaths and 500 injuries, many after opponents warned the FDA, led to the partial ban. Other chemicals are seen as potential health risks, for example, nitrites (cancer), brominated vegetable oils (heart), HVP or hydrolized vegetable protein, and MSG (neurological).

Consumers seeking safe food must remember that scientists present what they *know* about food chemical harm, not what is actually happening. A chemical causing harm does so whether the scientists know it or not. If saccharin causes cancer, sulfites lead to suffocation, and aspartame, MSG, or HVP cause brain damage, they are doing it now, even though scientists haven't "proved" it.

Conceptual Summary.   Safety is relative. Data is limited and commercial. Disorders caused by food chemicals occur whether scientists "know" it or not. These facts set the framework for food safety choices.

Consumers who knowingly accept the risks inherent in this framework—the exceptionally healthy, confident of science or with more pressing demands on their resources—gamble that they will not develop cancer, heart disease, or brain or genetic damage caused by food additives. By inference, they believe that if they do become ill, the gamble will have been worth it.

Policymakers call these individuals *risk accepting consumers*. If you are one of them, if you realize the risk and accept it, read no further since by definition you accept the current system. If you are not accepting risk, then policymakers call you *risk averse*. What follows is for you.

SELF-KNOWLEDGE

Risk averse people break into two groups: those who know they are risk averse and those who do not. Matching food safety behavior with desires begins with knowing into which group you fit. If you assume food additive consumption entails no risk, you are probably risk averse and do not know it. You are probably unwilling to accept risk and therefore deny it exists. If you want to avoid risk, you are consciously risk averse. In either case you would like to avoid personal food chemical sensitivity. Pursuaded by existing evidence that a chemical is harmful, you try to avoid it. You also try to avoid any personal food chemical risk discovered by applying your time, energy, and money. Here are some guidelines to self knowledge:

Biochemical Individuality. Individuals are chemically different. Dr. Roger Williams, University of Texas nutritionist and National Academy of Sciences member, first applied biochemical individuality of nutrient needs. Each individual, he argued, needs different amounts and combinations of nutrients.

Individuals also respond differently to chemical exposure. A chemical that causes cancer, genetic damage, seizures, or other harm will affect only some people exposed to it. A person interested in efficient personal responses to food chemicals can begin by learning his or her own biochemical individuality.

Begin by collecting a careful personal and family medical history. Learn which, if any, disorders run in the family. Remember and note all personal disabilities and disorders, treatments and results, including reactions or side effects. This information should already be part of medical or insurance records.

Develop a personal "normal" health profile. Individual heart beat, blood pressure, temperature, and other health measures vary in a normal range. Knowing your personal statistics will help you steer away from unique personal dangers and detect early warning changes.

Be alert to how you feel. Headache, depression, fatigue, and other debilitating conditions so much a part of our lives do have causes. But you will never detect the causes if you are unaware of the conditions. If you are *really* serious, record your emotional behavior in a journal or daily calendar.

Personal Environmental Context. Food, with its chemical additives, is a major part of your personal environment. Observe it carefully. Keep a food record as part of your daily routine. Habits go unnoticed. There is a pattern to what you eat that will surprise you.

Doctors, dieticians, insurance companies, and devotees of the fitness movement, among others, are turning the food diary into a contemporary fad, if not a necessity. Most are designed to develop calorie control eating patterns. Yours should include notations on the consumption of food chemicals.

Also keep track of where you spend time—inside or out, working or resting, asleep or awake, and where you eat. When you connect behavior patterns with personal reactions, the places where you spend time will be important. For instance, bad indoor air quality in tightly sealed, energy efficient homes has caused illness in some families.

If you are up to it, keep track of significant events and activities. Pumping gas, exercise, time spent in crowds, smoking, weather, television, stressful events—births, deaths, accidents, and disease involving friends and family all affect your health and the way you feel.

Being conscious of these influences on your health will help you identify and address specific aspects, like food chemicals, that interest you.

The Personal Environment/Biochemical Matrix. If you regularly and systematically look at your biochemical indicators and your personal environment, including food chemicals, correlations will appear. Over time you might actually see food chemical causes for an otherwise unexplained malaise or disability.

One conscientious diarist tracked his descent into suicidal depression in daily entries that included his food. He noticed that his deterioration paralleled his use of diet sodas flavored with NutraSweet. He stopped consumption and his condition reversed. The government's Center for Disease Control noted that 25% of NutraSweet complainants could stop and start their symptoms by stopping and starting NutraSweet consumption.

Increasingly, doctors, dieticians, and other health professionals look to diet for explanations of malaise. The more data you can supply, the more fruitful their observations and advice. The matrix of information looked for includes how did I feel; when did I feel that way; and what was I doing at the time. This approach is central to the preventive (as distinct from the corrective) approach to health.

Detailed self-knowledge is the first step toward controlling your personal environment. The next step is control over time.

A TIME ALLOCATION PLAN

Time is more than money. The way a person uses time defines his life. If you think the relationship between food chemicals and your health deserves some of your time, then it is worth planning how to use that time. It is more important how you use the time than how much time you use. Balance, routine, and duration are more important than the amount of time used. Two hours a week used effectively will show a greater return than 10 times that amount used compulsively or erratically.

Balance means being alert and not compulsive. It means accepting the food chemical environment, including the fact that it entails risk, as a given. It means setting a goal to reduce exposure to food chemical risk, not trying to totally eliminate that risk.

Routine means working regularly. Add 10 minutes for food chemical consideration to each shopping trip. Look for nitrite or MSG free meats on one trip, BHT and BHA free cereals on another. Seek alternatives to products containing NutraSweet, to canned goods containing sulfite, or to baby food containing modified starch, or

hydrolyzed vegetable protein (HVP), or salt, if you are avoiding them.

Duration means keeping up the routine over a long period of time—months or even years. If you set aside 2 hours a week to consider your food chemical environment (adding 1 hour to shopping and 1 hour for reflection away from the store), you will accomplish as much and possibly more than in the same 104 hours over 3 or 6 months and with more ease.

Your time for considering food chemical safety (2 hours a week for one year) needs to be divided into four categories: labels, advertisements, research, and action.

Labels work emotionally, not rationally. Designed by experts and tested by psychologists, they are the handsome faces of merchandising meant to seduce, not to convince.

Ordinary shoppers spend six-tenths of a second making each food buying decision. In this atmosphere of mercantile flirtation, pretty labels and cute packages have the advantage. American food shopping has the quality and commitment of sex in a singles bar.

Labels are a powerful, intrusive force. They affect your life. Crude rules of thumb give some control over their efforts.

Esther Peterson, consumer advisor to Presidents Johnson and Carter and to the Giant Food chain in Washington, D.C., says, "If you can't pronounce it, don't eat it." Similarly, the longer the chemical list, the better to avoid the product. Avoid "artificial," but do not necessarily embrace "natural."

More subtly, chemicals are listed in order of predominance, although this is sometimes misleading. If you are avoiding salt, notice that sodium and MSG (mono*sodium* glutamate) are not salt substitutes. Fructose, glucose, and sucrose are all sugars. Watch for colors listed as artificial or, by more sensitive companies as FD&C (Food, Drug, and Cosmetic) colors. Flavors can be natural or artificial, though this distinction for *flavors* is arbitrary and dubious.

For label reading information, see sources in the information section. Preparing before shopping saves time.

Advertisements are bright, loud, and pervasive—gobs of frothy clutter obscuring the realities of eating in America. A 10-year-old sees 25,000 TV ads (mostly for food) in one year. Where labels tend to be seductive, advertisements approach rape.

Rule of thumb: the more intrusive the ads, the more chemicals to watch for. Advertised foods—selling convenience, taste, and improved appearance made possible by food technologists, with higher markups and more processing, use more chemicals. A penny's worth of vitamins added to corn flakes creates a totally fortified cereal, raises the price 19¢, and leads to massive advertising.

Research

The plan is to focus 2 hours weekly on food chemicals, 10 extra minutes during 6 shopping trips, 30 minutes on research, 30 minutes on action.

Research means gathering good food-buying information. Daily newspapers and general circulation news and information magazines give good early warnings. Take seriously any food safety problem they mention. Cautious in reporting (we won't report on it until it's banned), tied to advertising with limited news space, their report of a food safety problem is a red flag.

To follow up and discover what has not made the news, look for information from government, health, and science associations, and professional dieticians. Again, these are cautious sources whose food safety concerns should be taken seriously. Next consider consumer, environmental, and public interest groups and advocates who try to publicise safety problems early in their development.

Finally consider the health, natural, and alternative food marketplace, which has a record of being first to highlight a number of food safety concerns ultimately adopted by the rest of society. None of these sources has the "truth." Each must be taken on its own terms, evaluated, and then integrated or rejected into your information bases as they make sense to you.

Spending 30 minutes a week gathering and sorting food chemical safety information that comes through these sources will, over time, build a strong body of information on which you can rely.

Action

Spend the final 30 minutes on action. Time spent learning your biochemical individuality and your personal food chemical environment can be considered research or action. You might consider including time spent with your health care professional. Doctors, dentists, psychologists, and chiropractors are increasingly receptive to the idea that chemicals in the food environment can undermine an individual's health.

Influencing food manufacturers, sellers, and regulators is action, not research. Interested people can exert influence. Again, try grafting time onto already scheduled activities. Church groups, PTAs, women's and men's clubs, and health and fitness groups, among others, have taken on food safety issues and, with urging of their members, will take on more.

Direct action can also mean writing individual letters to food and additive manufacturers and regulators and to retail stores. The record built up over time by such action can influence food safety policy.

The ultimate action is buying or not. Your primary goal is assuring the availability of food safe enough for you to buy. This means getting manufacturers and regulators to create and allow choices you want, ensuring availability of information about inherent food risks, and finally, in extreme cases, lobbying to take unsafe products off the market.

Over time, 30 minutes a week efficiently spent on actions of this kind will have an effect.

INFORMATION

The effectiveness of the foregoing approach depends on the quality of the information you can locate *and use*. How you assimilate the information you find will determine how effectively you use it.

Assimilation. Apologists for food chemicals (knowingly or unknowingly) present a series of arguments designed to protect their economic investment. Understanding what they are saying and why they are saying it will allow you to use your information most effectively.

They say: a food chemical cannot be proven absolutely safe. They mean that risks proven to our satisfaction are outweighed by benefits, including our economic benefits. A good response: consumers should be told directly—perhaps on labels or in ads—whenever food contains potentially harmful ingredients. A bad response: banning any food containing a risky substance.

They say: just because a chemical harms an animal does not mean it will harm a human. They mean that test animals have been harmed by a chemical they are defending. A good response: just because a chemical does not harm animals does not mean it will *not* harm people; we need a better way to test food chemicals. A bad response: if it harms animals, get rid of it.

They say: this chemical has been used 10 (25, 50, 100) years with no harm to people. They mean that, even though test animals are harmed by the chemical, there is no evidence that people have been harmed. A good response: since virtually all chronic risks and most acute risks are of unknown origin, we do not know whether this or that food chemical has caused harm, so let's organize epidemiological studies that will focus on human consumption as it has been and will be. A bad response: food chemicals cause most acute and chronic human diseases.

They say: the American food supply is the safest in the world. They mean that any conceivable improvement in health that might come from a more restrictive use of food additives will be too expensive (particularly to them) to make it worthwhile. A good response: the potential for improvement in American health is great, and food chemicals should be considered a possible areas of focus. A bad response: the American food supply is not safe.

They say: the amounts of chemicals added are too small to cause any harm. They mean that while the chemical in question inflicts demonstrated harm at high doses, it is only present in small doses. A good answer: pricking a finger with a pin causes only small harm; doing it 20 or 30 times a day, day in and day out, will cause serious harm. A bad answer: a little bit of chemical is as bad as a lot of chemical.

They say: our chemical is less risky than many chemicals that occur naturally in food. They mean that, since you accept the "natural" risk, you should accept the added risk. A good answer: the more natural risk in the food supply, the less added risk that should be accepted. A bad answer: natural risks should be treated (banned, for example) in the same way as added risks.

"Good" and "bad" responses in these do not mean the content is good or bad. Perhaps any chemical that harms an animal should be banned. It means that, in response to the point they are making, you will probably lose the argument if you give the "bad" answer.

These are examples of a way of thinking that has confused the food safety debate. Most of these statements have been made so often that people using them do so unthinkingly. A thoughtful response often will lead to useful exchange. Food chemical apologists are not setting out to purposely harm food consumers, and many (if not most) are open to thoughtful exchanges.

The biggest challenge is refusing to allow a thoughtless assertion to trap you into a thoughtless response. This is true whether you are in an exchange or you are responding in your own mind to something you have heard or read.

Sources. As already mentioned, watch for articles concerning safety in your daily newspapers. Items mentioned there have already reached a level of debate requiring your attention.

To follow up leads gleaned from the press, pay attention to advocate groups who follow food chemical safety issues, including:

Center for Science in the Public Interest, Washington, D.C.

Natural Resources Defense Council, Washington, D.C. and New York, N.Y.

Environmental Defense Fund, Washington, D.C.

National Institute for Science, Law and Public Policy, Washington, D.C.

Community Nutrition Institute, Washington, D.C.

If these groups are unable to help, they may be able to send you to others who can.

Each of these groups produce regular and special publications dealing with food safety issues. There are various books that can help orient persons with a food safety interest:

Eaters Digest by Michael Jacobson

Food Additive Dictionary by Ruth Winter

The Chemical Feast by James Turner

Working on the System by Ralph Nader (the Food and Drug Administration section)

Each of these books will lead to others. With a regular application of time to following up food safety questions, you can make the choices best suited to you and your views.

CONCLUSION

Intelligent people ask: Which is safer, saccharin or NutraSweet? The answer depends on whether you prefer the risk of eye and brain damage now or the risk of cancer in the future. Questions like this one are examples of the problem. How would *you* answer the question of which is safer, cyanide or strychnine? Remember, he who asks the question controls the debate.

In the food safety debate, those with the economic interest in selling food chemicals have the resources to control who does the asking and what they ask. With massive advertising, research, and lobbying budgets, they will try to convince society to accept the risk of any chemical that they believe will make money in the market. They will start this campaign to change the law to allow risks in the food supply currently not allowed by saying they will be outweighed by benefits (including the economic benefits to chemical and food manufacturers).

The next big round will be an effort to change the law to allow risky chemicals to be added to food. Hopefully this short essay will help interested individuals ask the right questions, understand the answers given, and act—personally and socially—to increase rather than diminish the chemical safety of the food supply.

21

DIET, NUTRITION, AND WEIGHT CONTROL

Anne M. Fletcher, M.S., R.D., is a nutrition writer and educator, currently writing a book for Harper & Row, Publishers, Inc. She is a former executive editor of the *Tufts University Diet & Nutrition Letter*. Ms. Fletcher gained her expertise in weight management as assistant director and clinical nutritionist for a private practice specializing in obesity treatment.

Dieting in America is probably a more popular sport than baseball, football, or basketball. Dieting *is* America. There are surprisingly few women's magazines that don't publish a new diet method in every issue. So one might conclude that Americans are either fat and anxious to reduce their bulk or they are an obsessed race. Whichever the case may be, dieting is clearly a national obsession and the question of who should diet and why and when and how is open to anyone who cares to offer an opinion. Anne Fletcher lends real credibility to the subject. Hers is not a "how to" piece but rather a "what's it all about" survey, one much needed amidst the multitude of diet noisemakers.∎

Covers of women's magazines aptly capture two American obsessions that are in direct conflict: the desire to be thin *and* a passion for eating rich foods. Indeed, the weight loss plan-of-the-month is invariable juxtaposed next to page after page of sumptuous desserts and calorie-laden entrees. Such confusing messages have many women and men alike bouncing from one weight loss scheme to the next, often to little avail.

But a great deal of confusion and distress could be alleviated if individuals could rationally determine whether they really need to lose weight. If so, the next step is to decide upon a reasonable, healthy, and lasting way to accomplish the task. If not, the goal is to accept body weight as it is and learn how to maintain that healthy level.

CLASSIFYING BODY WEIGHT—WHAT'S "IDEAL"?

Some people live in dread of a trip to the doctor's office for fear that stepping on the scale will lead to admonitions about getting down to what the charts say they should weight. Others balk at the values listed on the familiar Metropolitan Life Insurance Company weight tables, believing that they would be "fat" if they ever weighed in at the ranges specified for their heights.

However, the most common means that medical experts employ to evaluate an individual's weight is a comparison with the Metropolitan charts that list weight ranges for which people of given heights tend to live the longest. (See chart below.) Someone whose weight is 20% or more than the specified value is considered to be obese. "Overweight," however, is often considered as a scale reading of up to 20% above the chart values. It is important to note that someone can be overweight without being fat. Consider, for example, a body builder or a football player whose weight is greater than charted number by virtue of having much more muscle tissue than most people.

Compared to people with small frames—a reflection of bone size and thickness—those who are larger can carry more weight without having

1983 METROPOLITAN LIFE INSURANCE COMPANY HEIGHT—WEIGHT TABLES*

Men					Women				
Height		Small Frame	Medium Frame	Large Frame	Height		Small Frame	Medium Frame	Large Frame
Feet	Inches				Feet	Inches			
5	2	128-134	131-141	138-150	4	10	102-111	109-121	118-131
5	3	130-136	133-143	140-153	4	11	103-113	111-113	120-134
5	4	132-138	135-145	142-156	5	0	104-115	113-126	122-137
5	5	134-140	137-148	144-160	5	1	106-118	115-129	125-140
5	6	136-142	139-151	146-164	5	2	108-121	118-132	128-143
5	7	138-145	142-154	149-168	5	3	111-124	121-135	131-147
5	8	140-148	145-157	152-172	5	4	114-127	124-138	134-151
5	9	142-151	148-160	155-176	5	5	117-130	127-141	137-155
5	10	144-154	151-163	158-180	5	6	120-133	130-144	140-159
5	11	146-157	154-166	161-184	5	7	123-136	133-147	143-163
6	0	149-160	157-170	164-188	5	8	126-139	136-150	146-167
6	1	152-164	160-174	168-192	5	9	129-142	139-153	149-170
6	2	155-168	164-178	172-197	5	10	132-145	142-156	152-173
6	3	158-172	167-182	176-202	5	11	135-148	145-159	155-176
6	4	162-176	171-187	181-207	6	0	138-151	148-162	158-179

*In shoes with one-inch heels and clothing weighing five pounds for men and three pounds for women.

Reprinted with permission from the Metropolitan Life Insurance company.

an increase in the risk of mortality. But it's not enough to simply go by a person's appearance to determine frame size. Accordingly, the Metropolitan Life Insurance Company offers the following guidelines for arriving at frame size: extend one arm, bending the forearm straight up, at a 90 degree angle. Keeping the fingers straight, turn the inside of the wrist toward the body. Then place the thumb and index finger of the other hand on the outer edges of the two protruding bones of the bent elbow. Pull the fingers away, maintaining the space between them. With a measuring tape or ruler, measure this space and compare it with the values for a medium-frame size person, listed below. Lower measurements indicate a small frame; higher values suggest a large frame.

HEIGHT IN 1" HEELS

Men	Elbow Breadth
5'2" — 5'3"	2½" — 2⅞"
5'4" — 5'7"	2⅝" — 2⅞"
5'8" — 5'11"	2¾" — 3"
6'0" — 6'3"	2¾" — 3⅛"
6'4"	2⅞" — 3¼"
Women	
4'10" — 4'11"	2¼" — 2½"
5'0" — 5'3"	2¼" — 2½"
5'4" — 5'11"	2⅜" — 2⅝"
6'0"	2½" — 2¾"

Although the Metropolitan charts are useful in evaluating weight, there are a number of reasons why they should not be considered as listing ideal values for which everyone should strive. In the first place, the charts are based on studies that showed weights associated with the lowest death rate for a group of people, predominantly men, insured by Metropolitan Life. Thus, the values are based on a relatively small group. Furthermore, insurance companies are only aware of a person's weight at the time a policy is issued; weight could be different when death occurs. Besides, even if the weight listed on the charts is associated with a lower death rate, it doesn't mean that value is ideal for preventing chronic ailments, such as hypertension.

Another shortcoming of the Metropolitan charts is that they fail to account for age, lumping together weights associated with low death rates for young adults with those of older folks. In fact, independent analyses of the same data by Reubin Andres, M.D., of the National Institute on Aging suggest that, when age is considered, the charts list weights that are appropriate only for people in their forties. Since the weight range associated with the lowest death rate progressively increases with age, the values appear to be too high for young adults and too low for individuals in their fifties and sixties.

The message here is that height and weight charts only offer general guidelines for optimum weight, not hard and fast values for what any individual should weigh. A person's ideal weight, according to my personal definition, is one at which he feels good about himself and has no major medical problems, as well as one that can be maintained without undue psychological suffering. For someone who has been 100 or more pounds overweight for many years, that value may be much higher than the listing on the Metropolitan charts. For others who have a weight-related medical problem, such as hypertension or diabetes, ideal weight may be lower.

WHAT CONSTITUTES A WEIGHT PROBLEM?

Defining a weight problem depends on whether the standards are medical or societal. From a medical standpoint, nearly everyone agrees that people who are 40% or more overweight are in jeopardy. In this category, for instance, the incidence of arthritis doubles and that of gall bladder disease triples compared to the risks for normal weight individuals. In fact, it came as no surprise when the 1985 National Institutes of Health Consensus Development Panel on the Health Implications of Obesity concluded that obese adults are at risk for high blood pressure, adult-onset diabetes, and high blood cholesterol. In addition, compared to nonobese women, the obese are more likely to die as a result of cancer of the gallbladder, ovaries, breast, and uterus. Obese men carry a higher mortality rate from cancer of the prostate, rectum, and colon than their normal weight counterparts.

What remains unclear is the cut-off weight that places someone at risk for developing these problems. The NIH panel somewhat arbitrarily designated a hazardous weight as one that is 20% or more above the Metropolitan Life Chart values, using the midpoint of the range for a medium-build person. Going by these values, well over 30 million Americans are at medical risk because of excess body fat. However, some experts believe that the NIH panel's criteria are too stringent in light of evidence suggesting that mildly obese people—up to 30% overweight—who have no other medical problems, may have the same life expectancy as average weight individuals. On the other hand, as expressed earlier, individuals who already have medical ailments that are aggravated by extra weight may jeopardize their health with just 10 or 15 extra pounds.

Where people are overweight may be as important as *how* overweight they are. It now appears that individuals with abdominal fat in the form of "spare tires" or "beer bellies" are at higher risk for heart disease, stroke, and death than those whose fat is distributed primarily in the hips and buttocks.

Placing aside medical definitions, many people have a weight problem only because they *think* they have one. For some, an obsession with 5 or 10 pounds becomes life-controlling. This may stem from society's disdain for excessive body fat, apparent at an early age from a study in which young children described silhouettes of obese youngsters as "lazy, dirty, stupid, and ugly." Some experts believe that this prejudice against "fatness"—coupled with condoning of excessive thinness on the part of some physicians and parents—are in large part responsible for today's rapid increase in eating disorders, specifically anorexia nervosa and bulimia.

The blame for eating disorders and what I term weight obsessions, in which normal weight people who don't fit the psychological criteria for eating disorders gear their entire lives around food and weight, may at least partially be placed on perpetual media portrayal of unrealistic body images that many individuals feel they should strive to attain. Indeed, a recent study revealed that more than three quarters of average weight girls had dieted in the past year. Fortunately, understanding the causes of overeating as well as developing helpful strategies to gain control can be helpful for any type of weight problem.

WHAT MAKES PEOPLE OVEREAT?

People in all weight categories tend to overeat from time to time, usually for the same reasons: habit and emotions. Hunger, of course, is a factor determining how much people eat. But the physiological mechanisms controlling appetite are complex and not clearly understood. Besides, hunger often has little to do with overeating when, in fact, the "extras" that people eat are commonly consumed when they're full. Consider, for instance, how easy it is to find room for a favorite dessert after a big meal. Conversely, people can often teach themselves to tolerate hunger. It is thought that some formerly obese people learn to keep their weight down by eating very few calories in the face of frequent hunger pangs.

Longstanding habits are probably a more powerful determinant of overeating—that is, eating more calories than the body needs to maintain itself at a certain level, ultimately resulting in weight gain. Such habits, also called behaviors, can become so ingrained that they're automatic. As a case in point, a man who goes to the refrigerator the minute he comes home from work may, with time, have a desire to eat anytime he walks through the door to his house. For someone in the habit of having a donut each morning at coffee break, seeing 10:00 AM on the clock may spell "time to eat," even after a large breakfast.

Sight and smell of food can be powerful cues for overeating, too, particularly in a society with widespread availability of high calorie foods. The desire to eat something sweet, for example, may not present itself until a shopper hits the candy rack at the check-out counter. And there's little more enticing than the smell of fresh-baked bread to lure someone into a bakery. Emotional situations that lead people to overeat include depression, frustration, anger, and psychological stress. Think about the message "Eat this, you'll feel better," that is often relayed to small children in unhappy situations. By the time adulthood rolls around, the habit of soothing the ravages of a "bad day" by indulging in food is one that is well entrenched. Overeating can also be brought on by recurring, self-defeating thoughts such as "I'll never be thin. Why bother?" Or "It's not worth it to lose weight so slowly." These kinds of negative thoughts can become strong triggers for binge eating because they've led to this behavior so many times in the past.

The fact that many thin, normal weight, *and* obese people will relate to all of these reasons for overeating serves as evidence that they do *not* explain why some people gain weight much more easily than others. In fact, current findings suggest that the obese are no more likely than normal weight people to overeat because of habits, sensitivity to food cues, or negative thoughts and feelings. According to Thomas A. Wadden, Ph.D., with the Obesity Research Group at the University of Pennsylvania, a number of studies have arrived at the "somewhat surprising conclusion that there are greater similarities than differences in the eating behaviors of obese and normal weight adults."

WHAT MAKES SOME PEOPLE FAT—BUT NOT OTHERS?

Most people know the weight gain equation by heart: you gain weight when you regularly consume more calories than your body burns off each day. Until recently, the focus in understanding obesity was on the intake side of the equation, assuming that excessive body weight was the result of overindulgence. Given that, compared to their thinner counterparts, heavy people are not necessarily more likely to eat for behavioral or emotional reasons, could it be that obese people simply go overboard with food?

The answer in many cases appears to be no. One recent study on the calorie intake of more than 6000 adults suggested that the obese consume no more than the nonobese. In fact, another study showed that the heaviest subjects actually ate 300 to 400 calories less each day than the thinnest participants.

Since the signs seem to point away from the notion that obesity is the result of an intake problem, researchers began focusing on the output side of the weight gain equation. Below are some of the current theories—all of which are equal contenders for being right—that may explain why heavy people don't burn off enough calories for some metabolic reason. No one theory accounts for all cases of obesity; for many individuals more than one factor is likely to be at play.

The Setpoint Theory. There is some evidence that each individual has a biologically predetermined weight that his body "fights" to maintain; for obese people, that setpoint appears to be higher. The setpoint theory may partially explain why many dieters get stuck after losing a certain amount of weight, as well as why weight is often gained back after dieting. It is thought that exercise helps to lower setpoint.

The Fat Cell Hypothesis. This theory suggests that the more fat cells someone has, the greater the propensity for storing body fat and gaining weight. It makes sense in light of the fact that severely obese people have up to five times more fat cells than normal weight adults. And individual fat cells have the potential to increase in volume hundreds of times if provided with excess abuses. In part, the number of fat cells a person has is genetically predetermined. But consistent overeating appears to trigger the formation of new fat cells in both adults and children. Unfortunately, it's difficult or even impossible to get rid of fat cells once they're formed.

The Brown Fat Theory. The body has two types of fat: the familiar white fat that *stores* excess calories and brown fat that actually *gives off* calories as heat. The theory goes that some obese people have less of the efficient brown fat, thereby explaining why some individuals can only eat half the number of calories as others who weigh the same and are equally active. At this time, there is no known way to stimulate brown fat to burn off more calories.

Genetic Explanations. Given that the chance of a child becoming obese is 10 times higher if both his parents are obese than if neither parent has a weight problem, it seems logical to assume that heaviness is inherited. But it's also possible that "fat" habits—love of rich foods and aversion to physical activity—are passed on through generations. Although nature and nurture may interact in breeding obesity, current evidence indicates that inheritance is a more powerful influence. A study published in the *New England Journal of Medicine* revealed that adult weights of people who were adopted are significantly closer to those of their biological parents than to the weights of adoptive parents.

Inactivity and age. In general, obese people are less active than thin individuals. But it is not clear whether this is the cause or the result of overweight. The physical strain of excess weight would become obvious if you filled a suitcase with 50 pounds of books and carried it around for a day! Nevertheless, it is believed that inactivity is largely responsible for 15 to 25 pounds the average American accumulates between the ages of 25 and 50. Usually creeping on slowly, in 1- to 2-pound yearly increments, the gain probably stems from the tendency for older people to engage less often in purposeful exercise, such as tennis or exercise classes. It is also a likely reflection of having the kids assume family chores like mowing the lawn and taking out the trash.

HOW NOT TO LOSE WEIGHT

Many overweight people are reassured to learn that the cause of their heaviness may, indeed, be faulty metabolism. But that knowledge does little to help them lose the excess weight when, regardless of the cause, the only way to shed pounds is to consume fewer calories than the body burns off each day. There are any number of ways to accomplish this task—some 30,000 different weight loss approaches exist, according to one estimate! Although many of these schemes are unsound, they lure obese people, as well as normal weight individuals who think they need to lose, into spending billions of dollars each year.

Here are some tip-offs for spotting the weight loss remedies that are least likely to work:

Eat only....Don't eat any.... Grapefruit diets, high protein diets, the Rice Diet—they all have something in common: boredom. If only a handful of foods are allowed each day, weight loss is bound to occur. But how long can a dieter keep this up? Chances are, when normal foods are eaten again, weight will be gained back.

Eat All You Want. When diets allow unlimited amounts of certain foods, skepticism is in order. Any food, if eaten in excess, can lead to weight gain. It's also wise not to be swayed by claims that certain foods have the ability to "cancel out" the calories in other foods. There's no such thing. Invariably, when people lose weight on such diets, it's because, other than the low calorie "eat all you want" foods, many foods are forbidden.

"Sensitivities" Are Responsible. Some diets encourage avoidance of particular foods based on the notion that food "sensitivities," similar to allergies, are responsible for weight gain. Not only is there no sound evidence that overweight is caused by allergic or sensitivity reactions, but restricting favorite foods often heightens desire for them.

Guaranteed, Forever. When even the most reputable of programs cannot promise success, it should be clear that there are no guarantees in the weight loss business. Sadly, statistics have it that in general, about 95% of those people who lose weight gain it back within the first 5 years.

Secret, Breakthrough. If a breakthrough in weight control were to occur, obesity experts would surely know about it. To date, there are no miracle remedies, and none appear to be on the horizon. If such an event were to occur, scientists would not be likely to release the good news by means of an advertisement in a magazine!

Burns Off Fat. The only way to "burn off fat" is to eat less and/or exercise more. Touting a particular food for fat-burning capabilities is fraudulent in the eyes of the U.S. Food and Drug Administration. As far as the claims that certain amino acids such as L-carnitine, or hormones such as cholecystokinin are concerned, there is no evidence that they'll eliminate excess fat.

Overnight, Immediate. Since people don't gain weight overnight, how is it possible to lose detectable amounts of fat in just hours? One popular "overnight" approach suggested taking the amino acids arginine and ornithine. But they have not been shown to be effective. Certainly, laxatives and diuretics could lead to overnight weight loss, largely through the excretion of fluids and body waste, not through fat loss. Abuse of these drugs could involve serious medical risks such as electrolyte and fluid imbalance.

Kills Hunger Pangs. Sure, there are appetite suppressants that can help people eat less. The problem is that, even with powerful prescription drugs, most people regain the weight they lose when they stop taking the medication. Moreover, appetite suppressants can be risky for certain individuals. For instance, phenylpropanolamine, the active ingredient in many over-the-counter preparations, is not recommended for people with hypertension, diabetes, thyroid disease, or kidney problems. "Bulk producers," such as methyl cellulose, bran supplements, and glucomannan (from a plant root), have also been demonstrated to help people eat less. But their effectiveness has not been demonstrated.

Effortless. The ploy that a weight loss scheme involves no effort is unfair because no easy means of shedding excess pounds has ever been found. When put to the scientific test, such claims don't pan out. Take the case of starch blockers that supposedly prevent carbohydrate adsorption: studies have shown that they don't work. Grapefruit extracts, taken in pill form, are another example of products that supposedly allow people to eat as they please while shedding fat. However, there's nothing special in grapefruit that facilitates weight reduction. If weight loss occurs, it's probably the result of following the low-calorie diet that often comes with the pills.

"I lost 50 pounds in just 8 weeks." Ads for weight loss gimmicks, as well as best-selling diet books, often carry dramatic testimonials based on "success stories." But testimonials are not sci-

entific proof that a remedy will work for most people. Assuming that "if it's in a book, it must be so" is a mistake because authors are allowed by law to express weight loss opinions without having to substantiate them. The best bet is to go by the Council of Better Business Bureaus' motto: "If the promotion or plan sounds too good to be true, it probably is."

A QUESTION OF ADEQUACY

Not only are many popular loss schemes ineffective, they often set the stage for nutrient deficiencies. In fact, a recent survey on the nutritional adequacy of a number of popular diets, published in the *Journal of the American Dietetic Association* revealed that the Beverly Hills, Richard Simmons, and Stillman diets provide less then 70% of the U.S. Recommended Dietary Allowances for more than half the vitamins and minerals studied.

High protein, low carbohydrate diets, such as the Atkins and Stillman plans, have their own set of problems. Not only do they have the potential for raising blood uric acid levels (a particular problem for someone predisposed to gout), but the survey described above found both diets to be high in fat and cholesterol. The large weight loss often found on these types of diets is predominantly water that is excreted when the body's carbohydrate stores are depleted. Much of the weight is regained when people start eating "carbos" again.

At the other extreme are low protein regimes, such as the Beverly Hills Diet and the Rice Diet. While the Beverly Hills plan has been shown to provide less than 50% of the Recommended Dietary Allowance for protein, the early stages of the Rice Diet (which dieters are encouraged to follow indefinitely) provide no more than one third of the RDA for the nutrient. And protein deficient diets can lead to tearing down of body protein from the muscles and vital organs, such as the liver.

One of the clues that a diet is nutritionally unbalanced is the omission of a major food group. If a plan avoids dairy products, fruits and vegetables, grain products, or protein foods (meat, poultry, fish, eggs, and cheese), then it's likely to be lacking some important nutrients. Another signal that a diet is inadequate is a calorie level of less than 1000. At that level, the amount of food is limited, making it difficult to meet nutritional needs. Furthermore, with prolonged dieting at a very low calorie level, the body's response is to slow down metabolism in an effort to protect against "semi-starvation."

CALORIES DO COUNT

"One more sliver won't hurt. Crumbs don't count. Just a spoonful more. It doesn't count if you eat in the dark or when you're standing up." These "indiscretions" that dieters often joke about really can add up to a weight gain when it only takes an extra 100 calories per day more than the body needs in order to put on 10 pounds in 1 year. That gain can result from just a tablespoon of peanut butter or mayonnaise, a tiny piece of cake, or a small handful of nuts. The good news is that cutting back here and there by "spoonfuls and slivers" can have a cumulative effect, too, eventually leading to weight loss.

Weight reduction is not likely to come about quickly by "cutting back" because a 3500-calorie deficit is needed to lose a pound of fat. Therefore, to lose a pound a week, people have to eat 500 calories less per day; to lose 2 pounds a week, 1000 fewer calories have to be consumed each day. Fewer than what? Fewer than the number of calories needed to maintain current weight.

Determining maintenance calorie needs entails two steps. The first is to estimate basal metabolic rate (BMR) by multiplying current weight by 10. That figure represents the approximate number of calories requires to support normal bodily processes, including breathing and blood circulation, while the body is resting. The next step is to calculate physical activity calories which, for a typical sedentary person, can amount to about 30% of BMR calories. So for a 150-pound woman:

$$150 \times 10 = 1500 \text{ BMR calories}$$
$$1500 \times .30 = \underline{\;\;450 \text{ activity calories}\;\;}$$
$$1950 \text{ daily maintenance calories}$$

In addition to total calorie intake, it's also important to consider *where* those calories come from. Specifically, fats and fatty foods have two strikes against them for someone trying to lose weight. On one count, fats have more than double the calories of pure carbohydrate or protein on an ounce-for-ounce basis. In addition, accumulating evidence suggests that fat calories are more "fattening" than carbohydrate calories. While the body expends some calories in processing any nutrient eaten, it appears to burn off fewer calories in handling fat than it does with carbohydrates.

All of this adds up to the wise approach of consuming less fat while eating proportionately more carbohydrate—whether following a low-calorie diet or just trying to maintain weight at a certain level. You should avoid using butter, oil, margarine, mayonnaise, and regular salad dressing. Fatty meats and cold cuts should be replaced with lean red meat, fish, and skinless poultry. Substituting skim milk or low-fat dairy products for whole milk versions will eliminate fat, too.

To increase carbohydrate intake, most veteran dieters already know that eating more fruits and vegetables helps to "fill up." But many have trouble with the concept that it's okay to eat "carbos," including bread, pasta, potatoes, and rice, when trying to lose weight. Once again, too much of anything can lead to weight gain. And slathering carbohydrate foods with butter, creamy sauces, or sour cream defeats the purpose.

As for sweets, the advice for people limiting their calorie intake is to "go easy." Sugar is not any more fattening than other carbohydrates, but foods rich in table sugar and corn sweeteners often provide "empty calories." This means they provide carbohydrate—and often fat—calories but very little in the way of other nutrients.

None of this is to say that weight conscious people can't enjoy a bowl of ice cream, a prime steak, or french fries once in a while. The trick is to regard them as occasional treats. The same applies to alcoholic beverages since they, too, provide largely empty calories.

THE MAKINGS OF A SOUND WEIGHT MANAGEMENT PROGRAM
Picking the "Right" Diet

People who choose to follow a diet without medical supervision should be certain, as stated earlier, that it contains at least 1000 calories. Men are better off with several hundred calories more because their nutrient needs are higher. Anyone who consumes less than 1200 calories for more than a few weeks should consider taking a multivitamin/mineral supplement that provides levels within the RDAs. To avoid the complications of low carbohydrate diets, about 100 daily grams of carbohydrate are sufficient. That amount would be supplied by three small pieces of fruit, two cups of low-fat milk, two slices of bread, plus a cup-and-a-half of most vegetables. To meet the RDA for protein, women should consume 44 grams daily; men need 56 grams. Either level would be easily exceeded by adding 5 ounces of lean meat, poultry, or fish to the carbohydrate sources listed above.

Looking at the diet concept another way, however, one could argue that people who need to lose relatively small amounts of weight—say, 5 to 20 pounds—are better off not following any diet at all. Indeed, a connection between chronic dieting and the tendency to binge eat has repeatedly been demonstrated, even in normal weight people. Individuals with modest amounts to lose, as well as those trying to maintain a weight loss, may be more successful if they focus on eating fewer fatty foods, changing their food habits, and getting more exercise.

At the other extreme, it's understandable that someone who is faced with losing 50 pounds or more can become easily discouraged on any plan that allows for a loss of 1 or 2 pounds a week. Therefore, individuals who are more than 40% above their desirable weight often do well on what nutritionists call protein-sparing modified diets. These diets consist of 300 to 600 daily calories provided by controlled portions of high quality protein foods (meats, eggs, poultry, and fish). Sometimes high protein liquid formulas are used, instead. The idea with protein-sparing diets is to provide the body with just enough dietary pro-

tein to prevent it from breaking down its own muscle protein. The average loss is 45 pounds in 12 weeks. Because medical complications may occur and special supplements are needed, protein-sparing diets should only be followed under close supervision by a physician who has experience with such regimens.

CHANGING FOOD HABITS—BEHAVIOR MODIFICATION

Be it a 1000-calorie or protein-sparing diet, no diet works if old habits are resumed when dieting stops. That's why sound weight loss programs incorporate a behavior modification component, based on the notion that ingrained counter-productive food habits can be unlearned and replaced with more productive behaviors.

The first step is to figure out what the problem habits are by keeping a detailed diary of everything eaten, noting time of day, location, and other activities engaged in while eating. Soon, patterns start to emerge. For instance, a woman might become aware that she eats half a box of crackers every week on her way home from the grocery store. Or a salesman might notice that he eats a "fourth meal" on the 2 days each week that he passes his favorite fast food restaurant en route to an account. Another problem people commonly encounter is the constant availability of tempting foods—on kitchen counters, for example, or in social situations.

As soon as people identify habits associated with overeating, they can start to change them. The woman who eats in the car could benefit by transporting her groceries in the trunk, rather than on the seat next to her. She might also try shopping after a meal when she's not hungry. A solution for the salesman would be to find another route that doesn't go by a fast food restaurant.

Behavior modification also involves learning to eat more slowly, so people appreciate what they're eating and feel more self-control. Tempting foods are to be kept out of the house or, if that's not possible, out of sight. When social situations involving food are encountered, it's helpful to preplan what will be eaten', "saving up" some calories for the occasion and consciously deciding not to stand next to areas in which food is served. People who tend to engross themselves in other activities, such as reading, while eating may find that they feel more satisfied with their meals if they concentrate on making it "pure" activity.

Does behavior modification work? Yes, according to hundreds of scientific studies, behavior modification is more effective for mild obesity than drugs, nutrition education alone, psychotherapy, and self-help approaches. Since the average loss of 25 pounds in 25 weeks may be frustrating for someone who needs to lose large amounts of weight, behavior modification is often coupled with a protein-sparing diet. It's encouraging to note that many people who lose weight in behavior modification programs maintain their loss 1 year after the training ends.

Using Your Head—Thought Restructuring

Behavior modification is often combined with learning how to change negative, self-destructive thoughts, as well as developing productive ways to cope with stress and emotions. Once again, it's helpful to keep a diary—in this case, of thoughts and feelings that occur when the urge to eat strikes. Negative thoughts associated with overeating, such as "It's not fair. No one else has to eat like this" or "I ate a piece of candy. Now I may as well eat the whole bag" can be replaced with more helpful statements. These two thoughts can be restructured as "It doesn't help to feel sorry for myself. Lots of people have to watch their weight. I'm not alone," and "One piece of candy doesn't wreck my diet. I shouldn't feel guilty for having a treat once in a while."

One way to avoid negative thinking in the first place is to establish realistic goals that don't set the stage for failure. Attainable goals such as allowing dessert once a week or exercising every other day are more realistic than rules like "I'll never eat dessert again" or "from now on, I'm going to exercise every day."

Learning how to cope with stress, anxiety, and depression without binge eating typically entails generating a list of alternative activities that will really make a person feel better. After all, turning to food may temporarily soothe the soul, but overeating invariable leads to eventual feelings of guilt and doesn't solve the problem. Helpful substitutes include going for a walk, listening to some relaxing music, engaging in a hobby, or calling a friend.

Using Your Body—The Value of Exercise

Exercise offers a positive perspective for people who are sick of focusing on what they can't have. Becoming more physically active places the emphasis on something people can do to take control of a weight problem. Witness to results of a study in which obese women walked at least 30 minutes a day. Without dieting, they lost an average of 20 pounds at the end of a year. Exercise also enables people who are trying to maintain their weight to eat more. For example, walking two miles in an hour can burn off the number of calories in a dish of ice cream.

Another value of exercise is its ability to counteract the drop in metabolism that occurs when calorie intake is restricted. Research with obese people revealed that following a 500-calorie diet for 2 weeks resulted in a 9% drop in basal metabolic rate (BMR). But adding 20 to 30 minutes of exercise daily raised BMR 7% above predieting levels within 2 weeks. In contrast, a group of sedentary people on a similar diet for four weeks experienced a 19% decrease in BMR. Another bonus for dieters is that exercise helps minimize the loss of protein tissue that often occurs. Finally, physical activity has been shown to have psychological benefits, including improved self-esteem.

It's a mistake to think that exercise has to be intense or highly structured to be of value. As mentioned earlier, walking can be very beneficial and is safe for most people. Another way to get more exercise is to work it into a daily routine by taking stairs instead of escalators and elevators, walking instead of driving to do local errands, parking at the far end of lots, and getting off the bus one stop away from your destination.

PUTTING IT ALL TOGETHER

The best way to lose weight is to combine sensible eating habits—or dieting, if necessary—with behavior modification, cognitive restructuring, and exercise. Not only are these techniques valuable for obese people, but they're helpful for overweight individuals and those with "food obsessions." Granted, it's not always easy to do it on your own, and many people benefit from professional weight loss programs as well as self-help groups.

PART VI EXERCISE

22 **The Relationship of Fitness To the
Prevention of Disease and
the Promotion of Health**
John W. Farquhar, M.D.,
and Christine L. Farquhar, M.A.

23 **Exercise and Reduced Risk of
Coronary Heart Disease**
Ralph S. Paffenbarger, Jr., M.D.,
and Robert T. Hyde, M.A.

24 **Which Sport Is For You?**
Joan Ullyot, M.D.

22

THE RELATIONSHIP OF FITNESS TO THE PREVENTION OF DISEASE AND THE PROMOTION OF HEALTH

John W. Farquhar, M.D., is director of the Stanford Center for Research in Disease Prevention, which is actively pursuing research in social, psychological, and medical issues relevant to cardiovascular disease prevention. He is the author of *The American Way of Life Need Not Be Hazardous to Your Health* and more than 100 papers. In 1983 he received the James D. Bruce Memorial Award from the American College of Physicians for outstanding contributions in preventive medicine.

Christine L. Farquhar, M.A., is a writer and former teacher. She holds degrees in English and Education from Stanford University.

Regular exercise can dramatically reduce the risk of heart attacks and strokes, reduce high blood pressure, and benefit diabetes patients. Exercise can also help us maintain strong bones and may prevent the onset of osteoarthritis. It may even help lifelong cigarette smokers kick the habit. In this article, John and Christine Farquhar explain their belief that "personal behavior is the only trustworthy source of disease prevention."▪

When Freud said the ultimate purpose of life was to love and to work, he forgot to mention what it takes for a fellow to do either one. You have to feel good. There is almost a mystical quality to that concept of feeling good. We all know what it is when we have it, but finding it in our busy lives has not had top priority. Recognizing the need to feel good and arranging our daily habits around that pursuit is something that has only recently appeared in our culture.

What I mean by feeling good is, of course, that sense of well-being that comes from fitness. The person who is fit is like a well-tuned piano. Everything he does resonates in concord with all parts of his being. He sleeps well, he works efficiently, he plays happily, and he loves generously. By taking care of himself, this fellow is giving to others. He makes a place for himself in the world and he enhances that world.

When two young people get married, they vow to keep one another "in sickness or in health." Along with the marriage certificate, they should also receive a crystal ball to show them what they will look like in 30 years. If they live in one style, they will be keeping one another in sickness; if they live in another style, they will be keeping one another in health. For as we know today, ill health is not an isolated event; it is the result of an accumulation of abuses or a series of patterns of behavior that, heaped together, create sickness. Conversely, good health, generally speaking, is also the result of an accumulation of patterns of behavior. Given their druthers, everyone with any sense would choose the good health picture in the crystal ball.

Our role as physicians and health educators is to help our patients find the right path to good habits. Chief among those habits is exercise and its attendant benefits. The bottom line to exercise, or the chicken in the pot pie, is "feeling good." Let's talk about exercise, what it is, how to make it part of our life, what it does for you, and what you'll become as a result of it. Fitness won't make you rich and it won't make you young, but you'll feel rich and you might look younger. What it will do is make you healthy and that, as a personal commodity, grows in value with age.

There is a decided relationship between fitness and the prevention of disease. Riding tandem with that fact is the free bonus: exercise actually promotes health. Nature obviously intended us to be active. "Play" to a child means to run, jump, skip, throw balls, climb trees. To an adult, those same activities are similar to jogging, tennis, golf, skiing, mountain climbing. The child's play is instinctive and natural, and it gives him pleasure. When the child becomes inactive, the parent worries that he is ill. Yet by the time most Americans are parents, they themselves are slowing down into inactivity. Something seems to happen in adulthood. We suppress our fundamental need for physical activity. (And I think we cover up our need for natural pleasure and feeling good.) For thousands of years our everyday existence, even our survival, depended on physical exertion. Then along came the Industrial Revolution and automation. The paradox of modern living is that we are killing ourselves with our own sophistication. In highly industrialized countries, physical inactivity among the bulk of the population has become the rule, not the exception. What used to be a necessary part of daily living, physical activity, must now be artificially inserted into one's daytime hours. As we all know, the interest in physical fitness is happily on the increase. Ten years ago a Gallup Poll reported that 47% of all adult Americans participated in some form of regular physical exercise. That was twice the percentage reported in 1961. The same poll today might well report an additional increase. We Americans spend more than $65 million annually on home conditioning equipment. That sounds like a lot of money for taking care of ourselves, but when you compare it to the $500 million spent annually for cigarette advertising one must still ask if we are doing enough.

Even though the message is finally getting out that we don't have to have disease descend upon us like locusts, still many of our citizens accept as normal the concept that our neighbor Fred had a heart attack and his wife's diabetes is a problem in her life. We humans seem to adapt to most realities around us rather than digging in our feet and saying such physical indignities need not occur.

If every day of the year four jumbo jets crashed, killing more than 900 persons per day, by the end of one year 350,000 decent folks would have met a sudden end. That is the total number of premature deaths from heart attacks and strokes. Yet we humans adapt to what we read and tolerate such outrages. To continue the analogy, 700,000 more decent folk are involved in nonfatal "crashes" each year. The total cost in lost earnings and medical care is about $70 billion. This figure is the estimated annual lost earnings and medical expenses of heart disease and stroke patients in the under-75 age group alone. How much does it cost to buy a good pair of comfortable shoes and take a brisk 20-minute walk three or four times a week? A lot less.

We know beyond any doubt that lack of exercise contributes to heart attacks and stroke. Other risk factors in the development of heart disease and strokes are a high level of LDL cholesterol (the harmful kind of cholesterol), a *low* level of HDL cholesterol (the protective kind of cholesterol), smoking, high blood pressure, being overweight, and stress and tension. All these risk factors can be controlled, and each to some measure is affected by the amount of exercise one does.

Smoking causes lung cancer and increases the rate of atherosclerosis (the gummy deposits inside our arteries). Of all the risk factors to poor health, smoking and faulty diets are the very worst. According to surveys, over two thirds of the current 46 million adult smokers in the U.S. would like to quit. We know that smoking and not smoking involves a complicated system of behavioral cues and habits. We know that smoking stands in the way of fitness. We also know that as a person, with patience and support, abandons smoking and adopts exercise, his desire to smoke decreases.

High blood pressure, or hypertension, is a stubborn problem. Over 10% of middle-aged Americans have elevated blood pressure. That figure includes more women than men. High blood pressure is caused in part by too much salt, by being overweight, and by the lack of exercise. It damages the heart muscle itself and increases the risk of stroke.

Once again, the importance of exercise, of

using one's body, strikes like a clarion bell. If lack of exercise raises blood pressure, then increased exercise lowers blood pressure. It does so mainly because exercise is the most effective way to keep from being overweight (obese).

Obesity almost always is caused by a sedentary lifestyle and a high caloric intake. There are three ways to lose weight: (1) become more physically active; (2) reduce your caloric intake; (3) exercise and eat less. Fortunately, for people with a weight problem, information about calorie intake through the foods one eats and caloric expenditure through assorted sports and physical activities is readily available in popular magazines at the check-out counter of most grocery stores. It's no secret that whipped cream is more fattening than a carrot, or that a 40-minute brisk walk will expend more calories than reading a book. What does seem to be a secret is that obesity can create serious health problems. It increases the risk of high blood pressure and diabetes. It also raises the amount of cholesterol in the blood. Some people feel that watching calories is a *negative* way of dealing with being fat; holding back from favorite foods can feel too *punitive* for success. If that is the case, a *positive* way of watching one's weight is through exercise. The truth of the matter is that if a fellow begins an exercise program and sticks to it, he'll notice that his weight will start to fall without a constant dose of nagging himself to eat less.

Diabetes, which runs in families, is greatly benefited by exercise. The benefit comes in two ways. First, the exercise itself makes the body more efficient in metabolizing sugar, so blood sugar doesn't get as high. Second and most important, exercise helps create the lean state that scares diabetes away. Adult onset diabetes (now called Type II diabetes) is the most common kind, and for this problem exercise and weight control is often the only treatment needed. For the Type I diabetic, who requires insulin, some benefit of exercise exists but the fundamental problem of needing extra insulin will persist.

A high level of cholesterol in the blood is a serious risk factor in heart disease and in stroke. The artery plugging, called atherosclerosis, is composed of deposits of cholesterol. It has recently been discovered that exercise sufficient to produce cardiovascular conditioning causes a slight decrease in low density and very low density lipoproteins, which are the cholesterol fractions in the blood that have been shown to produce atherosclerosis in man and in experimental animals. This change was also associated with a large fall in plasma triglyceride levels since this blood lipid is carried in the very low density fraction. It has also been established that exercise increased another cholesterol fraction, the high density lipoproteins. This high density fraction is associated with lowered cardiovascular death rates. The greater the proportion of high density lipoproteins in the blood, the greater protection one has against developing atherosclerosis. Research studies have led to the idea that high density fraction is the body's own roto-rooter systems for shuttling cholesterol out of tissues, including arteries, and back to the liver where it gets broken down. One can conclude that exercise is in fact a protective device available to the human body against atherosclerotic pollution.

We like to say that life in the 1980s is full of tension and that ours is a particularly stressful time to be living. We don't know if that is true. We suspect all generations of mankind have had their share of stresses. Ours, however, is probably the noisiest and certainly the most chaotic. Clearly, stress does exist and it is something very real that each of us must cope with. Stress creates feelings of anxiety which create muscle tension. Learning to relax those muscles is an antidote to stress. We now know that a more powerful drug than tranquilizers is exercise. One study measured muscle tension at two different times in stress-affected adults and showed that a 15-minute walk produced a greater change in muscle tension than a tranquilizing pill.

Exercise provides many psychological benefits. It improves body image and makes one feel more attractive to others. It generates more energy for daily living and improves one's general sense of well-being. It makes people feel happier. It reduces the feelings of stress, tension, and pressure associated with daily life. And most important, exercise makes people feel that they are

in charge of their own health. It gives them the satisfying sense that they are doing something positive every day to improve and maintain their good health, the natural condition for living. Recently, we have been bombarded by advertisements claiming that calcium pills can prevent thinning of the bones (osteoporosis) which particularly affects thinner women and which becomes more severe following the menopause. Such is the consumer response that calcium supplements have even been added to antacids and breakfast cereals. Less publicity has been given to exercise, even 20-minute daily walks, as a preventive measure. The public should know that the benefits of increasing dietary calcium (using nonfat milk so as to avoid artery clogging from butterfat) are additive to the effects of exercise in producing stronger bones that help prevent bone fractures of older adults. Exercise works by providing repetitive mechanical forces to the bone through muscle contraction. Even ordinary household activity as well as walking and gardening are enough to keep bones healthy. Older people need active encouragement and opportunities to avoid the calcium loss resulting from inactivity. This loss is particularly severe during prolonged bed rest or after immobilization of any part of the body.

The best exercise should require continuous exertion, rather than frequent stops and starts. The intensity should remain about the same throughout the exercise period. Examples of uninterrupted exertion are best seen in running, walking, swimming, and bicycling where the intensity can be held constant. Tennis, basketball, and calisthenics, for example, are less suitable because of the frequent stops and starts and changes of exertion intensity. Ideally, one should exercise at least three times a week for at least 15 to 20 minutes. As a general rule, the less intense activity of walking should be done daily and for 30 to 50 minutes, whereas more intense activities, such as jogging, are better done every other day and for 20 to 40 minutes. The activity level should be sufficient to make you feel "almost tired" while exercising; enough to produce sweating and to reach the magical aerobic goal of exercise at 50% to 85% of your "maximum aerobic capacity" (the punishing level reached in exercise electrocardiogram tests on treadmills). Pulse rate goals and intensity of exercise should be lower for older people, leading again to walking as an excellent way to go for those aged 50 and above.

An exciting new concept, as yet quite unproven, is that exercise may actually prevent rather than cause the kind of arthritis called "osteoarthritis" previous thought to be partly due to "wear and tear." This novel thinking is that a certain amount of exercise is *beneficial* to the health of the cartilage surfaces of joints. Evidence for this is based on an apparent higher rate of osteoarthritis among sedentary as compared to active people. The flow in the studies is that a self-selection bias may be present; those with early symptoms of arthritis may "slow down." This argument therefore pits exercise as a potential destructive force against a role as a constructive force in cartilage and joint function.

If the "pro-exercise" argument wins, it will be another bonus. If the "anti" argument wins, it will lead toward low impact activities (swimming, bicycling, walking) as preferred over higher impact activities (jogging). Avoidance of hard surfaces and use of well-padded shoes will still be advised, no matter how the argument is resolved, as measures needed to make us comfortable and to avoid some of the tendon injuries that runners experience.

The important factor in establishing exercise in one's life is to keep the resolve long enough to get hooked. After exercise becomes a comfortable necessity for one's well-being, one can be faithful to meeting that need. Personal behavior is the only trustworthy source of disease prevention.

Remember this. Exercise is to fitness as caring is to love. The one begets the other. To love, to work, to feel good means living life to the fullest. From the physician's point of view, it's better to prevent a disease than to try to cure it. From a fellow's point of view, it's more wonderful to tap into the universe with energy than to close down in disease.

Now is the time to close this book, put on your shoes, and go out for a nice, brisk walk.

23

EXERCISE AND REDUCED RISK OF CORONARY HEART DISEASE

Ralph S. Paffenbarger, Jr., M.D., is professor of epidemiology at Stanford University. He studies the determinants of disease in large population groups. Previously concerned with identifying the means by which poliomyelitis and other infectious diseases were transmitted, he now confines his research to chronic disease, including heart disease and cancer. He is particularly interested in identifying personal characteristics and lifestyle elements that affect life expectancy and reduce the risk of developing coronary heart disease.

Robert T. Hyde, M.A., is an epidemiologist with the Stanford University School of Medicine. He has been studying host and environmental influences on chronic diseases, seeking to identify trends, associations, and causal relationships of personal characteristics and lifestyles elements and their effect on health, aging, and longevity.

For 22 years, Dr. Ralph Paffenbarger monitored the strenuous work of longshoremen on San Francisco loading docks. He discovered that cargohandlers suffered half as many heart attacks as their less active supervisors. They were also more likely to survive heart attacks than sedentary workers. Robert Hyde and Dr. Paffenbarger review various studies of occupational groups and the evidence that lifelong vigorous exercise habits, whether on the job or at home, may prevent coronary heart and extend longevity. The authors note that this beneficial effect is only associated with year-round strenuous activity, not with sporadic or seasonal efforts, but that the effects of exercise are at least partially independent of the influences of smoking, hypertension, and obesity.▪

Since ancient times exercise has been recognized as being important to the preservation of sound health and good mood, and its influences on various body systems have long been postulated. Hippocrates warned against both the lack of exercise and overexertion. Ramazzini noted that seventeenth-century tailors sitting cross-legged on the floor all day developed ailments escaped by fleet-footed messengers. English poet John Dryden declared that sportsplay afield far better medicine than any "naseous draught" prescribed by eighteenth-century physicians. Nineteenth-century studies of British mortality data by Guy and Smith corroborated these observations in a somewhat more methodical fashion.

Thus the early lore of healthful exercise can be documented, but only in our present century has scientific evidence for the benefits of adequate physical activity been obtained. When modes of transportation and labor shifted from muscle to machine, many patterns of habitual exercise were drastically reduced. Automation and electronics further hastened the trend toward unprecedented sedentariness among large populations. The public health implications of this situation became more visible as other new developments cut down infectious disease incidence. Research interest began to focus on coronary heart disease, which had been clinically defined by J.B. Herrick in 1912. Later, as statistics rose to alarming levels, heart attacks were termed "a twentieth-century epidemic," "executive's disease," and the like. In 1939, O.F. Hedley published an analysis of 5116 deaths from cardiovascular disease in Philadelphia between 1933 and 1937. Rates were higher among managers and professional men than among laborers, but the contrast was not attributed to differences in exercise. Important relationships of physical activity levels and coronary heart disease were yet to be recognized.

For some time, indeed, strenuous activity was considered bad for the heart, but by the 1950s, Paul Dudley White of Boston was advocating regular exercise as a preventative against heart attack. He personally led a bicycling crusade for young and old. When his most famous patient, President Eisenhower, was recovering from a myocardial infarction, White advised him to resume golf. White also contributed to reports on the heart of marathoner Clarence DeMar and to a 1958 study of former football players. Of the latter he said, "The most interesting findings concerned the amount of exercise taken habitually during the lifetime of these men. Those in coronary group engaged in less vigorous exercise than did the others, and no individual in this study who maintained a heavy exercise program happened to develop coronary disease."

A detailed 1957 monograph by Montoye and associates at Michigan State University analyzed the characteristics and health histories of 628 of 1129 former athletes who had earned letters there prior to 1938. Using a 1950 questionnaire designed for a never-completed national survey of athleticism, morbidity, and longevity, this pilot case/control study tackled many provocative questions but was too diversified to reach firm conclusions. A 1977 follow-up found that athletic status might extend life span. Surviving athletes and controls tended to have a history of more years of sportsplay than did decedents.

The accepted landmark study documenting the inverse relationship of habitual physical activity and coronary heart disease was published in England in 1953 by Professor J.N. Morris and associates. Among London busmen, active conductors had fewer heart attacks than their sedentary drivers. Morris conducted further studies of these men and of the leisure exercise and coronary heart disease patterns among thousands of British civil servants. The findings repeatedly supported his provisional hypothesis that "Physical activity of work is a protection against ischaemic heart disease. Men in physically active jobs have less ischaemic heart disease during middle age, what disease they have is less severe, and they tend to develop it later than similar men in physically inactive jobs."

Global concern about heart attacks was so great that Morris's views drew quick attention. Many other studies were soon underway. Letter carriers were compared with sorting clerks, farmers with city businessmen, railroad truck walkers with dispatchers, cargohandlers with warehousemen, active Israeli kibbutzim workers with those less active. Most reports showed inverse relationships of physical activity level and heart attack rate—but some did not. Definitions and methods of determining exercise levels varied widely. Confounding influences of cigarette smoking, blood lipid profile, dietary habits, socioeconomic status, and other characteristics were being overlooked or overplayed. When the interactions of important variables such as these were not appropriately taken into account, findings were likely to be inconclusive, misleading, or missed altogether. Justified criticisms (and some less admirable) were soon advanced. Out of all this came much confusion, but also improved study programs, better understanding of problems, more sophisticated analyses, and a greater respect for the social implications of what soon became known as the "exercise revolution." Not only White and Morris but many other epidemiologic investigators of patterns of coronary heart disease became sportsplay evangelists urging revision of exercise habits of sedentary individuals. Some promoted marathons, some developed formulas for aerobic exertion, some published programs of various kinds of fitness, and some established clinics and salons for physical rehabilitation.

It may never be clear, however, whether the extraordinary boom in personal sports activity and health consciousness observed since 1970 actually resulted from such medical leadership or sprang spontaneously from other causes. Perhaps the human species that evolved from eons of required physical agility could not adapt immediately to the sedentary pattern of modern occupations. If so, the twentieth century urge to ski, swim, run, and cycle, hike, climb, sail, skydive, bowl, do gymnastics, pump iron, disco-dance, aerobicize, et cetera, may have sprung from an instinctive urge to be physically active. Such may be the most likely explanation of why this modern enthusiasm for exercise is emerging as a bona fide social upheaval and not a mere fad. Fortunately, it has been accompanied by several fringe benefits such as reduction in cigarette smoking, revision of diet, improved health awareness, and better health care. Many observers now believe this trend of recreational activity will continue into the twenty-first century and will have lasting effects.

REPRESENTATIVE STUDIES

Here it is appropriate to summarize a few representative contemporary studies and their implications. In the aggregate they do afford considerably understanding, although all show that the door is still wide open for further research. Many questions remain as to the type, frequency, duration, and intensity of exercise that should be recommended for various individuals. The mechanisms by which exercise produces its beneficial effects are very much under study. Methods of assessing physical activity are still being developed and in turn are dependent on answers to problems of definition and measurement.

Occupational Physical Activity

Studies of occupational physical activity have been based on job categories, job descriptions, simple or complex questionnaires and interviews, or measurements and estimates of energy output. One of the more intensive was a 22-year study of 3686 San Francisco longshoremen who worked long hours at heavy jobs in the warehouses, wharves, and shipholds on the waterfront. These men were given a multiphasic screening examination in 1951 and evaluated in 1972. Their exercise levels were assessed on the basis of energy output measurements on actual job tasks, plus union records of their work assignments, which were checked annually. Coronary heart disease mortality rates were computed from official death certificates and man-years of observation.

Longshoremen working as cargohandlers expended over 8500 Kcal/week, in contrast to warehousemen and checkers who had less demanding jobs. However, union rules required all men entering the industry to serve as cargohandlers for at least 5 years; the average was 13 years, and many continued in that category. Therefore, regardless of job assignment, few if any preselected weaklings were likely to have been present in the starting population of the study.

During the 22-year period there were 395 deaths from coronary heart disease (11%), but the rate per 10,000 man-years for cargohandlers was about half that of their less active fellow workers. The cargohandlers had much lower risk of sudden death from heart attack, whether because they were less likely to have an attack or more likely to survive one. Since sudden deaths would be less often heralded by premonitory symptoms conducive to a shift to an easier job assignment, this contrast in rates is not readily ascribed to self-selection. All in all, the longshoremen study presented strong evidence of the benefits of exercise for cardiovascular health.

Factoring out age, cigarette smoking, obesity, higher blood pressure, and history of coronary heart disease, it was confirmed that the risk of fatal heart attack was lowered progressively as work energy output on the job increased from 4750 to 9500 Kcal/week, being halved when output was twice the baseline level. A sampling check had shown that recreational exercise by the longshoremen was minimal compared to their unusually high physical activity at work. The beneficial effect of cargohandling job status was greatest at the younger ages but evident at all ages. Shifting trends, including changes in technology such as mechanization and containerization, are some reasons why the protective effect of vigorous exercise at work was seen chiefly in the younger two of the four 10-year cohorts born between 1877 and 1916. As demands for muscle power on the job continued to diminish, recreational exercise habits would become as important for longshoremen as for workers in traditionally sedentary occupations. The effects of historical changes such as these may be considered further evidence for the inverse relationship of coronary heart disease and adequate exercise.

Recreational Physical Activity

Research under Morris in England surveyed effects of recreational exercise on the rate of coronary heart disease among workers whose desk jobs did not require nor even permit vigorous energy output. On a Monday morning 17,944 middle-aged men in the civil service were asked to log on a standard diary form their physical activities by 5-minute intervals for the preceding Friday and Saturday, constituting one work day and one leisure day. These detailed recall reports were subjected to extensive analysis along with 1138 first clinical attacks of coronary heart disease that occurred in the study population during 8.5 years of follow-up. Men who had reported vigorous leisure activity had an attack rate of 3.1%, in contrast to 6.9% for those lacking such exercise. Fatal first attack rates were 1.1% and 2.9% respectively, and of sudden deaths (that is, not preceded by sick leave) 0.65% and 1.60%. Similar results were found among retirees. Morris noted further that the rise of coronary heart disease morbidity with age occurred chiefly among men in the nonexercising groups, there being relatively little increase among men who reported engaging in vigorous physical activity such as sportsplay.

Meanwhile, in the United States a long-range study has been underway of recreational exercise and other favorable and unfavorable aspects of lifestyle in relation to chronic diseases, particularly coronary heart disease, and also to mortality and longevity. The data relate to some 50,000 former students from Harvard University and the University of Pennsylvania who entered college in the years 1916 to 1950. Records of their case-taking and physical examinations at matriculation have been obtained from the college archives, plus data from athletic files, follow-up examinations, personal questionnaires returned by alumni at various intervals since 1962 with the assistance of alumni offices, and official death certificates of decedents.

In effect, this body of information spans the experience of the twentieth century. The younger alumni represented are now in their 50s, the older survivors are in their 80s or 90s, and all have been the subjects of epidemiological reports for more than 25 years. The investigations have concerned their family health histories, their personal characteristics and athletic status of college days, their present-day exercise patterns and other habits, and their current health status, including physician-diagnosed coronary heart disease. These analyses have shown consistently that current and continuing adequate exercise, not history of hereditary vigor or youthful sportsplay, is related inversely to risk of coronary heart disease in all age ranges and various other subsets of these college alumni.

By the end of 1972 there were 572 first attacks of coronary heart disease among 16,936 Harvard alumni who had returned completed questionnaires in 1962 or 1966 and again in 1972. Rates per 10,000 man-years for the 6- to 10-year interval declined as energy expenditure increased, which was assessed by reported walking distance, stair climbing, sportsplay, and a composite physical activity index derived from the combination of those activities and totalled in kilocalories/week.

The index was intended to serve as an indicator rather than a measure of total energy expenditure. When a convenient breakpoint was chosen at 2000 Kcal/week, 60% of the man-years represented alumni who scored below that index level and had a 66% greater risk of coronary heart disease than the 40% whose exercise rated 2000 + Kcal/week. Risk continued to decrease as physical activity index increased to about 3500 Kcal/week, beyond which the influence of exercise appeared to stabilize.

That energy output is noticeably lower than was found for the San Francisco longshoremen at work, but when an appropriate allowance is assumed for occupational or other activities not included in the alumni index, the difference between the two populations in estimated total output is reduced. The remaining contrast might explain a divergence in sudden death patterns still under study, but otherwise the inverse association of exercise level and risk of coronary heart disease is paralleled in both populations, although the alumni findings are derived from subjective data and the longshoremen experience from objective measurements and records.

As in the longshoremen study, the Harvard alumni analyses included adjustment for various characteristics other than exercise—age, weight for height, net gain since college, cigarette smoking, history of hypertension, and parental history of coronary heart disease. The cardiovascular health advantage of continuing adequate exer-

cise held good over a wide range of lifestyles and at all ages studied. Coronary heart disease risk patterns were similar in each 10-year age group from 35 through 74 years, and the saving effect of current exercise was heightened by vigorous sportsplay (which seemed to taper off at about age 65). Alumni who engaged in strenuous activities plus at least 1000 additional Kcal/week of stair climbing, walking, and other light activities had less than half (42%) the coronary heart disease incidence of their nonathletic, sedentary classmates with low activity index.

Relative risks of first attack of nonfatal or fatal coronary heart disease are shown in Table 17-1 for the presence versus absence of each of five beneficial characteristics, adjusted for differences in age, follow-up interval, and each of the other characteristics listed. Thus, men with adequate exercise were at 67% of the risk for men less active; nonsmokers had 77% the risk of cigarette users; men who kept their weight for height at modest levels had 76% the risk of hypertensives; and men without parental history of coronary heart disease were at 78% the risk of men whose parents had such history.

TABLE 23-1

RELATIVE RISKS OF FIRST CORONARY HEART DISEASE ATTACK, FATAL OR NONFATAL, AMONG 16,936 HARVARD ALUMNI, 1962–1966–1972, BY PRESENCE/ABSENCE OF COUNTERING CHARACTERISTICS

Characteristic	Relative Risk* (1 SE)	P
Adequate exercise**	67%(0.08)	<0.001
Nonsmoker	77%(0.08)	0.016
Limited body mass #	76%(0.08)	0.010
Normotensive ##	43%(0.06)	<0.001
No parental CHD /-	78%(0.09)	0.024

* Risk with characteristics as % of risk without characteristic, adjusted for age, followup interval, and each of the other characteristics listed.
** Physical activity index = at least 2000 Kcal/week.
# Less than 20% over 1959 MLIC standards.
No physician-diagnosed hypertension.
/- Alumnus questionnaire reported.

Whether assessed positively or negatively, each of the five characteristics contributes independently to coronary heart disease risk. The impact of adverse traits is estimated by their respective attributable risk percentages in Table 2. Hypertension is the strongest predictor clinically but the least prevalent. Sedentary lifestyle is the most prevalent and contributes the greatest share to risk of coronary heart disease in the community or population of alumni. The clinical risks are not additive, but if adverse levels of all five characteristics could be eliminated in the community, first attacks of coronary heart disease among the alumni might be cut by 67%. In comparison, the longshoremen might have achieved an 88% reduction by eliminating low work activity, cigarette smoking, and hypertension.

With increasing interest in athletic energy output as a regimen for maintenance of cardiovascular health, attention has sharpened on both the benefits and the hazards of endurance exercise (Table 23-3), which has been defined as "sus-

TABLE 23-2.

CLINICAL AND COMMUNITY ATTRIBUTABLE RISKS OF FIRST CORONARY HEART DISEASE ATTACK, FATAL OR NONFATAL, AMONG 16,936 HARVARD ALUMNI, 1962-1966-1972, BY PRECEDING CHARACTERISTICS

| Characteristic | Prevalence % | Attributable Risk* of CHD, % | |
		Clinical	Community
Sedentary**	61	33	23
Cigarette user	52	23	13
Obese category #	38	24	11
Hypertensive #	9	57	10
Parental CHD history /-	39	22	10

* Theoretical risk attached to presence of adverse characteristic over risk in its absence. Adjusted for differences in age, followup interval, and each of the other characteristics listed. the other characteristics listed.
** Physical activity index = 2000 Kcal/week.
\# 20% over 1959 MLIC standards.
\#\# Physician-diagnosed.
/- Alumnus questionnaire reported, either or both parents.

tained, rhythmic, large-muscle movement for 30 or more minutes, at three-quarters estimated maximum heart rate, four or more times weekly." Basic precautions for this exercise are: (1) avoid unaccustomed strain on an untrained system, (2) start slowly, (3) exercise prudently, and (4) taper off.

As the table shows, neither the benefits nor the hazards of exercise are limited to the cardiovascular system. For an average individual the benefits are likely to be spread over nearly all body systems, while hazards might affect chiefly a weakest point, such as skeletal porosity in the elderly person. Overstress is unwise for anyone but is especially inadvisable in the presence of known or probable cardiovascular abnormalities. Body thermal and psychologic excesses may be more subtle in onset than musculoskeletal or cardiorespiratory overstress events, but they too are very common and should be avoided.

Recent Supporting Studies

In Norway, risk of coronary heart disease among all Oslo men aged 40 to 49, and a 7% random sample aged 20 to 39, was studied relative to both occupational and leisure-time physical activity. A 1975 report by Leren and associates showed that risk was higher for men who were physically active at work than for sedentary job holders more active in their leisure time. While the former might be blue-collar class and the latter white-collar men with other contrasts in lifestyle, a suggestion is offered that leisure-time exercise may be more beneficial than job-required exertion because it can be selected and performed to suit the health needs of the individual.

Kannel and Sorlie in 1979 described the results of a 14-year follow-up of 1909 men and 2311 women in the Framingham Heart Study. This involved a predominantly sedentary population assessed by a brief interview questionnaire regarding hours of rest and occupational and leisure activity classed as light, moderate, or heavy and weighted as to estimated oxygen consumption needed. This approach resembled the Harvard alumni study, but perhaps from lack of contrasts the findings as to exercise were not impressive or uniform. Coronary heart disease mortality was related inversely to exercise index level in the men but not in the women. However, the investigators recommended development of vigorous habits as a counter to aging tendencies.

In 1980 Dawber reassessed the data with similar conclusions.

In 1979 Magnus and associates reported on a case-control study of walking, cycling, gardening, and first attacks of coronary heart disease, conducted in Holland from 1970 to 1974. Interviews

TABLE 23-3.

BENEFITS AND HAZARDS OF ENDURANCE EXERCISE WITH REGARD TO CORONARY HEART DISEASE AND OTHER CHRONIC DISEASES

Body Systems Involved	Beneficial Effects	Potential Hazards
Cardiovascularrespiratory	Enhances physical work capacity, hemodynamic function, hematologic action, and cardiovascular fitness Reduced risks of hypertensive-atherosclerotic disease Increase maximum breathing capacity	Increases risk of sudden death in overstressed susceptible individuals Initiates asthmatic attacks Contraindicated for paitents with acute coronary occlusion, acute myocardial infarction, myocarditis, dissecting aneurysm, severe aortic stenosis, or uncontrolled hypertension
Endocrinemetabolic	Stimulates metabolic processes Influences hormone production Decreases fat body mass and increases lean body mass Improves plasma lipid and lipo-protein fraction profiles Enhances fibrinolytic activity Reduces risk of adult-onset diabetes	Induces temperature imbalance (effects of hyperthermia)
Musculoskeletal	Enlarges and strengthens muscle fibers Increases oxygen utiliztion Strengthens connective tissues Eases low back pain syndrome Retards osteoporosis Reduces rheumatoid- and osteo-arthritic trends (?)	Produces acute and chronic injuries of cartilage, muscle and bone Falling injuries "Overuse syndrome" Induces traumatic arthritis (?)
Gastrointestinal	Promotes peristaltic and mixing action of intestine Shortens enteric passage time Modifies appetite	Induces electrolyte imbalance
Neurologic	Influences neuromyocardial action Enhances mood, thought, and psychological behavior	Initiates dysrhythmia Induces compulsive-reactive syndrome (?)

This research supported by Grant #'s HL24133 and HL34174 of NHLBI, U.S. Health Service, Marathon Oil Foundation with 473 patients or survivors and 875 controls free of coronary heart disease in 1972 assessed physical activity as habitual (9 + months per year), seasonal (4 to 8 months), or occasional (less than 4 months), and by hours per week. Only habitual exercise associated inversely with coronary heart disease attack, and hours per week and intensity of effort showed no added effect. Death within 4 weeks of attack was most frequent among the occasionally active group. An implication is that cardiovascular health maintenance requires year-round exercise, and benefits may be lost by months of inadequate activity.

An extensive structured interview was used by Karvonen and associates in a 15-year follow-up extending Finnish observations originated in the Seven Countries Study. Sedentary habits and atherosclerotic trends were definitely associated by prevalence in men aged 50 to 69. Coronary heart disease mortality and total mortality were inversely related to physical activity among 1310 men if they had been diagnosed with the disease at the beginning of a 5-year study; otherwise, total mortality showed no relation to exercise level in this 1982 report.

An 8.5-year study by Garcia-Palmieri and associates in Puerto Rico of 2585 farmers and 6208 townsmen aged 45 to 65 found a strong inverse relation between exercise level and coronary heart disease risk. These conclusions, issued in 1982, paralleled those described earlier for the British civil servants, San Francisco dock workers, and Harvard alumni. Highest activity lowered risk for nonsmokers but increased it for cigarette smokers. Otherwise, exercise effect was independent of other influences. The results for exercise in this study were of special interest because the incidence rate of coronary heart disease in Puerto Rico is only half as high as on the mainland. The investigators considered vigorous activity to be a long-time custom in rural areas of the island.

Pomrehn and associates studied 62,000 deaths in Iowa in 1982 among men aged 20 to 64. Coronary heart disease mortality was about 10% lower in physically active farmers than in non-farmers or townspeople. The favorable effects of exercise on diet, body composition, tread-mill fitness, HDL-cholesterol level, and personal habits were also noted in a sample population. The farmers were healthier despite higher caloric intake, which they evidently needed because of their higher physical activity. These findings suggest that a diet matched to a vigorous exercise program is preferable to reduction of energy intake without adequate exercise.

Results of bicycle ergometer tests required of 2779 firemen and law officers of Los Angeles County in 1983 were used by Peters and associates to study thus-measured physical fitness and risk of myocardial infarction during an average follow-up of 5 years and a total of 13,317 man-years. The men aged 35 to 54 were divided by median levels of fitness, blood pressure, serum cholesterol, weight and body composition measures, habitual physical activity, smoking, and family history of heart disease. Men below median fitness had more than twice the likelihood of having an infarction, but these men also usually had higher blood pressure and cholesterol and the smoking habit, combinations of which increased their risk up to six times.

Risk of sudden death from heart attack was markedly lower among vigorously active men in England and San Francisco, though such a benefit was less evident among the Harvard alumni. In Seattle in 1982, Siscovick and associates found the probability of primary cardiac arrest was lower by more than 50% among persons whose habitual recreational exercise reached at least 60% of maximum oxygen uptake, in contrast to persons lacking such intensive activity.

A 7-year study in 1982 by Salonen and associates in Finland of 7666 men and women aged 30 to 59 showed that relative risks of acute myocardial infarction for low versus high physical activity at work were 1.5 for men and 2.4 for women. The risk of stroke and other causes of death were also altered. Results for leisure-time exercise were less consistent, perhaps being more subject to confounding influences. Data were adjusted for differences in age, cholesterol, blood pressure, height, body mass, and smoking. However, adjustments for cholesterol may have factored out some of the influence of exercise instead of revealing it, since exercise alters cholesterol profile.

SUMMARY OF CONSIDERATIONS

In the past 30 years, epidemiological and other investigations have gathered strong evidence that the inverse association of adequate contemporary exercise and coronary heart disease risk signifies a genuine protective effect that reduces incidence of the disease. Among the important observations supporting this view are the following:

1. Findings of reduced risk of nonfatal or fatal coronary heart disease relate to both occupational and leisure-time exercise, including various kinds of physical work activity, walking, sportsplay, programmed aerobic and endurance exertion, and so on. Risk reduced because of energy output at any level is further reduced if the exercise pattern at that level includes vigorous activity or successive peaks of strenuous exertion.

2. The beneficial effect of exercise is dose-dependent over a considerable range of practical effort, in which increased energy expenditure progressively lowers coronary heart disease morbidity, recurrence, case-fatality, and mortality.

3. Findings are similar in subsets established by age, sex, other personal or lifestyle characteristics, or by clinical category of disease, i.e., angina pectoris, myocardial infarction, sudden unexpected death, or total death from coronary heart disease.

4. The beneficial effect is associated with contemporary, year-round activity rather than prior, sporadic, or seasonal effort; therefore, it requires a maintenance of cardiovascular health and physical fitness that is dose-dependent to appropriate levels. The process functions through many systems of the body, as physical activity not only improves cardiopulmonary fitness but favorably alters biochemical and physiological processes such as blood lipid profiles, fibrinolytic activity, endocrinologic influences, and hematologic action.

5. Findings persist in successive increments of time and in varied populations and circumstances.

6. The observed effects of exercise are at least partially independent of the influences of other host and environmental characteristics, e.g., smoking, hypertension, weight-for-height, prior disease status, family history of coronary heart disease, etc.

7. Risk of coronary heart disease is increased in formerly active individuals if they do not continue sufficient vigorous exercise through their adult years. Conversely, persons formerly sedentary acquire decreased risk if they take up habitual adequate exercise as adults.

8. Although appropriate exercise does benefit all systems of the body, its influence against hypertensive arteriosclerotic diseases appears to be paramount. Comparatively little evidence of relationships to other causes of death has been found so far, despite a clear inverse association of physical activity level and all-cause mortality. Be that as it may, further study of exercise processes is surely warranted.

9. Studies of exercise, diet, and atherosclerotic patterns in primates have furnished direct experimental evidence that long-term moderate exercise inhibits the development of coronary heart disease.

24 WHICH SPORT IS FOR YOU?

Joan Ullyot, M.D., is a sports medicine specialist and a nationally ranked masters distance runner. A graduate of Wellesley College and Harvard Medical School, she is a well-known lecturer and consultant on physical fitness, sports injuries, and women in sports. Dr. Ullyot has written three books about running, and she serves as the women's editor for *Runner's World* and as medical editor for *Women's Sports and Fitness* magazine.

Few of us should attempt to scale Mount Everest or play professional football. Even long-distance running is beyond the realm of most potential athletes. But we can all enjoy vigorous exercise—if we choose appropriate activities. Sports provide enormous psychological and social benefits. They should also be fun for the individual. The trick is in finding a sport that strengthens your cardiovascular system, enhances your social life, and relieves tension and anxiety. Joan Ullyot examines the physical and psychological benefits of aerobic exercise and how you can build a fulfilling personal fitness program that is guaranteed to bring vim and vigor back into your life.■

The human body is built for movement. Our legs are suited for walking and running, our arms for catching, holding, throwing. It is natural then for us to crave physical activity, and we see this impulse expressed in children's spontaneous games. Tag, dodgeball, and kick the can all involve plenty of running and movement, and all are done for fun.

As we grow older, such play is frowned upon. We turn to more serious—and usually more sedentary—pursuits. Our bodies are denied their natural action, and our psyches suffer as a result. But adults gradually learn that they feel better if they make time in their lives for recreation—a time to relax, enjoy vigorous movement, and thus "recreate" their natural selves.

Sports have evolved over the centuries in response to this human need, and they are most important in those populations which have sufficient leisure time to play and socialize. There is little sport in wartime or in those societies where backbreaking toil is needed to earn a living. But even in such adverse circumstances, the psychosocial benefits of sport are sought under the guise of drinking, socializing, even watching others play. The popularity of spectator sports—football, soccer, hockey etc.—rests on this universal impulse toward recreation.

Not all forms of sport and exercise are equally beneficial to our bodies. Some of the most enjoyable sports in terms of mental relaxation and socializing—for instance, bowling or golf—are widely practiced but do little for physical fitness. Such sports lack the vigorous movement that our bodies crave. Conversely, there are many sports which are very demanding physically but which do not promote health, such as sailing and weightlifting. There is no single ideal sport. So how do you choose the right sport for yourself? First you must decide upon your personal fitness goals.

The various benefits sought from sport include the psychosocial—relaxation, sociability, and enjoyment—and the purely physical—cardiovascular fitness and endurance, muscular strength, coordination, and flexibility. Of these desirable physical benefits, only cardiovascular fitness and endurance are considered vital to optimum health. Sports that promote these benefits are called aerobic (with oxygen), a term coined by Dr. Kenneth Cooper (in his 1968 book, *Aerobics*) to emphasize that such activities require and promote the utilization of large amounts of oxygen.

Research in exercise physiology in the past 30 years has shown that the best single physiological indicator of fitness is the ability to utilize oxygen. In everyday terms, a person with high aerobic capacity is able to perform work (or sport) for longer periods of time without undue fatigue and at a lower effort level (measured by heart rate) than an unfit person. Thus, fitness correlates well with a subjective feeling of strength and energy.

But aerobic fitness is now recognized as important to optimum health as well as physical work capacity. As little as 20 minutes of jogging three times a week has beneficial effects on the body's fat and cholesterol metabolism, lowering blood fats (triglycerides) and raising the percentage of HDL cholesterol associated with lowered risk of coronary heart disease. Epidemiological studies by Dr. Ralph Paffenbarger have shown a direct correlation of vigorous exercise (equivalent to jogging about 3 miles per day) with lower incidence of stroke and heart attacks.

Exercise also serves as a major method of weight control, because muscular activity burns calories. There is considerable evidence that aerobic activities regularly performed for an hour or so also enhance the body's ability to metabolize fat, which is utilized as fuel in endurance sports. Therefore, doctors recommend such sports, in conjunction with a moderate reducing diet, for permanent weight loss. Pounds lost by exercise are pounds of fat, whereas pounds shed by diet alone are mostly water and muscle.

Almost as important to health as these physical benefits of aerobic exercise are the psychological benefits. Sports like running have been called positive addictions because they soon become a daily necessity for one's optimum mental health. Psychological studies vividly show that habitual exercisers feel less anxiety and tension and experience improved self-esteem and optimism after their daily workout. So vivid are these effects that some psychiatrists use running as an important therapy for depression. It has been suggested that this mood elevation induced by regular, rhythmic exercise is caused by the rise in serum endorphin levels. Whatever their physiological basis, the psychological effects of fitness are beneficial and real.

Because of these diverse health benefits, aerobic sports (such as running, bicycling, or swimming) are the most desirable for basic recreation. But there are numerous goals besides improved health that can be achieved in sport. Individuals in pursuit of a perfectly sculptured body, a better slap shot, or the relaxation that only a fishing trip can provide must supplement their aerobic sport with other activities tailored to their own needs. In this context, the accompanying chart rating the recreational values of various sports should prove useful. Keep in mind, however, that the aerobic component is the only one vital to optimum health. (See table 24-1.)

As a practical matter, how much aerobic exercise is enough? How frequently, how intensely, and for how long should you work out? To a large extent, the answer depends on the sport you choose. But there is general agreement among doctors and exercise experts that health and fitness can be improved and maintained by a very moderate amount of aerobic exercise, provided it is done regularly.

To qualify as aerobic, the exercise must cause a steady elevation of the pulse above a minimum level (dependent on age) of 110 to 140 beats per minute. In practice, this level of exertion translates to a "perceived effort" sufficient to cause deep breathing and sweating (after the first 5 to 8 minutes) without great discomfort. Experts disagree about how much of this exercise is enough, but their recommendations range from a low of 20 minutes every other day to an hour every day. The advantage of exercising daily rather than every other day is that it's easier to incorporate into the daily schedule and harder to skip or get the days mixed up. After all, you wouldn't brush your teeth every other day.

Given these general guidelines, which exercise is best for you? First, if there's any exercise you are currently doing and enjoy, get a copy of Dr.

Kenneth Cooper's *New Aerobics* or *The Aerobics Way* and find out how much your chosen exercise is worth in terms of "points." You need about 30 of these points weekly, distributed over at least 4 days, to become fit and stay that way. Since points are awarded for a combination of duration and intensity factors, you'll need many hours of aerobically less demanding sports, such as golf, to get the same number of points earned by 20 minutes of jogging.

The number one criterion for choosing your sport is to do something you enjoy enough to do *regularly*. The next consideration is practicality: do you have enough time and are facilities available? Cross-country skiing is terrific aerobic exercise, but it doesn't work during summer months or in Florida. If you have a pool in your yard or a nearby bike trail, you're in luck. City dwellers are more limited in their options, which accounts for the popularity of jogging in New York's Central Park: it's accessible, cheap, and about all there is!

The "Big Three" of aerobic exercises, according to Cooper, are bicycling, swimming, and running or jogging. These sports give you your needed points in the shortest amount of time when performed at a moderate level. (Tennis, which is often more strenuous, is done in short bursts rather than steadily, so it ranks much lower in aerobic benefit. Hours of play are the equivalent of a short run.)

Whereas swimming requires a pool and bicycling a vehicle (and preferably bike paths as well), only good shoes are needed for jogging. This economy and convenience (you can run almost anywhere), plus its high aerobic point value, make jogging one of the most popular sports for men and women of all ages. But women just beginning to exercise, as well as many older people, may be hesitant about jogging. They feel a little silly, perhaps, or would rather stroll through the woods at a more leisurely pace rather than dash along attracting attention. This is fine; walking is excellent exercise. But you need to spend more time on it than on jogging. An hour of jogging daily at a pace of 15 minutes per mile (fairly brisk) will enable you to cover 4 miles and earn 7 aerobic points. If you're ambling along more slowly, tak-

TABLE 24-1.

ACTIVITIES AND SPORTS RATING CHART

	Aerobic Fitness	Muscular Strength	Coordination	Flexibility	Relaxation	Accessibility	Economy	Safety	Sociability	Family Involvement
Archery	2	5	5	5	6	2	4	9	5	4
Badminton	6	6	8	6	4	5	6	4	7	5
Baseball	4	5	6	6	3	4	5	8	6	4
Basketball	8	6	7	6	3	5	8	7	5	1
Billiards/Pool/Darts	1	2	5	2	9	6	5	9	9	3
Bowling	2	3	5	2	6	6	7	9	8	2
Boxing	10	10	8	6	1	5	8	1	4	1
Canoeing	7	9	6	7	3	2	3	4	6	2
Cricket	4	5	8	5	6	5	3	5	9	6
Cycling	10	9	6	3	9	9	4	4	4	9
Dancing	7	8	9	10	10	8	6	6	10	2
Fencing	5	9	9	9	6	3	4	3	6	4
Fishing	1	1	3	1	10	8	6	10	4	7
Football (American)	5	10	6	3	2	2	5	1	3	2
Football (soccer)	6	9	8	6	5	5	6	3	7	3
Golf	4	3	7	5	6	6	8	2	7	6
Gymnastics	2	9	10	10	8	3	7	2	3	1
Hockey (field)	6	6	6	6	5	3	7	6	7	3

Activity										
Hockey (ice)	8	6	10	9	8	3	4	3	4	8
Judo/Karate	3	6	9	9	6	5	7	2	6	8
Lacrosse	8	9	8	8	6	2	7	6	6	1
Mountaineering	7	10	8	5	4	2	3	1	6	3
Orienteering	6	7	7	2	6	6	7	6	5	3
Riding (horse)	2	7	7	2	8	4	2	3	6	8
Rowing	10	10	6	2	6	2	3	6	8	1
Rugby	6	9	6	2	4	2	6	2	9	2
Running	10	9	3	3	8	10	7	5	5	4
Sailing	2	6	6	2	9	1	1	3	8	8
Skating (ice)	5	5	10	8	8	2	3	2	5	9
Skating (roller)	5	5	9	8	9	7	7	3	3	9
Skiing (cross-country)	10	9	8	7	6	2	2	4	2	5
Skiing (downhill)	5	8	9	8	8	2	1	2	9	9
Skipping	9	4	6	3	9	9	10	8	1	8
Squash	6	7	9	7	3	5	6	4	5	5
Swimming	10	10	9	9	9	6	7	8	2	10
Table Tennis	5	3	8	5	6	5	7	7	6	8
Tennis	6	8	8	6	6	7	5	6	7	7
Volleyball	7	9	9	7	5	6	8	7	5	2
Walking (Brisk)	6	3	2	2	9	10	10	10	6	9
Water Skiing	3	9	8	2	5	2	2	2	4	4
Weight lifting	2	10	8	5	2	7	7	5	3	2
Climbing Stairs	8	5	7	6	2	10	10	9	1	0
Do-it-yourself repairs	3	3	2	5	7	10	7	8	2	6
Gardening	6	6	6	6	9	7	8	9	1	7
Housework	3	5	2	5	3	10	10	10	1	10

ing 1 hour and 20 minutes or more to cover the 4 miles, you'll only earn 4 points and will have to spend more time getting your total of 30 for the week. The choice is yours. Many walkers compromise: they wear good running shoes for walking, and by inserting short jogs (1 minute or so) into their walk every 5 minutes, such people keep their heart rate up in the beneficial range and do their daily stint fast enough to chalk up more points.

The same considerations apply to cycling and swimming. If you have plenty of time, you can go along at a more leisurely pace, whereas if time is limited, you have to work harder. Those who have never learned to enjoy the sensations of moving along briskly, on foot or by bike, with heart pumping strongly and the warm glow of perspiration making them feel well oiled like a fine car, may never learn what fitness is until they retire. Then, with days of leisure available, they can get out in the fresh air, walk or bicycle ever farther afield, and by sheer duration of activity achieve better conditioning.

A few hints for those who choose to swim or bike: you have to swim steadily for at least 15 minutes, not just paddle around and socialize in the club pool. If your neighborhood pool is too crowded for lap swimming, it's not a good place for an aerobic workout. Cyclists seeking aerobic benefits need not be agile or coordinated enough to dash around on a fancy 10-speed model. I have seen several older men and women using adult tricycles to get around golf courses, explore bike paths, or even do their shopping.

But what does one do in winter to keep fit? Again, convenience and enjoyment determine the answer. When snow is on the ground, cross-country skiing is an obvious substitute for walking and jogging. It should be done for the same amount of time as your usual exercise. If you're a cyclist in the summer months and the roads become dangerous and the paths impassable in winter, try an exercise bicycle or a rowing or skiing machine indoors.

Boredom is the chief enemy of any exercise program. It is best avoided by getting out of doors and meeting with friends for your daily run, bike ride, or other workout. When you socialize on the go, you can forget about time and pace. Indoors, boredom can set in fast if you're staring at the walls or counting the seemingly endless minutes. You might try watching your favorite TV program or listening to music while you work out. I know one man who cycled himself into excellent aerobic condition during Monday Night Football.

Aerobic dancing is an increasingly popular indoor activity. It attempts to incorporate aerobic conditioning into a program that focuses more on muscle strengthening and flexibility than the classic aerobic trio of running, cycling, and swimming. Dance classes have the advantage of being inherently social. Despite the expense and inconvenience of taking a class, most people prefer working out in a group to dancing to the same music alone at home.

Vigorous and popular ball sports such as tennis, squash, handball, or racquetball are not as beneficial to health as their advocates often believe. Because the exercise involved is intermittent, seldom raising the pulse for more than a few minutes at a stretch, it is hard to achieve an aerobic effect unless the total playing time is an hour or longer. Other disadvantages include the necessity of finding a partner and a free court. For these reasons, and because aerobic conditioning improves stamina for all sports, most good ball players like to supplement their game with steady running on alternate days.

One word of caution is in order. Some of the more vociferous believers in aerobic exercise may feel that fitness protects them against heart disease and all other ailments. Alas, such is not the case, as the sudden death in 1983 of Jim Fixx, a seasoned marathoner, reminded us. Aerobic fitness is statistically associated with a decreased incidence of heart disease and stroke, but it is by no means a panacea. Other risk factors such as smoking, high blood pressure, or high cholesterol levels can be as lethal as a sedentary life style. For this reason, doctors generally recommend that anyone with chest pain (or pressure), a family history of heart problems, or any of the known risk factors mentioned should have a physical exam with a maximal exercise stress test periodically. The aim of sport, after all, is to enhance the quality of life, not to endanger it!

PART VII SPECIFIC HEALTH ISSUES

25 Caffeine, Cocaine, "Crack," Alcohol, Heroin, Marijuana and Other Mind-Affecting Drugs
Edward M. Brecher

26 Patients and Pills: The Consumer's Role in Assuring Safe and Effective Drug Use
Philip R. Lee, M.D., and Helene Levens Lipton, Ph.D.

27 The Future of Pharmaceuticals
Clement Bezold, Ph.D.

28 Can Health Promotion Enable People to Live Healthier Lives into Later Life?
James F. Fries, M.D.

29 Exercise and the Aging Process
Ralph Paffenbarger, Jr., M.D., and Robert T. Hyde, M.A.

30 Some Myths and Realities About Aging
Ruth G. Newman, Ph.D.

31 Social Networks and Social Isolation Among the Elderly
Meredith Minkler, Ph.D.

32 Motivating the Adolescent: Special Needs and Approaches
Dale C. Garell, M.D.

33 Crisis in Adolescence: An Unexpected Opportunity for Growth
James S. Gordon, M.D.

34 Varities of Integral Cancer Therapies
Michael Lerner, Ph.D.

35 What You Should Know About Smoking
Tom Ferguson, M.D.

25

CAFFEINE, COCAINE, "CRACK," ALCOHOL, HEROIN, MARIJUANA AND OTHER MIND-AFFECTING DRUGS

Edward M. Brecher is senior author of *Licit and Illicit Drugs: The Consumers Union Report on Narcotics, Stimulants, Depressants, Inhalants, Hallucinogens, and Marijuana—Including Caffeine, Nicotine, and Alcohol*. He has participated in other drug studies under both governmental and private auspices, and he has written and lectured widely since 1972 on numerous aspects of this country's chronic (and continuously worsening) drug problem. He has served on the Ad Hoc Committee on the Treatment and Prevention of Drug Addiction and Drug Abuse and on the Advisory Panel on Evaluation of Drug Treatment Programs.

There are few of us who haven't come close to abusing at least one potentially harmful drug, even if it's simply a matter of drinking too many cups of coffee in the morning. And it is just this factor, our personal familiarity with the most commonly available drugs, that creates a mythology about their effects on our health. Edward Brecher discusses the history of drug abuse and society's attempts to solve the problem— attempts that have often met with less than satisfactory results. He debunks a few theories concerning the consumption of coffee, cigarettes, and mind-affecting drugs, and shares his knowledge of a topic that has provoked much public hysteria and political opportunism.▪

Drugs such as heroin, cocaine, and marijuana have for many decades been "the drugs we love to hate." They have been the target of intense emotional hostility—an emotional reaction so intense that even the simplest facts about these drugs have commonly been obscured.

One psychoactive (mind-affecting) drug, however, has escaped this emotional zealotry: the addicting stimulant caffeine. In this chapter, accordingly, we shall first seek to explain the facts about caffeine as they have emerged both from laboratory research and from everyday experience. Against this relatively calm background, the other psychoactive drugs of major current concern will then be reviewed in turn:

- Stimulants other than caffeine (especially cocaine and the amphetamines).
- Alcohol and the alcohol-like drugs—such as the barbituates (Barbital, Nembutal, Seconal, Pentothal, and many more); and the minor tranquilizers (Librium, Valium, Tranxene, Sera x, and many more).
- The opiates (chiefly morphine, heroin, and methadone).
- Marijuana—a drug in a class by itself.

Nicotine, like marijuana, is a psychoactive drug in a class by itself.

The medical data on which this chapter is founded are drawn largely from the fifth (1978) edition of the authoritative medical textbook, *The Pharmacological Basis of Therapeutics*, edited by Louis S. Goodman and Alfred Gilman (hereafter referred to as "Goodman and Gilman's textbook"). The historic and other nonmedical data and the underlying philosophy are drawn from my own *Licit and Illicit Drugs: The Consumers Union Report on Narcotics, Stimulants, Depressants, Inhalants, Hallucinogens, and Marijuana—including Caffeine, Nicotine, and Alcohol*, by Edward M. Brecher and the Editors of Consumer Reports.

This chapter will conclude with a review of alternatives to the drug experience—that is, nonchemical ways of achieving precisely or approximately the same mood-altering and consciousness-altering effects most Americans seek through psychoactive drugs. Included among these non-

chemical techniques are vigorous exercise of many kinds; meditation and other relaxation techniques; creating or responding to literature, music, and the visual arts; fasting and sleep deprivation (vigils); dancing; the sauna and the hot-tub; the cinema, television, and radio; skiing, parachute jumping, and the roller coaster; sexual activities; and perhaps even (for infants) the cradle and the pacifier.

CAFFEINE

Americans get their caffeine mostly from coffee, tea, and cola drinks. The psychoactive effects of these beverages are described by Dr. J. Murdoch Ritchie, professor of pharmacology at the Yale University School of Medicine, in Goodman and Gilman's textbook:

Caffeine stimulates all portions of the [cerebral] cortex. Its main action is to produce a more rapid and clearer flow of thought, and to allay drowsiness and fatigue. After taking caffeine one is capable of greater sustained intellectual effort and a more perfect association of ideas. There is also a keener appreciation of sensory stimuli and reaction time to them is appreciably diminished. . . . In addition, motor activity is increased; typists, for example, work faster and with fewer errors. However, recently acquired motor skills involving delicate muscular coordination and accurate timing may . . . be adversely affected. These effects may be brought on by the administration of 150 to 250 milligrams of caffeine, the amount contained in one or two cups of coffee or tea.

Caffeine, Dr. Ritchie adds, also stimulates the human metabolic rate; three of four cups of coffee or tea can raise basal metabolism "an average of 10% and occasionally 25%." The peak effect occurs from 1 to 3 hours after consuming the beverage.

Decaffeinated coffee brands and caffeine-free cola drinks, of course, are as readily available as beverages containing caffeine—but they are far less popular. This is one of several lines of evidence demonstrating that most Americans consume beverages containing caffeine in order to secure the psychoactive effects of the caffeine. Coffee drinkers themselves confirm this conclusion. When asked why they drink their morning cup of coffee, they give replies such as these:

REASONS FOR DRINKING COFFEE	PERCENTAGE
Helps you wake up	46%
Gets you going in the morning	42%
Gives you a "lift"	28%
Stimulates you	24%
Gives you energy	21%

After a few hours, the stimulant effect of a cup of coffee wears off and depression sets in. Habitual caffeine users are not in the least inconvenienced, however. They simply reach for another cup of coffee or tea or another can or bottle of cola.

Caffeine As an "Evil Drug." We Americans are accustomed to dividing all psychoactive drugs into three main classes: good drugs, evil drugs, and nondrugs. The three most popular psychoactive drugs—caffeine, nicotine, and alcohol—are commonly classified in popular thinking as nondrugs—supposedly quite different from marijuana, cocaine, or heroin, for example, But caffeine, strangely enough, has only recently acquired its privileged status as a nondrug; for centuries it was deemed among the most evil of all drugs.

Coffee originated in Ethiopia; its spread to other countries aroused a deep sense of moral outrage and intense efforts to suppress its use. Thus in Arabia, where coffee was first used to help Mohammedan worshippers stay awake during prolonged religious vigils, the newly imported beverage "stirred up fierce opposition on the part of the strictly orthodox and conservative section of the priests. Coffee by them was held to be . . . prohibited by the Koran, and severe penalties were threatened." An Arabic writer of that era reported that "the sale of coffee has been forbidden. The vessels used for this beverage . . . have been broken into pieces. The dealers in coffee have received the bastinado [whipping on the soles of the feet], and have undergone other ill treatment." Nevertheless, "the coffee-drinking habit spread among the Arabian Mohammedans, and the growing of coffee and its use as a national

beverage became as inseparably connected with Arabia as tea is with China."▪

In Egypt similarly, a recent commentator adds that "the 'coffee bugaboo' . . . caused almost as much fuss as the 'marijuana bugaboo' in the contemporary United States. The sale of coffee was prohibited; wherever stocks of coffee were found they were burned. . . . All this fuss only had the result of interesting more people in the brew and its use spread rapidly." Efforts to ban coffee in England proved similarly self-defeating.

In the United States as recently as 1902, a leading psychiatric authority continued to class coffee addiction, along with morphinism and alcoholism, among the "narcomanias." Young people were warned against coffee with the sad story of "a prominent general in a noted battle in the Civil War; after drinking several cups of coffee he appeared on the front of the line, exposing himself with great recklessness, shouting and waving his hat as if in a delirium, giving orders and swearing in a most extraordinary manner. He was supposed to be intoxicated. Afterward it was found that he had used nothing but coffee."▪

Another early twentieth-century warning against coffee resembles a current warning against marijuana: "Often coffee drinkers . . . turn to other narcotics, of which opium and alcohol are the most common."▪

Whether coffee became this country's most popular beverage in spite of or because of such warnings is a question difficult to answer. For many young people, the peril warned against is a part of the lure; witness the popularity of skiing.

▪ Albert Barton Rendle, D.Sc., F.R.S., F.L.S., Keeper of the Department of Botany, British Museum, and William George Freeman, B., Sc., A.R.C.S., in *Encyclopaedia Britannica*, 11th ed. (1911), vol. 6, p. 646.

▪ T.D. Crothers, M.D., superintendant of the Walnut Lodge Hospital in Connecticut, editor of the *Journal of Inebriety*, and professor of nervous and mental diseases at the New York School of Clinical Medicine, in his book, *Morphinism and Narcomanias from Other Drugs* (1902)

▪ Idem. There is, of course, some slight truth in this allegation. A teenager today who scrupulously refrains from tasting coffee, tea, or cola drinks, and who never lights a cigarette or samples an alcoholic beverage, is in little danger of succumbing to marijuana, cocaine, or heroin use.

Should Caffeine Be Reclassified? Let us suppose for a moment that the governmental agencies, private organizations, and mass media that are currently waging crusades against marijuana, cocaine, and heroin should decide that their predecessors were right—that caffeine is also an "evil drug" and should be banned. What reputable scientific evidence could they marshal to support that view?

First of all, they might correctly warn that coffee and tea, even in modest doses (a few cupfuls) can adversely affect the heart rate, the heart rhythm, the supply of blood to the heart muscle, the blood vessel diameter, and the blood pressure—in short, the entire cardiovascular system. These effects cause many physicians to warn patients with heart problems against consuming caffeine.▪

Further, a campaign against caffeine might describe the adverse effects of caffeine (and other coffee ingredients) on the stomach lining.

But an effort to reclassify caffeine as an evil and dangerous drug would no doubt lay primary stress on its terrifying psychological effects. The authentic case history might be told and retold, for example, of the young woman who took several caffeine tablets, each tablet equivalent to less than a cup of coffee, in order to pep herself up for a party. "Shortly afterward, she became silly, elated, and euphoric. As hours passed she took more and more of the tablets" until she had taken the equivalent of 15 cups of coffee. "She became confused, disoriented, excited, restless, and violent, shouted and screamed and began to throw things." She was admitted to a general hospital in "an irrational state varying from wild, manic screaming, kicking, and biting, to muttering semistupor." After remaining wildly manic for several days, she was transferred to a psychiatric hospital where, over a period of almost 2 months, she slowly recovered from her caffeine-induced psychosis.▪

▪ However, Dr. Ritchie adds a caveat: "Most authorities take the attitude that the complete denial of coffee to an individual who enjoys it is apt to be more disturbing than any stimulation he may receive from the beverage."

▪ Margaret C. McManamy and Purcell G. Schube, writing in the *New England Journal of Medicine* in 1936 (215:616-620).

Even a single gram of caffeine (seven to ten cupfuls of coffee) may produce acutely toxic psychological and behavioral effects. "Insomnia, restlessness, and excitement are the early symptoms which may progress to mild delirium," Dr. Ritchie reports. "Sensory disturbances such as ringing in the ears and flashes of light are common. The muscles become tense and tremulous."

Is this really the kind of drug, anticaffeine crusaders might ask, that we want to have sold by the pound at urban supermarkets and country crossroads stores—as well as by the cupful at restaurants and coffee shops?

Addiction To Caffeine. The case against caffeine could next be enormously buttressed by demonstrating that it is an addicting drug.

The term "addicting" as commonly used has lost most of its meaning in recent years; it has come to be merely a synonym for evil or dangerous. Actually, an addicting drug differs from other drugs in two specific ways:

- It produces tolerance. This means that the daily dose needed by an addict is large enough to overwhelm a novice.
- It produces dependence. This means that an addict deprived of his drug experiences adverse symptoms—an abstinence syndrome or hangover.

The addict knows, of course, that the sovereign cure of his hangover is another dose of the drug, and he develops a craving for the drug that is most intense during his first few drug-free days or weeks. This craving may return in powerful waves months or even years after he has become abstinent. Driven by this craving, the addict engages in drug-seeking behavior, sometimes with an intensity that might be described as obsessive and compulsive. His entire life may be devoted to seeking the drug he craves.

Studies demonstrating that coffee is an addicting drug were reported back in 1969 by Dr. Avram Goldstein and Dr. Sophia Kaizer at the Stanford University School of Medicine. They first distributed a questionnaire to all of the housewives living in a housing project for married graduate students; 239 of the 250 questionnaire recipients (96%) responded. More than three-quarters of these women were coffee drinkers. Among the coffee drinkers, more than one-third drank three or four cupfuls daily and an additional third drank five or more—enough to ward off their withdrawal symptoms throughout the day. More than one third of these housewives, moreover, frankly recognized their addiction to their morning cup of coffee; they reported that they drank it because they "feel the need for it."

Some of the housewives drank their first cup *before* breakfast. Among these, 60% reported that they did so because they "feel the need."

Among those who drank three or more cups daily, and especially among those who drank five or more cups, skipping their morning coffee was reported to produce a well-defined syndrome or coffee hangover: "headache, irritability, inability to work effectively, nervousness, restlessness, and (curiously) lethargy."▪

To check these questionnaire reports, Drs. Goldstein and Kaizer next prepared coded vials containing specially compounded instant coffee. Some of the vials were caffeine-free, some contained 150 milligrams of caffeine, and the remainder contained 300 milligrams (equivalent to two or three cups of brewed coffee). The three types of vials and the coffee they contained could not be distinguished by appearance, taste, or aroma. Both coffee drinkers and nondrinkers were then supplied with nine vials, three of each kind. They were asked to score their mood before drinking their first morning cup and at half-hour intervals thereafter for the next two hours. The 9240 mood scores thus secured were analyzed with the aid of a computer.

The experimental results strikingly confirmed the women's earlier questionnaire reports. Those who drank five cups a day or more felt less alert, less active, less content, and more sleepy and irritable before their first morning cup. On days when their coffee contained no caffeine, they continued to feel that way through the subsequent 2 hours; indeed, they felt increasingly nervous, jittery, and shaky as the caffeineless hours dragged by. On days when their coffee contained caffeine, however, the withdrawal syndrome was dramatically relieved. These heavy drinkers also reported fewer headaches on caffeine mornings. The favorable effects were more marked with the 300-milligram dose. Since the experiment was double-blind—neither the participants nor the experimenters knew which vials contained caffeine until after the experiment was concluded—there remained no room for doubt that people who drink five cups a day are physically dependent on caffeine.

The other requirement for an addicting drug, tolerance, was also demonstrated in this study. The same caffeine doses that alleviated the hangovers of the addicted coffee drinkers made non-coffee-drinking housewives *more* jittery and nervous, and produced unpleasant gastrointestinal effects.

Note, however, that caffeine addiction does relatively little harm in our culture, for the drug is readily available, at relatively little cost, day and night. This is in marked contrast to heroin addiction (see below). Heroin addicts may devote their entire lives to securing the money for heroin—and then to finding a supply.

"Caffeine Can Kill You!"   Using animal data, an anticaffeine campaign might also popularize the slogan "Caffeine can kill you."

"A fatal dose of caffeine given to an animal," Dr. Ritchie notes in Goodman and Gilman's textbook, "produces convulsions because of the central stimulating effect. Early in the poisoning, these are epileptiform in nature; as the action of the drug on the spinal cord becomes manifest, strychnine-like convulsions may appear. Death results from respiratory failure." (The fatal dose for humans is estimated by Dr. Ritchie at about 10 grams—roughly the amount contained in 100 cups of coffee or tea.)

Caffeine-Crazed Rats on TV.   An anticaffeine crusade would also call attention to animal evidence indicating that caffeine damages chromosomes—the hereditary carriers of the DNA genetic code. But the climax of the campaign would no doubt be a prime-time television program

▪ Avram Goldstein, Ph.D., and Sophia Kaizer, Ph.D., of the Department of Pharmacology, Stanford University School of Medicine, writing in 1969 in *Clinical Pharmacology and Therapeutics*.

enabling viewers to see for themselves the psychoactive effects of caffeine on rats.

Several research teams have confirmed that rats fed massive doses of caffeine become aggressive and launch vicious physical attacks on one another. Much more remarkable, a caffeine-crazed rat may bite and mutilate *itself*. "Automutilation was so acute and intense in some rats that the animals died of hemorrhagic shock"—that is, they bled to death from self-inflicted wounds. What an anticaffeine TV show that would make!▪

Here, however, many readers may be moved to protest that the bizarre behavior of rats fed massive doses of caffeine is irrelevant to the lives of human coffee drinkers, few of whom are likely to bite themselves to death or to kill themselves by consuming 100 cups of coffee at a gulp. Let us wholeheartedly agree. Let us remember to be similarly critical, however, when reviewing the evidence (see below) concerning drugs currently labeled evil—notably heroin, cocaine, and marijuana.

Caffeine is potentially a dangerous drug. But our culture has successfully domesticated it—that is, we have found and made use of many techniques for minimizing its damaging potential:

First and foremost, we dilute each 100-milligram dose of caffeine with 180,000 milligrams (a cupful) of water. This ensures that our kidneys and bladder will serve as an automatic check on overdosing.

For the most part, we also drink our coffee *after* meals; this further dilutes the drug and tends to protect the stomach lining from adverse effects. We add cream or milk to the coffee as a protective buffer. We refrain from coffee at bedtime, thus minimizing its potential for producing insomnia. Finally, and of the utmost importance, we keep coffee legally available at moderate prices so that addiction to caffeine rarely leads to obsessive-compulsive drug-seeking behavior, crime, imprisonment, and other distressing effects of certain other addicting drugs.

▪ J.M. Peters, writing in 1967 in *Archives of International Pharmacodynamics.*

A Balanced View.   Americans are daily assailed both by unwarranted paeans of praise for many new "miracle drugs" and by exaggerated hymns of hate against drugs currently classified as evil. In place of these familiar approaches, we shall attempt both here and elsewhere in this chapter to conclude each section with a balanced point of view.

- Because caffeine is a stimulant to the central nervous system, millions of people find that it helps them do their jobs and adds to their enjoyment of life.
- Because caffeine has adverse effects on the cardiovascular and digestive systems, however, some people— notably those with high blood pressure or other cardiovascular problems and those with ulcers—should drink coffee, tea, and cola drinks containing caffeine sparingly if at all.
- Many people go through life quite successfully and happily without caffeine.
- Because the potential hazards are dose-related, caffeine users should imbibe in moderation.
- Caffeine is an addicting drug. Its universal availability at moderate cost, however, minimizes the potential ill effects of caffeine addiction.
- Adverse effects can be further minimized by imbibing caffeine in the customary ways, diluted with plenty of water and with cream or milk, drinking if after meals, and refraining as bedtime approaches.

COCAINE, "CRACK," THE AMPHETAMINES, AND OTHER NONCAFFEINE STIMULANTS

Cocaine is derived from the leaves of a shrub known as *Erythoxylon coca*, which grows wild in the mountains of Peru, Bolivia, Ecuador, Chile, and Columbia. The mountain Indians there chew the leaves to secure cocaine, but since the cocaine content of the leaves is only 1%, it takes a lot of chewing to secure a modest dosage. Fatigue of the jaw muscles may protect against overdose much as the kidneys and bladder protect against coffee overdose. When consumed in this way, the beneficient effects of cocaine are quite similar to those of caffeine.

"All trustworthy travelers agree," an American physician summed up in 1886, "that the most notable effect . . . consists in a marvelous invigoration of the strength, both mental and physical. The native is enabled to undertake the most difficult and prolonged marches with little other sustenance."

The leaf-chewing custom still continues, enabling Indians of the high Andes to survive the rigors of an incredibly harsh mountain environment— to the continuing amazement of European and American visitors. Dr. Jerome H. Jaffe comments in Goodman and Gilman's textbook:

It is reported that two million Peruvians who live in the Andean highlands, or 90% of the adult male population, consume . . . cocaine . . . in the form of coca leaves. In view of the fact that many of these highlanders, who have chewed coca leaves for years, abandon the practice when transferred to a lower altitude, it does not seem appropriate to call this use of cocaine an addiction.

Among the early entrepreneurs who sought to capitalize on cocaine was a nineteenth-century Corsican, Angelo Mariani, manufacturer of a cocaine-containing beverage he called Mariani's wine. "Among his clients," we are told, "were Gounot, Massenet, and Pope Leo XIII, who for years was supported in his ascetic retirement by Mariani's product." ▪ President McKinley also praised Mariani's wine. An American entrepreneur, John Styth Pemberton of Atlanta, Georgia, went a step further: he combined cocaine with its rival stimulant, caffeine, in a single beverage, Coca-Cola. Cocaine was dropped from the Coca-Cola formula in 1903, but the caffeine is still there (except in caffeine-free Cokes).

"The subjective effects of cocaine include an elevation of mood that often reaches proportions of euphoric excitement. It produces a marked decrease in hunger, an indifference to pain, and is reputed to be the most potent antifatigue agent known. The user enjoys a feeling of great mus-

cular strength and increased mental capacity and greatly overestimates his capabilities. The euphoria is accompanied by generalized sympathetic stimulation. As in the case with amphetamine, a disturbed personality is not a prerequisite for cocaine-induced euphoria, and the drug is quite effective in relatively normal personalities." ▪

In the United States today, cocaine is commonly "snorted"— inhaled through a straw or other tube. It can also be smoked or injected under the skin or directly into a vein. The effects depend in part on the route of administration. Excessive snorting can damage the mucous membranes lining the nostrils; injecting has hazards of its own. Where cocaine is cheap, cocaine smoking is popular, but at U.S. black market prices, few can afford it here. Since the cocaine effect is short-lived—commonly half an hour or less—repeated doses must be taken to maintain the effect through an evening.

In part because of the high price, cocaine use in the United States was for many decades a "Saturday night special," rarely indulged in more than once a week. More recently, however, a much more damaging pattern of cocaine use has surfaced: users who stay "high on coke," snorting or injecting large and increasing doses, hour after hour and even day after day until they keel over in exhaustion—then resume snorting or injecting when they awaken. This pattern of use is for economic reasons found primarily among three classes of users: the very rich, cocaine dealers who buy at wholesale, and the spouses, sexual partners, and friends of the very rich and of dealers. The long-term consequences, both physical and psychological, can be disastrous. When consumed in this way, cocaine is an addicting drug.

Cocaine has been subject to the same legal restraints as heroin since 1913. At the moment, the mere possession of cocaine is a Federal offense, punishable by up to a year in prison and a $5000 fine, even for a first offense. Dealing in cocaine invokes far stricter penalties, especially for repeat

---

▪ Jerome H. Jaffe, M.D., then professor of psychiatry, Columbia University College of Physicians and Surgeons and chief of psychiatric research, New York State Psychiatric Institute, writing in 1976 in *The Pharmacological Basis of Therapeutics* (Louis S. Goodman and Alfred Gilman, eds.).

▪ Dr. Hector P. Blejer, writing in 1965 in the *Canadian Medical Association Journal.*

offenders. Neither these penalties nor the guarding of the U.S. borders against cocaine imports has curtailed the American supply, however. More than four million Americans are said to use cocaine regularly. U.S. consumption for 1984 was estimated at 80 tons—roughly four *billion* 20-milligram doses per year.

From Cocaine To the Amphetamines. What did curtail the U.S. consumption of cocaine for a 25-year period (1945–1970) was the introduction of a new class of synthetic stimulants known as the amphetamines. More than 30 amphetamine-sedative, amphetamine-tranquilizer, and amphetamine-analgesic combinations were marketed. They were prescribed by American physicians for depression and other indications; they were used as an alternative to electroshock treatments for profound depression. The cost of the amphetamines was so low—as little as $7.50 per thousand doses at wholesale—that cocaine could no longer compete.

The psychoactive effects of the amphetamines, as described by Dr. Ian P. Innes and Dr. Mark Nickerson in Goodman and Gilman's textbook, are remarkably similar to the psychoactive effects of caffeine and cocaine described above:

The main results of an oral dose . . . are as follows: wakefulness, alertness, and a decreased sense of fatigue; elevation of mood, with increased initiative, confidence, and ability to concentrate; often elation and euphoria; increase in motor and speech activity. Performance of only simple mental tasks is improved, and, although more work may be accomplished, the number of errors is not necessarily decreased. Physical performance, for example, in athletics, is improved. These effects are not invariable, and may be reversed by overdosage or repeated usage.

Long-distance truck drivers, long addicted to caffeine, were among the first to discover that the amphetamines were even more effective in helping to keep them awake during 12-hour or even 24-hour stints at the wheel. Businessmen (and their secretaries) found amphetamines useful, too. Because the amphetamines suppress appetite, they were widely prescribed for weight reduction and obesity control. Obesity and depression often go together; the amphetamines were targeted against both components of this common syndrome. Following 1970, when the amphetamines acquired a reputation as "evil" drugs and physicians hesitated to prescribe them, new nonamphetamine drugs having the same combination of effects were marketed as prescription stimulants and as diet pills. Whether these newer central nervous system stimulants have any real advantage over the amphetamines remains in doubt. Some other new antidepressant drugs, however, achieve their effects without caffeine-like, cocaine-like, or amphetamine-like stimulation.

Many who used amphetamines occasionally in these or other ways found that they could do so year after year; the same dose continued to have the same effect. Others, however, began (like some cocaine users) to escalate their doses and to take amphetamines repeatedly to avoid depression and "letdown" as the stimulant effect wore off. Instead of taking amphetamine tablets one at a time, some were swallowing whole handfuls.

A 1942 Swedish study indicated the relative frequency of various patterns of use. Physicians at that time were prescribing some six million doses of amphetamines per year to 207,000 Swedes—about 3% of the entire adult population. Most of the 207,000 appeared to be using the new stimulants sensibly and in moderation:

- 140,000 were occasional users, taking four amphetamine tablets or fewer per year. No doubt, like Americans at the same time, they used amphetamines on rare days when they had to work longer than usual, or faced some extraordinary challenge, or woke up depressed and out of sorts and needed something to "pull themselves together."
- 60,000 others were also occasional users, but with somewhat greater frequency; their usage ranged from five times a year to twice a month.
- 4,000 users took amphetamine only once a week or so, but often took two or three tablets at a time—perhaps for a Saturday night "high."

- 3,000 users might be described as border-line. Their frequency of use varied from several times a week to daily—and they sometimes took from five to ten tablets in a single day.
- 200 users—less than 0.1%—could properly be labeled amphetamine abusers. They took from 10 to 100 or more tablets per day, more or less regularly.

These data suggest that amphetamines prescribed by physicians have only a modest potential for abuse. The amphetamine figures may be contrasted with the estimated 10% to 20% of alcohol drinkers who become problem drinkers or alcoholics, and the estimated 1% who end up as skid row alcoholics.

Few similar statistics are available for what I shall call the user/victim ratio with respect to other psychoactive drugs; yet without such data, it is impossible to weigh the benefits against the hazards of a particular drug. Clearly, the assembling of additional data of this kind for all psychoactive drugs should be a high-priority task of public and private agencies concerned with drug abuse.

Instead of consulting user/victim ratios, it is the American custom to focus attention on the worst-case scenario—like the young woman caffeine abuser hospitalized for her caffeine-induced delirium in 1936 by McManamy and Schube.■ U.S. authorities concerned with amphetamines, for example, focused in on an exceedingly small minority of amphetamine users known as speed freaks, who compulsively inject directly into their veins ("mainline") enormous quantities of amphetamines, hour after hour for days in a row until they fall exhausted in their tracks, resuming the injections when they awaken. The results, as might be expected, are disastrous to both mind and body. Much of the widely publicized violence—including rapes, mayhem, and homicides—attributed to the drug scene in the 1960s was generated by this minuscule minority of drug users, the amphetamine-mainlining speed freaks. These were the drug abusers who most closely fitted the popular stereotype of the drug addict as wild-eyed, uncontrollable, and doomed.

As might be expected, however, the speed freak epidemic was short-lived, not because of law enforcement efforts or antiamphetamine propaganda, but because newcomers to the drug scene saw for themselves what was happening to amphetamine mainliners and resolved not to follow *that* route. In this as in other situations, the truth about psychoactive drugs has proved far more effective in curbing drug abuse than either law enforcement or hysterical antidrug propaganda.

Law enforcement did play a role in the amphetamine problem, however, late in the 1960s. Physicians who prescribed these drugs to more than a few of their patients were visited by the narcotics police; some were arrested, tried, and convicted. This frightened the medical professional and cut off the legitimate supplies of many hundreds of thousands of people who found prescribed amphetamines helpful occasionally when they had to work long hours or faced unusually difficult challenges. But it did nothing to curb the unlimited illicit supplies available on the black market.

The narcotics police next sought to cut off illicit supplies by tightening the border controls against illegal imports and by internal controls to curb leakage of legitimate supplies to the black market. Black market operators responded by manufacturing their own amphetamines in bathtub "labs"— at a cost even lower than the $7.50 per thousand doses charged by legitimate manufacturers. The next gambit in the law enforcement game was an effort by the narcotics police to cut off the supply of the raw materials from which black market amphetamines were being manufactured. These and other ploys successfully curtailed the black market supply of amphetamines and thus opened the door once again to cocaine, the drug which cheap amphetamines had superseded a quarter of a century earlier.

More and more cocaine, worth millions of dollars, was being smuggled into the United States from Latin America, *The New York Times* reported on February 1, 1970. A narcotics police official

■ Margaret C. McManamy and Purcell G. Schube, writing in the *New England Journal of Medicine* in 1936 (215:616-620).

explained: "It's because younger users are beginning to find out about it. They are beginning to learn it's pretty much like speed." Year after year, as anticocaine efforts were mobilized, cocaine prices on the black market rose and larger quantities therefore became available. The 1984 statistics—four billion doses of cocaine imported for more than four million regular cocaine users—is at or close to the all-time record.

The changeover from the amphetamines to cocaine engineered by law enforcement after 1969 was hardly a change for the better. First, cocaine is a much shorter-acting drug. A moderate dose of an amphetamine will provide stimulation for seven hours or so on the average; even large doses of cocaine must be repeated more often than that. Second, the exorbitant price of cocaine (the street price per dose is more than 100 times the pharmacy price of a dose of amphetamine) has produced economic corruption and distortion on a colossal scale measurable in billions of dollars per year. The billions spent on imported cocaine contribute notably to the U.S. balance of trade problem; the billions reaped by black market cocaine entrepreneurs are corrupting our entire society, including the police and banking systems.

Enter "Crack." By preventing the importation of surplus cocaine, law enforcement successfully maintained high prices (and therefore high profits) for cocaine as for other illicit drugs from 1970 through 1984. In 1985 and 1986, however, price maintenance by means of law enforcement broke down. Despite the continuing strong demand for cocaine, a rising tide of cocaine imports resulted in a growing U.S. surplus which seriously threatened the price structure.

This country's free enterprise system of drug distribution proved equal to the challenge. The surplus cocaine was processed into alkaloidal cocaine, also known as cocaine freebase or "crack"—a simple conversion achieved by exposing cocaine to ammonia and sometimes baking soda. Crack cannot be snorted as cocaine is, but it can be smoked in a cocaine pipe or mixed with tobacco in a cigarette. The crack made of surplus cocaine could thus be marketed at cut rates to attract a new kind of customer, the "crack smoker," while the price of the pure cocaine preferred by cocaine snorters could be maintained at traditional high levels.

Crack distributors, of course, could not buy advertising for crack as other new products are advertised in the press or on radio and TV. But the media solved that problem for the crack trade by advertising it free of charge. Front page stories and newscasts about the dangers of crack, the deaths of famous athletes and rock stars who smoked crack, the highly addicting nature of crack, and its growing popularity throughout the country served to alert even elementary school students to the arrival of this new product—and sales soared. It was not yet possible to predict, late in 1986, whether crack would eventually supersede cocaine altogether or the two markets would continue to flourish side by side—or widespread antidrug publicity and law enforcement efforts for some even new stimulant would eventually enable it to supersede both it and crack.

The cocaine-amphetamine-cocaine-again-crack sequence briefly summarized here raises a question that is rarely asked in America and even more rarely answered: If our efforts to curb the availability of a drug like amphetamine or cocaine prove successful, what other drug or drugs will take its place? Weighing the pluses against the minuses, will this be a change for the better or for the worse?

A Balanced View. Taken occasionally in modest doses, caffeine, cocaine, and amphetamines can enhance intellectual and physical output, postpone fatigue, and produce a sense of well-being. Of the three, caffeine in modest doses is no doubt the safest. Caffeine is legal, the cost per dose is relatively low, and when diluted 1,800 to 1 or more with water and milk or cream it is the stimulant least likely to lead to disastrous dose escalation. Cocaine and crack are currently the most hazardous of the stimulants for legal, economic, and pharmacological reasons.

While chemical stimulants have their usefulness, nonchemical approaches to stimulation of the central nervous system are likely to prove more lastingly beneficial to most people under most circumstances.

ALCOHOL

No drug has precisely the same effect on all people at all times, but alcohol is by far the most dramatic example of the ways in which a given dose of a drug may have vastly different effects on different people—and even on the same person at different times and in different settings.

A cocktail or a glass of wine before dinner, for example, may serve as a relaxant and an appetizer, increasing enjoyment of the meal. An after dinner drink may induce a sense of contentment and enhance the happiness of the evening. A drink or two may also serve as a social lubricant, enabling acquaintances to feel more friendly and friends to enjoy a closer camaraderie. A drink at any hour may alleviate anxiety. A nightcap may serve as a sedative and a soporific, speeding the onset of sleep.

As the dose of alcohol is increased, however, quite different effects begin to make their appearances, varying from person to person. Some drinkers, for example, become garrulous, silly, and boisterous; they speak too loudly and say too much. They retreat into a corner and nurse their drinks alone. The same drinker may react in one way on one occasion and in another way on another occasion. After imbibing large enough doses, almost all drinkers either become "roaring drunk" or else lapse into a stupor. Nausea and vomiting are common.

Dr. J. Murdoch Ritchie describes these processes more technically in Goodman and Gilman's textbook. Following a large dose of alcohol, he notes, the cerebral cortex is

released from its integrating control. As a result, the various processes related to thought occur in a jumbled, disorganized fashion and the smooth operation of motor processes becomes disrupted. . . . The finer grades of discrimination, memory, concentration, and insight are dulled and then lost. Confidence abounds, the personality becomes expansive and vivacious, and speech may become eloquent and occasionally brilliant. Mood swings are uncontrolled and emotional outbursts frequent. These psychic changes are accompanied by sensory and motor disturbances. For example, spinal reflexes are at first enhanced because they have been freed from central

inhibitions; as intoxication becomes more advanced, however, this first phase . . . is succeeded by a general impairment of nervous function and a condition of general anesthesia [stupor or coma] ultimately prevails.

After the alcoholic binge ends and the alcohol content of the blood gradually falls, moreover, withdrawal symptoms set in—a phenomenon commonly known as the hangover. Dr. Jerome Jaffe describes an extreme hangover in Goodman and Gilman's textbook:

Tremulousness, which appears within a few hours after the last drink, is often accompanied by nausea, weakness, anxiety, and sweating. Purposive behavior directed toward obtaining alcohol or a suitable substitute is prominent. There may be cramps and vomiting. . . . Tremors may be mild or so marked that the patient may be unable to lift a glass. The subject may begin to "see things," at first only when the eyes are closed but later even while the eyes are open. . . . *Grand mal* [epileptic] seizures can occur, but they are less common in alcohol withdrawal than in barbiturate withdrawal. . . .

The tremulous state reaches peak intensity within 24 to 48 hours. . . . If the syndrome progresses further, insight is lost, the subject becomes weaker, more confused, disoriented, and agitated. He may be terrified by his persecutory hallucinations. They are often so vivid that the subject, even after recovery, sometimes doubts their unreality. This pattern of hallucinations and tremulousness is known as *delirium tremens.*

If the patient does not die, recovery usually occurs within five to seven days.

Chronic alcoholism leads to cirrhosis of the liver, a frequent cause of death among alcoholics. It also leads to a particularly devastating form of brain damage known as Korsakoff's syndrome, and to other damaging effects on mind and body too numerous even to list here. Alcohol's contribution to automobile accidents, including fatal accidents, is well established. So is its association with crimes of violence; in a substantial proportion of homicides, for example, both the perpetrator and the victim are under their influence of alcohol at the time of the crime. Alcohol is a disrupter of marriages and of parent-child relationships, and it is a major cause of firings and of subsequent unemployment. Hence the question insistently arises: *why on earth does anyone ever imbibe so ghastly a drug?* The answer, like the answer to the same question with respect to caffeine, cocaine, the amphetamines, and other psychoactive drugs, lies imbedded in the user/victim ratio.

Many millions of Americans consume alcoholic beverages with no unpleasant or hazardous side effects whatsoever. Some never take a second drink on the same day. Some drink only on special occasions—birthdays and New Year's Eve, for example. Some take only a cocktail before dinner, or a glass of wine with dinner, or a beer or two in the evening, or a nightcap. They may enjoy alcoholic beverages sparingly for decades without ever once getting drunk or suffering a hangover. Others, in contrast, get drunk, suffer hangovers, turn to alcohol before breakfast as a hangover cure or "eye-opener," and end up as alcohol addicts—alcoholics.

Why do some drinkers become alcoholics while others remain healthy social drinkers? The traditional view was that alcoholics, like narcotics addicts, suffer from "weakness of will." Freudians may trace alcoholism to childhood events within the nuclear family; others view alcoholism as a response to current stresses—a wretched marriage, oppressive career tensions, loss of a loved one. There is also a social explanation. Perhaps those who live in a subculture where heavy drinking is the accepted norm are more likely to become heavy drinkers and later alcoholics.

Most of the evidence available until recently supported psychological and social explanations such as these, but most researchers through the decades have been *looking* for psychological or social explanations, and it is therefore hardly surprising (or convincing) that they have found the kinds of evidence they sought. Recently, evidence has been accumulating for the view that variations in individual biochemistry—perhaps even genetic differences—may enable one person to remain a lifelong moderate drinker while another escalates his or her doses, develops an addiction to alcohol, and ends up a skid row alcoholic. Perhaps there is

a modicum of truth in all of these views.

What *is* known but rarely discussed is the relation between alcohol effects and *speed* of alcohol consumption. The human body metabolizes alcohol (that is, converts it into harmless substances) at a fixed rate, perhaps one ounce of whisky per hour (though this varies from person to person depending on body size and no doubt other factors). "If the intake is sufficiently spread out over the day," Dr. Jaffe explains in Goodman and Gilman's textbook, "the alcohol may be metabolized without any substantial increase in blood concentration. On the other hand, the ingestion of only moderately larger amounts but spaced so that the body's metabolic capacity is exceeded"—for example, four ounces instead of three ounces of whisky in three hours—"can produce much higher blood concentrations, which can induce clinically significant physical dependence within a few days."

It is the subsequent *fall* in blood alcohol concentration that triggers the hangover, the craving for another drink, and alcohol-seeking behavior. The moderate drinker, it is now believed, can continue his moderate drinking so long as he keeps his intake per hour below his body's hourly capacity to metabolize that intake.

This formula also explains the modest advantage of drinking light wines, beer, or generously diluted highballs rather than beverages with higher alcoholic content. While it is *possible* to exceed one's metabolic capacity with even light wine or beer, low-alcohol beverages make it at least a bit easier to stay within the metabolic limit. As with caffeine diluted in coffee, moreover, the kidneys and bladder may help to limit overdosing when diluted drinks such as beer are imbibed.

A Balanced View.   The vast majority of alcohol drinkers drink rarely enough, slowly enough, and in small enough amounts on most drinking occasions to enjoy the benefits of a before dinner appetizer, a dinner wine, an after dinner cordial, or a nightcap with little risk of harm. But 10% or 12% of all drinkers become heavy drinkers, and all of these are at risk of becoming alcoholics. For those who find they cannot hold their hourly alcohol intake below their hourly capacity to metabolize alcohol, this drug can rapidly become the most devastating of all psychoactive substances. Their only sane course is to abstain from alcohol altogether, before, rather than after, the disastrous effects set in.

THE BARBITURATES, THE TRANQUILIZERS, AND OTHER ALCOHOL-LIKE DRUGS

Prior to 1903, alcohol was often prescribed by physicians for a variety of purposes, especially the relief of chronic anxiety and insomnia—two of the most life-disrupting conditions to which we humans are subject. But a growing number of patients at the turn of the century were "teeto-tallers" who had "taken the pledge" to abstain alto-gether from alcoholic beverages, even for medic-inal use. Others detested the taste and smell of alcohol, and still others tended to escalate their alcohol consumption far beyond the doses prescribed. For all of these reasons, an intensive search was launched for a nonalcoholic drug with sedative and sleep-inducing effects.

The first to be discovered was barbital, a bar-bituric acid derivative introduced into medical practice in 1903. More than 2500 other barbitu-rates were subsequently synthesized, and some 50 of these were accepted for medical use. Their effectiveness was unquestioned. When a patient suffering from insomnia, for example, was given an appropriate dose of a barbiturate and told it would facilitate sleep, the patient promptly fell asleep. When nervous, anxious patients, unable to function through the day, were given smaller doses and assured that the drug would "calm their nerves," it did. The barbiturates remained there-after among the mainstays of medical practice until the coming of a newer class of drugs known as the minor tranquilizers—Miltown, Equanil, Lib-rium, Valium, and many more.

As experience with the barbiturates and minor tranquilizers accumulated, however, it became increasingly clear that they are not as different from alcohol as had been supposed. A classic experiment undertaken by Dr. Harris Isbell and his associates illustrated the similarities.

Five male volunteers serving sentences for nar-cotic law violations were given a large dose of a barbiturate. The result was "a marked degree of intoxication" that resembled alcohol intoxica-tion in almost all respects. All five became "dead drunk." As with alcohol, however, the effects were not uniform. Three of the five passed out cold; the other two did not. Before passing out, two "be-came garrulous, boisterous, and silly"— just like some alcohol drunks. Two others became quiet and depressed. In all cases, "signs of intoxica-tion began to diminish within 2 hours after the drug was administered." The patients slept poorly that night, however, and "on the subsequent day they were nervous and tremulous and complained of anorexia [loss of appetite] and headache. They compared these [withdrawal] symptoms to a 'hangover' after an alcoholic debauch."

Having thus demonstrated that acute barbitu-rate drunkenness is precisely like alcohol drunk-enness, Dr. Isbell then went on to reproduce with barbiturates the successive phases of *chronic* alcoholism. Given a barbiturate "eye-opener" before breakfast and larger doses periodically from 9 a.m. to 11 p.m. thereafter, day after day, these men became "unkempt and dirty, did not shave, bathed infrequently, and allowed their liv-ing quarters to become filthy. . . . All patients were confused and had difficulty in performing simple tasks." Though they had been good friends before the experiment started, they now "became irrita-ble and quarrelsome. They cursed one another and at times even fought"—all characteristics of some alcohol drunks.

The barbiturate's effects on mood, as with alco-hol, "varied from day to day and from patient to patient." One of the five, "though occasion-ally euphoric, garrulous, and pleasant, was usu-ally depressed, complained of various aches and pains, and continuously sought increases in med-ication, although he was so intoxicated he fre-quently could not walk." He would also "weep over his wasted life and the state of his family."

Alcoholics often "swear off"—until it's time for the next drink. Barbiturate drunks were like that, too. In Dr. Isbell' study, one patient "frequently asked to be released from the experiment, but would always change his mind within 30 minutes after missing a dose." In other words, he was addicted.

It was following withdrawal from barbiturates that the parallel with alcohol was most impressively demonstrated. These patients went through precisely the withdrawal syndrome described above for alcoholics, including *delirium tremens*.

Relatively few people got drunk on barbiturates before 1942, when the American Medical Association launched a campaign to warn the public against taking barbiturates unless prescribed by a physician. Barbiturate warnings began to appear in popular magazine articles with titles like "Waco Was A Barbiturate Hotspot" and "Thrill Pills Can Ruin You." States began passing laws against nonprescription barbiturates; arrests engendered newspaper headlines, and for the first time a black market in illicit barbiturates became profitable. Agents of the U.S. Food and Drug Administration sought to curb the leakage of legal barbiturates into nonprescription channels, generating more publicity, raising the black market price, and attracting more black market distributors. By 1950, a nation that for decades had used barbiturates for the most part sensibly, to calm the nerves or to induce sleep, had been persuaded by antidrug propaganda that they were "thrill pills."

The warnings served as lures. Young people who would have never thought of taking a barbiturate sedative or sleeping pill were now getting drunk on barbiturate "thrill pills." By 1969, Americans were consuming an estimated 10 *billion* barbiturate doses a year, half of them secured from the black market. (Although enormous, those 10 billion doses were, of course, only a modest fraction of the alcohol doses consumed each year.)

Fortunately, no similar drive is currently underway to warn against the newer tranquilizers such as Tranxene™ and Serax™. They are believed to have some advantages over the barbiturates and the first tranquilizers, but they remain alcohol-like drugs which can, on occasion, be abused. Let us hope that another well-meant but self-defeating antidrug campaign will not attract additional non-

prescription users to these drugs, too, and thus engender a black market for them.

A Balanced View.   Chronic anxiety and chronic insomnia are two of the most frequent and most disruptive illnesses to which the human mind is subject. Alcohol and the alcohol-like barbiturates and tranquilizers are highly effective in calming anxiety and inducing sleep. Of the available alternatives, the newer tranquilizers have at least a modest advantage over alcohol and the barbiturates. Even the safest of these drugs, however, can lead to intoxication and addiction if the size of dose and frequency of use are escalated, and the duration of use prolonged, beyond the medically recommended levels. For many people under many circumstances, nonchemical alternatives to these drugs may prove at least equally effective.

HEROIN AND RELATED SUBSTANCES: MORPHINE, METHADONE, AND THE ENDORPHINS

Among the chemicals which the human nervous system itself manufactures and uses in the self-regulation of mood and behavior, two of the most important are *dopamine* and *norepinephrine*. The two are closely related. Cocaine, the amphetamines, and many other stimulants achieve their effects primarily by influencing the body's internal dopamine-norepinephrine system.

In 1975, however, another kind of nervous system self–regulation was discovered, rivaling the dopamine-norepinephrine system in importance. It is based primarily on *beta-endorphin* and other closely related endorphins and enkephalins generated within the nervous system itself. Here are some of the known endorphin functions:

- They are nature's own means of securing pain relief (analgesia). When a football player, for example, sprains an ankle but goes on playing, oblivious to the pain, it is because generous quantities of an endorphin have been released. As the endorphin level falls when the game is over, the pain becomes intense. Studies suggest that acupuncture also secures its analgesic effects by triggering the release of endorphins when appropriate sites in the body are stimulated.

- In both animal and human experiments, the endorphins function as tranquilizers, relieving anxious behavior in animals and the feeling of anxiety in humans.
- The endorphins contribute to the normal sense of well-being (euphoria) of the healthy human being. A fall in endorphin levels may be associated with dysphoria (misery) and depression.

Clearly such potent substances might have major medical usefulness, and we would expect a rush by the pharmaceutical companies to find new drugs capable of influencing the endorphin system, just as many of the older psychoactive drugs influence the dopamine-norepinephrine system. But, in fact, primitive peoples in the Middle East had discovered an endorphin-like drug more than 5000 years ago, and such drugs were in common use in Western medicine centuries before the endorphins themselves were discovered.

The first of these endorphin-like medicines was opium, secured by drying the juice of unripe seed pods from the opium poppy.∎ The most important ingredient in opium is morphine; it was identified and extracted in pure form back in 1803. In 1896, scientists developed a drug very similar to morphine, known as diacetylmorphine, by exposing morphine to vinegar (acetic acid). The common name for diacetylmorphine is heroin.

Opium and morphine were legally available at low cost throughout the United States during the nineteenth century, and heroin was similarly available after 1896. They were sold without a prescription not only in pharmacies but at crossroads country stores and by mail order. They were active ingredients in literally hundreds of patent medicines, sold under such names as Mrs. Winslow's Soothing Syrup, Godfrey's Cordial, McMunn's Elixir of Opium, and many more. The poppies

that supplied all these opiates were grown initially in Vermont, New Hampshire, and Connecticut; later poppy culture moved south to Louisiana, Florida, Arizona, and especially California. Most opiates were taken orally, but during the Civil War morphine was injected to secure prompter and more complete pain relief for wounded soldiers, and some users continued thereafter to inject opiates either under the skin or directly into a vein.

"Among the remedies that it has pleased Almighty God to give to man to relieve his sufferings," the great English physician Suydenham wrote back in 1680, "none is so universal and so efficacious as opium." Opium was called the Great Tranquilizer (the first recorded use of the word tranquilizer) by Thomas de Quincey in 1822. Other physicians referred to opium, morphine, and heroin as G.O.M., which stood for God's Own Medicine.

Nineteenth-century physicians were aware, of course, that the opiates are addicting. After taking substantial doses continuously over an extended period, many patients suffered severely if the drug were suddenly withdrawn, and they craved it thereafter. Physicians were not too concerned about opiate addiction in those days, however, for supplies were readily available at low prices. Addicts avoided disaster by continuing to take their opiates, just as caffeine addicts today continue to take their caffeine.

Some nineteenth-century physicians treated chronic alcoholic patients by putting them on opiates instead; often the results were beneficial. The advantages of morphine and heroin over alcohol were explained in 1928 by Dr. Lawrence Kolb, Assistant Surgeon General of the United States Public Health Service and a psychiatrist specializing in problems of drug addiction: "More than any other unstable group, drunkards are likely to be benefitted in their social relations by becoming addicts. When they give up alcohol and start using [opiates], they are able to secure the effect for which they are striving without becoming drunk or violent."

The Harrison Narcotics Act of 1914 abruptly curtailed the availability of opiates, even on pre-

---

∎ Some studies suggest that alcohol, too, achieves at least some of its effects through a direct or indirect influence on the endorphin system.

scription, and a Federal antinarcotics police force was established. The initial effects were reported in the *New York Medical Journal* for May 15, 1915:

As was expected . . . the immediate effects of the Harrison antinarcotic law were seen in the flocking of drug habitués to hospitals and sanitoriums. Sporadic crimes of violence were reported, too, due usually to desperate efforts by addicts to obtain drugs, but occasionally to a delirious state induced by sudden withdrawal. . . .

The really serious results of this legislation, however, will only appear gradually and will not always be recognized as such. These will be the failures of promising careers, the disrupting of happy families, the commission of crimes that will never be traced to their real cause, and the influx into hospitals for the mentally disordered of many who would otherwise lead socially competent lives.

Six months later, an editorial in *American Medicine* added:

[The addict] is denied the medical care he urgently needs, open, above-board sources from which he formerly obtained his drug supply are closed to him, and he is driven to the underworld where he can get his drug, but of course, surreptitiously and in violation of the law.

In 1922, when British physicians were considering whether or not to outlaw the opiates, Dr. Harry Campbell came to the United States to see for himself how our Harrison Act was working. He reported in utter dismay:

In the United States of America a drug addict is regarded as a malefactor even though the habit has been acquired through the medicinal use of the drug, as in the case, e.g., of American soldiers who were gassed and otherwise maimed in the Great War [World War I]. The Harrison Narcotic Law was passed in 1914 by the Federal Government of the United States with general popular approval. It places severe restrictions upon the sale of narcotics and upon the medical profession, and necessitated the appointment of a whole army of officials. In consequence of this stringent law a vast clandestine commerce in narcotics has grown up in that country. The small bulk of these drugs rendered the evasion of the law

comparatively easy, and the country is overrun by an army of peddlers who extort exorbitant prices from their helpless victims. It appears that not only has the Harrison Law failed to diminish the number of drug takers— some contend, indeed, that it has increased their numbers—but, far from bettering the lot of the opiate addict, it has actually worsened it; for without curtailing the supply of the drug it has sent the price up tenfold, and this has had the effect of impoverishing the poorer class of addicts and reducing them to a condition of such abject misery as to render them incapable of gaining an honest livelihood.

The British resolved not to follow the American precedent. British addicts continue today to receive their heroin at low cost through government clinics and morphine and other opiates on prescription from any physician.

As enforcement of the Harrison Act escalated opiate prices on the black market, those who had formerly taken their drugs orally were forced to convert to a much more economical (and much more dangerous) route of administration: "mainlining" injections directly into their veins. Another effect of the Harrison Act was to convert American opium and morphine addicts into heroin addicts. The reason was simple: an effective dose of heroin weighs less and occupies less space than an equivalent dose of opium or morphine. Heroin is thus the *smuggler's* favorite opiate; he can bring in more doses per pound and per cubic foot. The change from morphine to heroin made little practical difference, but it had the effect on public opinion of associating the newer drug heroin with the new evils brought on by the Harrison Act. Heroin thus became the evil drug *par excellence*. Congress even banned its medicinal use for pain relief in terminal cancer cases and other painful conditions. The bizarre result is that while addicts and others today can readily secure their supplies on the streets, the one group successfully cut off from heroin pain relief is composed of hospital patients writhing in great pain.

As law enforcement raised heroin prices and curbed distribution, some addicts found it impossible to maintain their addiction and became ex-addicts. Others became ex-addicts during long terms of imprisonment. Dr. John A. O'Donnell made a thorough epidemiological study of such ex-addicts for the National Institute of Mental Health. He reported in 1969 that almost all of them soon became readdicted, and that most of those who did not become readdicted to heroin became alcoholics.

Readers will recall how our culture has successfully domesticated caffeine by making it as harmless as possible—by diluting it with vast quantities of water, drinking it after meals, adding cream or milk, and so on. In contrast, since 1914, we have been dedicated to *increasing* the damage done by heroin. One way has been through law enforcement, which drives the street price of heroin up to bankrupting levels. An addict may have to pay as much as $10 for a dose of street heroin; the equivalent of a dose of morphine is available at the pharmacy on prescription for as little as 35 cents. Another way we have escalated the damage done is by long terms of imprisonment. We have even made it a criminal offense to sell or possess a hypodermic needle without a prescription. As a result, addicts must reuse dirty needles and pass them from user to user, spreading hepatitis, AIDS, and other serious infections in the process. In Britain, where disposable single-use needles are available legally, free or at low cost, epidemics of needle-transmitted infections do not occur.

When it was discovered in the 1980s that AIDS was also being spread among U.S. heroin addicts by reusing infected needles, and that it was spreading from them to their spouses and other sexual contacts, some health authorities decided that the time had come for a change in U.S. policy. They perceived that the single most effective measure they could take to curb the spread of AIDS overnight would be to supply addicts with disposable needles for one-time use only. But this proposal was promptly rejected; U.S. policymakers preferred to encourage the spread of AIDS rather than make heroin use safer.

In these and numerous other ways, American policy has converted what was once a modest misfortune—addiction to opiates—into a ghastly disaster for addicts, for their families, and for society. But we have made one exception.

During the Nixon Administration, the United States government decided to make a synthetic opiate, methadone, available to heroin addicts at low cost or free of charge. Although its endorphin-like effects are generally similar to those of morphine and heroin, methadone has several important advantages. First and foremost, of course, it is legal. Next, its low cost frees the addict from the need to turn to crime to finance his addiction. Methadone is fully effective when taken by mouth, and it is much longer-acting; one oral dose a day can replace the repeated injections of heroin that an addict requires. Congress permitted the establishment of methadone clinics in the hope that methadone might cure addiction. It doesn't, but there is general agreement that a heroin addict is far better off, and society is far better off, when he or she switches from heroin to methadone.

A Balanced View

- The endorphins are essential chemicals generated within the human nervous system for self-regulation—pain relief, tranquilization, and maintenance of a sense of well-being.

- The opiates—including opium, morphine, heroin, methadone, and many more—are addicting drugs, useful for securing endorphin-like effects when the body's internally-generated supply system goes awry or proves inadequate.

- By deliberately enhancing the damage done by heroin through laws and law enforcement, we have made it by far the most "evil drug" in the entire pharmacopeia. The only advice that makes sense with respect to heroin in the United States today, accordingly, is very simple: keep away from it.

- There are numerous American programs designed to help heroin addicts overcome their addiction and remain drug-free. When these programs fail (as they often do), conversion from heroin to methadone can prove beneficial both to the addict and to society.

MARIJUANA

Marijuana in the United States is commonly smoked in the form of hand-rolled cigarettes called joints. The main psychoactive ingredient in the smoke is delta-9- tetrahydrocannabinol (THC). Dr. Jerome H. Jaffe describes the psychological effects of THC in Goodman and Gilman's text-book:

[Small doses] produce effects on mood, memory, motor coordination, cognitive ability, sensorium, time sense, and self-perception. Most commonly there is an increased sense of well-being or euphoria, accompanied by feelings of relaxation and sleepiness when subjects are alone; where users can interact, sleepiness is less pronounced and there is often spontaneous laughter. . . .

Marijuana smokers frequently report increased hunger, dry mouth and throat, more vivid visual imagery, and a keener sense of hearing. Subtle visual and auditory stimuli previously ignored may take on a novel quality; and the non-dominant senses of touch, taste, and smell seem to be enhanced. Altered time perception is a consistent effect. . . . Time seems to pass more slowly—minutes may seem like hours.

Another effect frequently reported is the sense of camaraderie among those who smoke "pot" together, quieter but in other respects resembling the camaraderie of a cocktail party.

With higher THC doses, Dr. Jaffe warns, very unpleasant effects may follow, including "frank hallucinations, delusions, and paranoid feelings. Thinking becomes confused and disorganized. . . . Anxiety reaching panic proportions may replace euphoria, often as a result of the feeling that the drug-induced state will never end. With high enough doses, the clinical picture is that of a toxic psychosis with hallucinations, depersonalization, and loss of insight."

Dr. Jaffe hastens to add, however, that "because of the rapid onset of effects when marijuana is smoked, and the low . . . THC content of marijuana grown in the United States, most users are able to regulate their intake in order to avoid the excessive dosage that produces these unpleasant effects; psychiatric emergencies as a result of smoking marijuana are quite uncommon."

Most smokers similarly learn to avoid unpleasant overdosing when smoking the more potent imported and American-grown marijuana currently available.

One adverse effect of chronic marijuana smoking is well established: it is associated (like chronic smoking of nicotine cigarettes) with asthma and bronchitis. The U.S. government invested heavily during the 1970s in efforts to demonstrate other ill effects, including damage to the brain and to hereditary material in chromosomes. Not surprisingly, some studies based on laboratory and animal research using massive doses of THC did show such effects. These findings (unlike similar findings for caffeine) were widely publicized, and a sad future for marijuana smokers and their offspring was predicted. The expected hordes of brain-damaged marijuana smokers have not turned up in mental hospitals, however—nor have epidemics of genetic damage among the children of marijuana smokers made their appearance.

In countries like India where marijuana has been smoked for centuries, it has never managed to equal alcohol in popularity except among the very poor who cannot afford alcohol. Its popularity among young people in the United States during the 1960s can also be traced in part to its low cost in those days as compared with alcohol, but other factors no doubt played a role. The marijuana effect is less violent than the alcohol effect, for example, and there is little or no hangover. Also, rebellious young people in the 1960s saw rebellion against the prime drug of the older generation (alcohol) as part of a pattern that included rebellion against the music, dances, hair styles, and other customs of the older generation.

One striking effect of the 1960s explosion of marijuana use among young people was little-publicized then and has now been forgotten: the concurrent decline in alcohol drinking among marijuana smokers at that time. "There is already data," Dr. John Kaplan of the Stanford University Law School pointed out in 1970, " . . . showing that a sizable percentage of marijuana smokers . . . cut down their alcohol consumption on taking up their new drug." In one college study, 89% of daily marijuana smokers had reduced their alcohol intake. A Denver beer distributor told a *New York Times* reporter in 1970, "Our retailers say they can tell when a big shipment of marijuana hits town. The [beer] sales go down."

A University of Wisconsin professor of psychiatry, Dr. Seymour Halleck, supplied some details: "Perhaps the one major positive effect of [marijuana] is to cut down the use of alcohol. In the last few years [the late 1960s] it is rare for our student infirmary to encounter a student who has become aggressive, disoriented, or physically ill because of excessive use of alcohol. Alcoholism has almost ceased to [be] a problem on our campuses."

As law enforcement progressively boosted the price of marijuana between 1970 and 1985, it became much more costly per evening of use than beer or cheap whiskey. Many student thereupon switched to the cheaper product, alcohol, as their primary mood-affecting drug. No doubt the nationwide campaign against marijuana and the exaggerated warnings of brain damage and genetic damage from marijuana also encouraged this return to alcohol. College infirmaries today are again treating many students who have "become aggressive, disoriented, or physically ill because of excessive use of alcohol."

If efforts to suppress marijuana use were successful, some observers might applaud—even though the suppression of marijuana was purchased at the expense of a rise in alcohol drinking and alcoholism. Others might think this too high a price to pay. But efforts to suppress marijuana either by law or by warnings have failed dismally. Marijuana use today is at (or very near) an all-time high, and alcoholism is also continuing uncurtailed.

A Balanced View. Marijuana smoked judiciously, one joint from time to time, is a pleasant, convival experience for many people. To the extent that it replaces alcohol drinking, it may even be beneficial. Larger doses produce unpleasant effects—motivating most marijuana smokers to keep their doses relatively low. Some users, however, as with caffeine and some other mind-

affecting drugs, do escalate their consumption by staying "high" or "stoned" on modest doses all day long, day after day. While the predicted epidemics of brain damage and genetic damage to offspring have not appeared, the effects of this pattern of chronic continued marijuana use are socially and perhaps also medically adverse, though hardly rivalling the adverse effects of continual alcohol drinking.

Efforts to curtail marijuana smoking via law enforcement and exaggerated warnings of ill effects have been universally followed by *increases* in the consumption of marijuana—as was the case of heroin and cocaine. Consumption of all of these illicit, "evil" drugs has mounted throughout the past decades and is now at or near an all-time high. The time is approaching, some observers believe, for a fundamental change in our national drug policies.

ALTERNATIVES TO THE DRUG EXPERIENCE

Although this is hardly the place to spell out in detail a new national drug policy, this chapter in this book is an ideal place to propose one feature of such a policy. Emphasis must be shifted at least in part from futile efforts to curtail the availability of psychoactive drugs, and from self-defeating propaganda exaggerating the damaging effects of these drugs, to programs designed to popularize nonchemical ways of achieving stimulations, sedation, tranquilization, a sense of well-being (euphoria), and the other effects sought and achieved by users of psychoactive drugs.

Consider, first of all, meditation. Back in the 1960s, Dr. Herbert Benson of the Harvard Medical School brought into his laboratory 20 young male volunteers aged 21 to 38 and taught them transcendental meditation—sitting and pondering quietly for 15 or 20 minutes twice each day—to see whether this might affect their blood pressure. In chatting with these men about their use of psychoactive drugs, Dr. Benson turned up facts so astounding that he reported them in a letter to the editor of the *New England Journal of Medicine* in 1969.

Dr. Benson learned that 19 of the 20 volunteers

had used psychoactive drugs—marijuana, barbiturates, amphetamines, and in a few cases heroin—before taking up transcendental meditation. Since they had begun meditating, however, all 18 erstwhile drug users "reported that they no longer took these drugs because drug-induced feelings had become exceedingly distasteful as compared to [their] experiences during the practice of transcendental meditation." Perhaps, Dr. Benson commented, "transcendental meditation should be prospectively explored by others . . . primarily interested in the alleviation of drug abuse."

In a subsequent large-scale study, Dr. Benson began with 1862 women and men who had practiced transcendental meditation daily for 3 months or longer; the average was about 20 months of meditation. In this population, marijuana smoking declined from 78.3% of the participants before entering meditation to 26.9% after meditating from 4 to 9 months, and to 12.2% after meditating for 22 months or longer. Only one participant who had meditated for 22 months or more reported that he was still smoking marijuana daily, as compared with 417 participants (22.4%) who reported smoking marijuana daily before entering transcendental meditation.

Another study of 484 students engaged in transcendental meditation reported similar results for barbiturates and amphetamines as well as marijuana, and also cited the reasons meditators gave for discontinuing drug use:

- 49% stated that their use of drugs changed after transcendental meditation because life became more fulfilling.
- 24% said that they drug use changed because the drug experience became less pleasurable.
- 8% said that their drug use changed because the desire for drugs disappeared.

Participants added such comments as these:

"Drugs have naturally fallen by. I didn't try to stop. After a while I just found myself not taking them any more."

"Life after meditation became more satisfying. I no longer needed drugs."

"[I stopped] because all aspects of my life have become better—in school, at work, my inner personal life— everything."

These studies are subject to numerous qualifications. Here are a few:

- The participants in these studies were volunteers; they were the ones attracted to transcendental meditation. There is no evidence that meditation would prove similarly effective among nonvolunteers.
- Participants were expected to refrain from drug use for 15 days or longer before entering transcendental meditation; this no doubt screened out most or all drug addicts.
- These studies do not establish the superiority of transcendental meditation as compared with other alternatives to drug use. Perhaps sensitivity training, or Yoga, or Zen, or fundamentalist Christianity might prove even more effective. No one knows.

Strenuous exercise (jogging, running, etc.) is clearly a source of psychoactive effects comparable to drug effects, including euphoria, stimulation (as with caffeine, cocaine, and the amphetamines), sedation (as with the chemical sedatives and tranquilizers), and a good night's sleep without drugs. Skiing, mountain climbing, parachute jumping, and roller coaster rides produce thrills which in all probability rival or exceed the most intense experiences available chemically.

Literature and the fine arts also produce psychoactive effects rivalling drug effects. There is the creative ecstasy of the writer, the visual artist, or the composer. Next come the psychoactive effects on those who participate in the theater arts, the song fest, the dance, and music—whether it is playing bach on a Stradivarius or just strumming a beat-up guitar. Finally, there are the psychoactive effects of reading that novel, watching that play or film, listening to that music—or simply enjoying the beauties of nature.

While the evidence is not yet in, I see no reason whatever to doubt that these nonchemical roads to euphoria, stimulation, tranquilization, and other altered states of consciousness achieve their beneficent effects in precisely the way that the effects of psychoactive drugs are achieved: by enhancing, curtailing, or otherwise modulating the flow of the natural substances that the human nervous system uses for self-regulation. It would be a mistake to conclude that these nonchemical approaches to altered states of consciousness are without adverse side effects. The adverse effects of excessive indulgence in overly strenuous exercise are noted elsewhere in this volume. Television is by far the most popular nonchemical means of securing thrills, sedation, diversion, and other psychoactive effects in our culture. I find it hard to believe that addiction to television 5 to 10 hours a day, 6 or 7 days a week, is free from adverse effects.

A Balanced View. We have sought decade after decade to curb the use of "evil" drugs by warning each other against them and by trying to enforce laws designed to curtail drug availability. The net effect is that the use of these drugs has risen year by year and remains today at an all-time high. For young people who have not yet started using drugs, such alternatives to the drug experience as games, exercise, music, art, drama, and meditation seem the most promising alternatives to futile law enforcement efforts and self-defeating antidrug propaganda.

26 PATIENTS AND PILLS: THE CONSUMER'S ROLE IN ASSURING SAFE AND EFFECTIVE DRUG USE

Philip R. Lee, M.D., is director of the Institute for Health Policy Studies at the University of California at San Francisco. He served as Assistant Secretary for Health and Scientific Affairs in the U.S. Department of Health, Education, and Welfare from 1965 to 1969. He is now Commissioner of Health for San Francisco County and serves on the Committee on Population, National Research Council, and National Academy of Sciences.

Helene Levens Lipton, Ph.D., is assistant professor of clinical pharmacology at the University of California at San Francisco. She is also senior research associate for the Institute of Health Policy Studies. As a medical sociologist, she has had a long-standing interest in the relationships between health care professionals and their patients and the implications for drug use.

Dr. Lee and Dr. Lipton are co-authors of *Drugs and the Elderly: Clinical, Social, and Policy Perspectives* (Stanford University Press, 1986).

In a Food and Drug Administration survey, almost 70% of those surveyed reported that their physicians and pharmacists had not told them about precautions or potential side effects of recent prescriptions or given them complete instructions for taking the medication. But 96% of these people also admitted that they had not asked any questions of the physician or pharmacist. Dr. Lee and Dr. Lipton attempt in this article to show consumers several ways of maximizing safe and effective drug use while minimizing its problems. "Because improper use of medications is an important cause of illness and death," state the authors, "consumers need to be informed about the drugs they use."▪

THE GREAT AMERICAN LOVE AFFAIR WITH DRUGS

Americans are prescribed and use an enormous quantity of drugs every year. Some explain the phenomenon in terms of an "overmedicated" society, while others note our cultural preference for "a pill for every ill." Statistics reveal the widespread extent of drug use in our society:

- Americans spent almost $16 billion on prescription drugs in 1984.
- Almost $1.5 billion in prescriptions are dispensed each year in the nation's drugstores.
- The average physician writes approximately 8,000 prescriptions annually.
- Estimates are that one prescription is written for each outpatient visit and in about two thirds of all such visits, drugs are prescribed.

BENEFITS OF DRUG THERAPY

The magnitude of drug prescribing and use reflects the fact that in the past 40 years more and more prescription drugs have been developed and marketed for a wider and wider range of conditions and diseases. Few doubt the benefits derived from these advances in drug therapeutics, which have contributed to virtually every area of medical treatment. The introduction of new drugs has resulted in remarkable improvements in the outcomes of medical care, particularly in the treatment of patients with bacterial infections, hypertension, peptic ulcer, coronary heart disease, diabetes, epilepsy, Parkinson's disease, asthma, adrenal insufficiency, hyperthyroidism, and certain types of cancer. Vaccines have eradicated smallpox and have come close to wiping out poliomyelitis in industrial nations. Today, they offer the promise of eradicating mumps, measles, and rubella. Oral contraceptives have proved remarkably effective in preventing unwanted pregnancy. New tranquilizers and other mood-altering medications have had an important impact on the care of the mentally ill and have opened up new vistas for research in neurobiology, neurochemistry, and neuropharmacology. Still other drugs, by permitting smoother and safer anesthesia, have facilitated a wide range of surgical advances.

Use of these new drugs has resulted in the prevention, cure, and improved management of disease. It has also contributed to a dramatic reduction in infant and maternal mortality, overall age-adjusted mortality, and increased life expectancy. Further, drugs have improved the quality of life for millions of patients, contributed to savings that some estimate in the billions of dollars in medical costs each year, and reduced the loss of income and productivity due to illness.

PROBLEMS ASSOCIATED WITH DRUG USE

Yet with all these benefits have come problems. The increase in variety as well as quantity of drugs in recent years has been much more rapid than the growth in scientific knowledge and patient understanding of the problems associated with their use. These include marketing of drugs of questionable effectiveness by the drug industry, inappropriate prescribing by physicians, and, most importantly, less than safe and effective drug use by consumers, often referred to as "noncompliance" (intentional and unintentional underuse, overuse, or inappropriate use of prescribed drugs).

The consequences of noncompliance can be nothing short of disastrous as the following examples amply illustrate:

- A patient with hypertension discontinues his medication because its side effects make him feel worse than when he is not on medication. His high blood pressure is no longer controlled, and he eventually has a stroke leading to prolonged hospitalization and permanent disability.
- A woman suffering from depression discontinues her antidepressant drug therapy because she sees no improvement in her condition after 1 week of therapy. What she does not realize is that some drugs for depression need to be taken for several weeks before their benefits become apparent.
- A patient on diuretic therapy and digoxin for congestive heart failure stops taking his potassium supplement because he finds it

unpalatable and his conditions seems to be under control without it. Eventually he becomes hypokalemic (low in potassium), which in combination with his digoxin creates heart rhythm disturbances, leading to an emergency room visit and subsequent hospitalization.

Similarly, overuse of medications, including the use of tranquilizers and sedatives with alcohol, can lead to serious, even fatal, consequences.

Adverse drug reactions are a growing problem because of the increasing use of drugs of all kinds. The consequences are particularly severe with potent drugs that may be toxic when taken in an inappropriate dosage. This is most common among elderly patients, who often require a lower dose than younger adults.

It is not widely appreciated that drug-induced illnesses account for a significant share of consumer use of health care services, especially hospitalization. Studies indicate that about 10 percent of drug-related hospital admissions result from poor patient compliance, which also leads to increased physician and emergency room visits.

Because improper use of medications is an important cause of patient illness and even death, consumers need to be informed about the drugs they take. The challenge that this chapter addresses is to describe mechanisms consumers can use to maximize the benefits of drug therapies while minimizing the problems associated with their use.

PATIENT NONCOMPLIANCE

Problems with taking medications appear to cut across all social classes, educational levels, and ages. About 50% of patients do not take prescribed medications according to physicians' instructions. The reasons behind noncompliance are complicated. But two factors are of paramount importance: (1) the extent to which patients know how to take their drugs safely and effectively, and (2) the extent to which they believe drug benefits outweigh their "costs" (drug prices, side effects, disruption to lifestyle, etc.). Given the high incidence of noncompliance, the complex reasons

behind it, and its untoward clinical consequences, some experts view noncompliance as the most serious problem facing medical practice today.

It is impossible for patients to take their medications appropriately if they are confused about specific aspects of the regimen. Yet an overwhelming majority of consumers are not told the names and purposes of their drugs, how often and how long to take them, whether to take them on a regular basis or only when symptomatic, possible side effects, and adverse consequences. This lack of information is not surprising when one considers that physicians' rapid-fire drug instructions usually symbolize the end of the physician-patient visit, thus discouraging dialogue about drug use. But this lack of information can have dangerous consequences. It can limit the effectiveness of drug therapy, it can lead to serious adverse drug reactions, and in some instances it can precipitate drug-induced hospitalization.

Many studies suggest that lack of doctor-patient communication about drugs contributes to their improper use. In one Food and Drug Administration study, almost 70% of those surveyed reported that their physicians did not tell them about precautions and possible side effects of recent prescriptions or about how to take their medicines and how much to take. An equal percentage reported the same experience with pharmacists. Only 6% of patients surveyed reported that they were given written information about prescribed medicines by their physicians, and only 15% reported receiving written materials from their pharmacists. Despite the fact that consumers in this study reported that they felt they were given inadequate information about their drugs, an astonishing 96% of those with new prescriptions asked no questions of either physician or the pharmacist.

How can this consumer reticence be explained? Despite the growth of the consumer movement in medical care, there remain many barriers to effective doctor-patient communication. Patients are often reluctant to ask "trivial" questions. Since drugs are relatively inexpensive (compared to other medical therapies) and are readily available, they often are not considered important enough to discuss. Patients hesitate for fear of looking unintelligent or medically unsophisticated, and they do not wish to run the risk of incurring physicians' displeasure by appearing to challenge their authority. They may have lots of questions and yet be unable to put them into words. Some patients are unwilling to assume an active role in their own therapy, believing that the traditional authority relationship between physicians and patients—in which physicians make medical decisions and patients have an obligation to obey them—is entirely appropriate.

For their part, physicians often do not invite questions or concerns from patients about drug therapy. When questions are asked, the physician's response may be so short that the patient's need for information remains unmet. So the conspiracy of silence between patients and physicians is maintained. Under these conditions many problems with drug therapy remain hidden, and the ultimate victim is the patient, whose therapeutic outcome is compromised.

INFLUENCE OF THE MASS MEDIA ON DRUG USE

The mass media, particularly television and radio, present some special opportunities and problems with respect to drug education and use. Consumers are informed almost daily of new developments in drug therapeutics. Yet there is seldom any discussion of precautions and side effects. Take the case of aspirin, for example. Rarely, if ever, are the potential side effects mentioned in radio, television, and magazine advertisements for the many drug products containing aspirin—in particular, the likelihood of gastrointestinal bleeding if alcohol and aspirin are mixed. The same is true for laxatives, nasal sprays, antihistamines, and many other drugs for which millions of dollars are invested in advertising each year.

Too often, drugs are touted as the answer. Researchers sometimes contribute to this problem by exaggerating preliminary findings. Drug companies often encourage reporting of these "breakthroughs," which a few years later prove to be of little or no benefit.

The year 1984 witnessed a major develop-

ment in the use of mass media for consumer drug information: prescription drug advertising directly to consumers. In that year, a number of drug manufacturers launched major advertising campaigns designed to encourage consumers to request certain drug products. Although particular brand names were not mentioned in the ads because of an FDA moratorium, specific diseases for which the company sold drugs were permitted to be discussed. These advertisements appeared in newspapers and on television stations across the country and spurred sales for specific drug products.

Proponents of prescription drug advertising directly to consumers contend that an informed consumer will be able to make more intelligent choices because of the information received in newspaper advertisements and television commercials. They argue that advertisements sponsored by drug companies help patients detect and manage their diseases by explaining symptoms and available drug treatments. Conversely, opponents argue that these advertisements create a reliance on drugs, when in some instances exercise, diet, and other lifestyle changes are safer and less costly alternatives. Further, they argue that patients lack the technical expertise to weigh the claims of prescription drug advertisements, and they are therefore vulnerable to sophisticated marketing programs designed only to increase consumption of particular drug products.

Regardless of how the issue is settled—if it is settled—advertising prescription drugs directly to consumers will be with us in the future. Late in 1985 the Food and Drug Administration lifted its moratorium on advertising of specific brand-name prescription drugs, apparently in response to favorable consumer reactions to two model prescription drug advertisements circulated nationwide.

QUESTIONING PHYSICIANS ABOUT SPECIFIC DRUGS

In order to maximize the benefits and minimize the costs of drug therapy, consumers need to learn how to question their physicians about drug regimens. In fact, the National Council on

Patient Information and Education (NCPIE), a non-profit organization representing health care professionals, consumers, pharmaceutical manufacturers, government agencies and other organizations, has launched a national "Get the Answers" campaign designed to encourage consumers to pose specific drug-related questions to physicians. These questions include:

- What is the name of the drug and what is it supposed to do?
- How and when do I take it—and for how long?
- What foods, drinks, other medicines, or activities should I avoid while taking this drug?
- Are there any side effects, and what do I do if they occur?
- Is there any written information available about the drug?

To these questions we would add:

- Are there any nondrug alternatives to the proposed drug therapy?

For example, studies suggest that drugs can be replaced by exercise in the treatment of certain kinds of depression, and that smoking cessation, dietary changes, and weight loss can be as effective as medications in controlling certain levels of hypertension. These are but a few of a growing number of examples of lifestyle changes that have been shown to serve as well as chemicals to control certain diseases. Of course, not everyone will be willing or able to adopt such changes. but at least the choice should be theirs to make.

This line of questioning should not stop with the initial prescription. Some drug side effects do not appear until months after the initiation of therapy. Unusual or serious symptoms should be reported to physicians because they could be the direct result of drug therapy. (For example, impotence may occur in men taking certain types of antihypertensive medication; weakness and fatigue may result from a variety of drugs, including corticosteroids; antihypertensive drugs may cause a loss of potassium.)

When side effects occur, some patients take matters into their own hands and discontinue drug use without consulting their physicians. In certain instances this behavior may be fortuitous, especially when the prescription was inappropriate in the first place. But unilaterally stopping or changing drug use can be counterproductive and even dangerous. The best course of action is close, continuous, and frank communication between patients and physicians concerning the promise and pitfalls of prescribed medications.

WRITTEN INFORMATION ABOUT DRUGS

Written material can provide invaluable information about drugs—how they work, indications for use, proper use, risks, necessary precautions, and side effects. The public's desire for this kind of information is evident in the purchase of written drug information from diverse sources. One striking example of this trend is demonstrated by the popularity among consumers of the *Physicians' Desk Reference (PDR)*. Distributed free to physicians every year and available to consumers for about $30, the PDR is composed of paid advertisements of brand name products supplied by drug manufacturers to the publisher of *PDR* (Medical Economics Company, Inc. in Oradell, New Jersey). These advertisements closely resemble the package inserts that accompany drugs when they are distributed to physicians. As a result, descriptions of drugs in the *PDR* contain technical terms not always comprehensible to the average consumer. For example, adverse drug reactions to the commonly prescribed drug Valium® include the following information:

Side effects most commonly reported were drowsiness, fatigue, and ataxia. Infrequently encountered were confusion, constipation, depression, diplopia, dysarthria, headache, hypotension, incontinence, jaundice, changes in libido, nausea, changes in salivation, skin rash, slurred speech, tremor, urinary retention, vertigo, and blurred vision.

Other valuable sources of drug and health care information for lay audiences can be found in monthly newsletters published by prestigious institutions, such as Harvard Medical School (*The Harvard Medical School Health Letter*, 79 Garden Street, Cambridge, Massachusetts 02138, available at $21 for an individual subscription) and the Mayo Clinic (*The Mayo Clinic Health Letter*, Mayo Clinic, Rochester, Minnesota 55905, available at $24 for an individual subscription).

Another supply of printed drug information intended primarily for the public is patient medication leaflets contained in the *United States Pharmacopeia-Drug Information* system. Considered by many experts to be the book of choice for consumer drug education, this resource contains a compilation of information about drug products, including indications for use, side effects, precautions, dosages, and instructions for administration. Individual leaflets are generally available at most pharmacies, and they can be ordered through pharmacists.

If good written resources are not readily available when consumers purchase prescription drugs, they can ask their pharmacist to provide a copy of a package insert on the drug. These informational leaflets produced by drug manufacturers primarily for physicians and pharmacists are written in technical language, some of which will be unfamiliar to the average consumer. However, most pharmacists are willing to review and interpret these materials, as well as to provide other drug information service.

THE ROLE OF THE CLINICAL PHARMACIST IN PATIENT CARE

Many consumers are unaware of the key role that pharmacists can play in assuring safe and effective drug use while containing drug costs. In the minds of many, pharmacists' activities are still limited to "counting and pouring and licking and sticking." But times have changed.

To appreciate fully the unique contribution that today's pharmacist can make, it is essential to understand the dramatic changes that have taken place in pharmacy education. During the past two decades, many pharmacy schools throughout the country have substantially reoriented pharmacy education in the direction of training "clinical" pharmacists—pharmacists who are patient-oriented as opposed to product-oriented. The training of these clinical pharmacists now includes patient care responsibilities, including assessment of patient responses to drug treatment, identifi-

cation of drug-induced adverse effects, and drug-drug interactions, as well as patient compliance to drug treatment, patient education, and monitoring of drug therapy.

Consumers can take advantage of this advanced training by seeking pharmacists' advice on a whole range of drug therapy topics, including:

- Whether a particular combination of over-the-counter and prescription drugs is safe and effective. (For example, it is dangerous to take aspirin or medications containing aspirin when a patient is taking prescription blood anticoagulants, because it may cause severe bleeding. Also antacids taken to relieve acid indigestion or gas can seriously impair the absorption of the broad spectrum antibiotic tetracycline.)
- How drugs react in the body and how the body responds to drugs—how many consumers know, for example, that many topical ointments or creams (e.g., Kenalog ointment or creams that are rubbed on the skin) are absorbed into the body just like tablets and capsules?
- Evidence of whether a patient is allergic to a prescribed drug.

Pharmacists can perform these expanded roles not only because they are more highly trained today but also because Silicon Valley has come to the community pharmacy. More and more hospital and community pharmacies are using computer-based drug information systems that permit them to maintain patient profiles. They record such information as the patient's health status, diagnoses, drug allergies, drug regimens (including both prescription and nonprescription drugs), health insurance status, when drugs were dispensed and the names and specialties of the patient's physicians. This information is generally obtained by pharmacists from patients by means of a brief drug history. Maintaining patient profiles is a useful way for the pharmacist to examine complex drug regimens in order to guard against adverse drug reactions, drug-drug interactions that may mitigate the effect of a prescription drug, and drug-food interactions that may enhance or inhibit drug effects.

THE ROLE OF THE CLINICAL PHARMACIST IN DRUG PRODUCT SELECTION AND COST CONTAINMENT

The clinical pharmacist is also in a position to play a key role in reducing the costs of prescription drugs for consumers through drug product selection, the authority given to pharmacists in 49 states to dispense the lowest-cost equivalent drugs to patients. Such products are generally generic drugs, those that are no longer protected by patent and thus are manufactured by multiple drug companies. In contrast, brand name drugs are protected by patent and sold only by one company. Patents on brand name drugs provide exclusive marketing rights to drug companies for a minimum of 17 years after they first gain FDA approval. Following this period, the drugs may be produced in generic versions by competing manufacturers. The FDA reviews information on generic drugs before they are marketed to assure that the generic versions are chemically, biologically, and clinically equivalent. A major advantage of most generic drugs is that most, but not all, are less expensive than brand name drugs.

Although the availability of many generic drugs provides an opportunity for physicians to prescribe the lowest–cost clinically effective drug product, this is seldom done. After a drug is placed on the market and promoted by its manufacturer, brand name familiarity is established, and many physicians continue to prescribe brand name products long after lower-priced equivalent drugs are available. Physicians are often unfamiliar with the availability of generic products that are chemically, biologically, and clinically equivalent. As a result, they often prescribe higher-priced brand name drugs, believing that they are protecting their patients from lower-quality generics. In this sense, physicians appear to accept the advice of large pharmaceutical manufacturers, who invest millions of dollars in advertising to promote their brand name drug products.

Not only are brand names better known to physicians than generic names, but generic names are often unpronounceable and thus not easily remembered by consumers. Valium, for example, is no longer protected by patent, but it is still frequently prescribed by physicians instead of diazepam, which is the generic product.

Like physicians, pharmacists are influenced by brand name manufacturers to select brand name products. Further, they do not wish to antagonize local physicians who might discourage their patients from patronizing pharmacies where generic drugs are substituted for brand name products prescribed by physicians. Finally, pharmacists are often able to make a greater profit from brand name drugs. Despite these pressures, pharmacists often encourage consumers to purchase generic drugs. As the health professional most knowledgeable about drug prices and drug effects, the pharmacist has a key role to play in containing drug costs.

By the end of the decade, some analysts predict that the market share for generic drugs will reach 40%, up from the current 15% to 20%. Enactment of the Drug Price Competition and Patent Restoration Act of 1984 will intensify competition between brand name and generic drugs because it provides a clear federal policy for FDA review of generic equivalent drug products. This law makes it unnecessary for each new generic equivalent drug product to pass through prolonged review, including the animal and human studies of safety and effectiveness that were required when the original brand name drug product was approved for marketing. As a result of these developments, the role of the clinical pharmacist in drug product selection will become increasingly important with each passing year, and the potential cost savings for consumers will be enormous if this role is exercised responsibly.

COMMUNITY-BASED DRUG EDUCATION PROGRAMS

As we noted earlier, the primary sources of drug information for consumers are mass media advertising (particularly of nonprescription drugs), information provided to individual patients by physicians about prescription drugs, and information on prescription and nonprescription drugs provided to customers by pharmacists.

A distinctively different avenue for consumer

drug education that has developed in recent years—designed specifically to improve consumers' understanding of the drugs they take—are community-based drug education programs. These programs are operating in a number of cities across the country. Most of them employ group teaching methods. Apart from its primary goal of giving information, group teaching also establishes a network to which elderly consumers can turn for help. Two innovative programs are described below. These programs are targeted primarily toward older consumers, but their methods and approaches are similar to those used among mixed-aged populations.

Baltimore, Maryland: The University of Maryland's Elder-Ed and Elder Health Programs. At the University of Maryland School of Pharmacy there are two drug education programs, representing two different educational models. In the first model, Elder-Ed, retired pharmacists are paired with pharmacy students to provide drug education at senior centers, apartment complexes, and other community sites where elderly citizens congregate. The program has been operating since 1979 with start-up funding provided by the Administration on Aging. Major program objectives are the safe and effective use of medicines, prevention of misuse and abuse of drugs, and involvement of elderly patients in their own health care.

In addition to providing student-pharmacist presentations at local senior organizations, Elder-Ed has developed innovative instructional materials to address topics of special importance to the elderly: nonprescription and generic drugs, nutritional and vitamin information and personal medication records.■

Although Elder-Ed has not been formally evaluated, its effectiveness is evident. Community response to the program has been so favorable that it has influenced development of similar projects in various cities throughout the northeast.

■ These materials are available, in quantity, from Elder-Ed at printing cost plus postage, by writing directly to: Elder-Ed, School of Pharmacy, University of Maryland, 636 West Lombard Street, Baltimore, Maryland 21201.

Program staff have advised pharmacists in Florida, Mississippi, and California on developing similar programs. Elder-Ed serves as a model for consumer-oriented drug education programs across the country.

One disadvantage of Elder-Ed is that it reaches only those older adults able and willing to attend sessions. Since a large number of elderly cannot be reached by Elder-Ed, a second educational model has been developed at the University of Maryland entitled Elder-Health, A Partnership in Care. Faculty, students, and retired pharmacists train caregivers—professionals and family members—to deliver services to the elderly in various settings, including the home. In this way, the non-ambulatory elderly can avail themselves of valuable information. The program may have another benefit: it is hoped that younger family members, acting as caregivers, will know more about safe and effective use of drugs when they themselves face health problems associated with older age.

Another aspect of Elder-Health involves pharmacy students in developing long-term relationships with elderly individuals. The pharmacy student locates an older person and forms a visiting relationship with him or her for 3 years. During that time, the student learns more about the life and concerns of older people, and the older person learns more about correct medication-taking and health care. Students meet with their faculty advisors in Elder-Health weekly to discuss experiences and interactions with their elderly associates.

Many other drug education programs across the country are sponsored by pharmacy schools. Each is notable for the fact that consumers serve not only as recipients of drug education but also as providers of such information. It is hoped that these innovative programs will bring about changes in pharmacy school curricula, alterations in the practice of pharmacy, and enhanced faculty and student perceptions and knowledge of consumers' drug problems.

San Francisco: SRx: Senior Medication Program. In San Francisco an innovative drug education program, SRx: Senior Medication Program, was developed in 1978 by two community health professionals. In 1980, the program was integrated into the San Francisco Department of Public Health and now serves as a model for a joint undertaking involving private and public funding sources. The program has four central objectives:

- Reduce drug misuse and abuse among the elderly through education on the safe and rational use of medications.
- Motivate the elderly to become knowledgeable consumers of medications, able to take active roles in making decisions about their own health care.
- Train health care providers to develop strategies related to these problems.
- Advocate program, policy, and legislative change.

In addition to educating individuals and agencies in San Francisco, SRx has expanded to other counties by establishing the Regional Outreach Educational Plan. The plan involves establishing an organization similar to SRx in six northern California counties and participating in resource exchange, intercounty use of volunteers, and promotion of regional advocacy. A central regional body governs the program and oversees consultation services, instructional activities, and educational materials. Each county contributes an "in kind" amount of resources, supplies, and financial and clerical support. Cost efficiency is a primary goal of the regional plan.▪

This discussion of community-based drug education programs is by no means complete. It is meant to demonstrate the diversity of efforts in

this area. Available programs differ with respect to organization, staffing, funding sources, sponsorship, and teaching methods. Yet all share an underlying characteristic: they are pioneering innovative efforts to address an important yet unmet educational need of the elderly. A comprehensive discussion of these programs, particularly those targeted to the elderly, is included in a book, *Drugs and the Elderly*, written by the authors, published by Stanford University Press in 1986.

CONCLUSION

The great American love affair with drugs continues unabated. As more and more drugs enter the market, the benefits of drug therapy will inevitably increase. And just as inevitable will be problems associated with drug use.

The purpose of this chapter is to try to convey some avenues available to consumers for maximizing safe and effective drug use while minimizing its problems. It is our firm belief that patients who question their physicians about the appropriateness and details of proposed drug therapies; who continuously give physicians information about their perceptions of the benefits versus the side effects of such therapies; who avail themselves of written materials describing the pitfalls and potentials of drug therapies; who utilize the capabilities of today's highly-trained clinical pharmacists; and who are able to sift the evidence provided through mass media discussions of drugs—such patients stand a good chance of realizing the full potential of modern drug therapeutics and not falling victim to its costs.

▪ For further information about the program, contact Kathy Eng, Director, SRx: Senior Medication Program, City and County of San Francisco, Department of Public Health, Room 204, 101 Grove Street, San Francisco, California 94102.

27 THE FUTURE OF PHARMACEUTICALS

Clement Bezold, Ph.D., is executive director of the Institute for Alternative Futures. A political scientist by training, he regularly advises state and local governments and their "futures commissions." In health care he has developed a series of "foresight" seminars for Congressional staff. He is a frequent speaker on the future of health care and a consultant to major health care companies. He has published books and reports on the future of pharmaceuticals, the legal system, the information revolution, and "anticipatory democracy." His book, *The Future of Work and Health* (co-authored with Rick Carlson and Jonathan Peck) received *American Health* magazine's Health Book Award in 1986.

How will we take our medicine in the year 2010? What new drugs will be developed and how will the pharmacist's role change? Will self-treatment, acupuncture, and herbal medicine replace traditional visits to the doctor's office? And will health care costs rise or fall? Dr. Bezold, an imaginative futurist, reviews some of the most important current developments in pharmaceuticals and offers his predictions of coming attractions in the neighborhood drug stores and clinics. He foresees dramatic changes in medical record keeping, health care providers, pharmaceutical research, and consumer advocacy. But first he takes us on a trip to the "Pharmacy of 2010."▪

This article will review the future of pharmaceuticals in relation to the changing health care system. It will begin with an image of a visit to the pharmacy in the first part of the twenty-first century, then review some of the key trends that will take us in that direction.

A TRIP TO THE PHARMACY IN 2010

John was sick, He knew it. His home health care monitoring system had diagnosed it as an viral infection and recommended a specific type of antiviral drug. John's home health care system was linked to his doctor's information system. The doctor's expert systems confirmed John's in-home diagnosis and facilitated a telephone consultation between John and the doctor. As was the case for most therapies, John and his doctor reviewed the treatment options. Bed rest for 4 to 6 days, augmented by visualization programs to enhance immune functions (unless other complications arose), would be one option, or he could take the recommended antiviral drug. John did not have the time to spend resting, so he chose the pharmaceutical approach.

John's home health care monitoring system placed an order with the pharmacy's information system for the appropriate antiviral. It would take several hours to prepare the drug because of the new approach to pharmacology that was adopted by most other pharmacies after the turn of the century. The pharmacy would biologically manufacture the antiviral. John's genetic sequence was on file in the pharmacy's information system. This would allow the preparation of the most specific drug for John. This process recognized John's "biochemical uniqueness" and prepared the pharmaceutical agent on that basis.

The antiviral drug was then placed in John's health care wrist watch at the pharmacy. This device monitored body function and delivered some of the electro-therapy that became common after 2000. (New research on "the body electric" merged with the traditional wisdom of acupuncture to produce a series of new or enhanced therapies that work by adjusting the body's energy fields.) The healthcare wrist watch (some had called it the "hospital on the wrist") also delivered the new pharmaceutical therapies, transferring the minute quantities of the antiviral stored in the device's reservoirs with micro injections through the skin. The watch monitored the effectiveness of the doses and ensured that the minimal appropriate dose was in the body.

John's pharmacy stocked all of the major new drugs developed over the last 25 years (or the ingredients and technology needed to manufacture the pharmaceutical). The most exciting, innovative drugs include vaccines for many cancers and definitive cures for many others; a "roto-rooter" pill that melts plaque build-up in arteries; drugs that cure or reverse the worst effects of Alzheimer's and other major dementias. These very effective high technologies compete with nutritional and behavioral approaches or "soft technologies" that in many cases are equally effective. The pharmacy's shelves also included health-enhancing high tech pharmaceuticals. Research on wellness and longevity showed what was most effective and the pharmaceutical industry responded.

The pharmacy also stocked a variety of self-health equipment. (John's basic home health monitoring system was given to him by his doctor as part of the annual fee John paid for care.) John's doctor was affiliated with one of the five national health care chains. Four of these chains provided very sophisticated equipment to their patients to facilitate health promotion and self-care. The financial incentives of the health care providers reinforced this sophisticated health care.

John could have had the antiviral delivered, as he did with many of his purchases. But John wanted to visit with the pharmacist and review some of the self-care materials in the pharmacy.

The pharmacist herself in John's pharmacy has changed. In the 1980s, the vast majority of pharmacists were men. By 2010, most are women. Their training includes not only more sophisticated pharmacology but also basic health care and health care communications skills. In many pharmacies, John's included, the pharmacist provides a variety of self-care courses related to biochemistry and pharmacology. The rise in interest in homeopathic and other natural remedies led pharmacy schools to return to pharmacognosy (the knowledge of the medicinal properties of plants) as well as homeopathic pharmacology. Pharmacy schools were also helpful in making students aware of communication skills and how to develop a better rapport with patients. Pharmacists often specialized, some into high tech pharmacology, some into merchandising/ management, some into alternative forms of pharmacology.

John was a member of the local consumer group's Committee on Health Care Monitoring, and the pharmacist was one of the group's advisers. John's committee maintained a sophisticated computer network that evaluated health care providers, software, and specific therapies. At any given time, 10% to 20% of the local community members used software from the local consumer groups to restructure their medical information, so that it could be shared and compared while still protecting their confidentiality. The aggregation of this at the local level told consumers who was successful. This local experience was then aggregated by groups such as Consumers Union, which produces a comparison of the five national health care chains, more than 100 regional health care systems, and hundreds of thousands of individual practitioners working in 2010. This system allowed for the comparison of alternative therapies and providers and led to significant changes in therapeutic practice. Medical therapies in 2010 are much better targeted to the illness, generally less invasive, and less expensive.

People now live longer with lower health care costs, but their additional years are more vigorous than in the 1980s.

Side effects of drugs, a serious problem in the 1980s, diminished significantly for several reasons. Large databases were developed during the 1990s that revealed the interplay between genetic factors, behavior and pharmacology, so the side effects of drugs could be well controlled Health care information systems ensure that information on side effects is well integrated into everyday practice, and consumers still review (or have their own home health care information system

review) the potential side effects of drugs and other therapy they may take.

The above optimistic image of the pharmacy and pharmaceutical use in 2010 is an entirely plausible forecast based on several specific trends. In the rest of this article I review some of the most important current developments that will take us toward this image. I acknowledge that there are other, less favorable possibilities, which I have dealt with elsewhere. I emphasize this image because it is one which you, the reader, could help make happen.

MEDICAL RECORD KEEPING AND HEALTH CARE OUTCOME MEASURES

Current medical record keeping systems are primitive in relation to what will be common within 10 years, much less by 2010. Sophisticated automated systems will monitor health conditions at home and in treatment settings. Facilitated by "smart cards" that will store and manipulate large amounts of information, as well as other new forms of storage, these systems will alter medical practice. There are a host of privacy issues these systems raise, some of which will be considered below.

This better record keeping will contribute to the development of better outcome measures of care, be it pharmaceuticals or other therapies. These outcomes measures will include various dimensions including physical condition, pain, side effects, direct and indirect costs. They will identify results produced from health care expenditures and as such will be a critical part of health care provider accountability. They will affect the purchasing behavior of individuals and third party buyers.

Consumers and their health providers will know the consumer's "biochemically unique profile" as a result of a variety of more sophisticated medical record keeping, body function monitoring, and genetic knowledge that will be inexpensive and accessible in the years ahead. Much of our medical care is "normalized" or standardized. This is especially true in our pharmaceutical use. Yet each of us has a chemical factory in our body whose operation is as different as our fingerprints are different. We will come to understand what these variations are and when they are significant.

Medical information systems will include expert systems software which incorporate aspects of the clinical decision tree of physicians and other health care providers. This will result in the decentralization of knowledge of medical specialists to nonspecialists, particularly nurses and consumers. These expert systems, sophisticated health condition monitoring, and miniaturized drug delivery mechanisms will combined by the first part of the twenty-first century to provide the "hospital on the wrist."

HEALTH CARE DELIVERY SYSTEM CHANGES

Our health care systems are beginning to provide incentives to consumers and providers to adopt health promotion and cost effective treatment. A growing percentage of consumes will participate in some form of capitated care system (e.g., HMO and IPA). These capitated deliverers will have incentives to provide more cost effective care, including better monitoring of outcomes, and more consumer service-oriented care.

They will also have incentives to use nurses and other nonphysician providers wherever appropriate. (Nurse practitioners can provide equivalent or better care than physicians in 73% of primary care contacts.)

Drug therapy in this setting will often prove more cost effective than surgery and there will be more cost effectiveness comparisons among drugs and comparisons of drugs with other therapies (see below). Formulary committees within HMOs will have increasing power over these drug purchasing decisions.

Health care providers, in order to be accountable to consumers and competitive in an increasingly real health care market, will develop their own methods for monitoring the comparative efficacy, cost, and outcomes of the care they deliver. Simultaneously, consumers will seek and competitive providers will provide high touch treatments and effective reassurance. The market will reward quality care.

Greater attention will be paid to those factors which we control through diet, stress management, and personal development techniques and their roles as therapies. The development of these "soft technologies" and certain new drugs will be stimulated by research in the field of psychoneuroimmunology, which will show better how the brain works and how we can shape our immune system's functioning.

PHARMACEUTICAL R & D

The pharmacopoeia at the disposal of health care providers and consumers at the beginning of the twenty-first century will be far more specific and potent.

Basic biomedical research offers promise in several areas. Research on immunomodulators, neurotransmitters, neurotropic hormones, mood altering drugs, monoclonal antibodies, prostaglandins, vaccines, and other genetic engineering areas are likely to provide new drugs for a variety of uses. Some of these areas will produce more sophisticated drugs requiring greater knowledge and skill on the part of providers and consumers. Some will produce a greater awareness of how factors such as nutrition affect our health conditions and the potential of nutrition as therapy. Within the next 25 years major breakthroughs are likely in the areas of cancer, heart disease, and neurological conditions, including Alzheimer's disease.

Pharmaceutical research will pay increasing attention to individual variations in relation to specific drugs. The recognition of the importance of "biochemical individuality" will direct more attention to genetic variations in the way our bodies deal with drugs (pharmacogenetics) as well as the way in which our lifestyle (particularly diet and stress) affects drug functioning in the body.

This will give rise to prospective epidemiology—the ability to target and warn individuals who have certain characteristics which increase the risk for specific adverse reactions to a drug.

Currently drugs are shown to be safe and efficacious before they are put on the market, but there are often no formal requirements of monitoring the safety or efficacy in actual medical practice. There has been increased discussion of Phase IV studies or increased postmarketing surveillance studies of drugs. This is critically important and the new health care system will make this far easier.

The market place monitoring of practice (on the part of consumers, employers, and providers) will become a much more important source of drug information and will be used by consumers and providers (especially formulary committees of hospitals and primary care chains, whose large patient populations will be among those being monitored). Dramatic advances in medical record keeping and changes in health care delivery system changes will accelerate this development.

The combination of new breakthrough potentials from biomedical research and a marketplace requirement for cost effectiveness will focus pharmaceutical R & D on the most effective new possibilities. Very significant changes in the drug marketplace are occurring, both as more generics enter the market and as information on the cost effectiveness of drugs is developed and used. There will still be significant opportunities to provide breakthrough drugs that are more effective to use. And it will become harder to put drugs with little therapeutic gain on the market and assume that they will capture enough market share to be profitable.

"Designer gene machines" and related devices will appear in the pharmacy. These will allow the pharmacist to develop drugs that are most compatible with each person's genetic makeup.

CONSUMER AND CONSUMER GROUP CHANGES

Self-care, both in treating illness and for health promotion and wellness, is one of the most powerful forces driving health care system changes. This includes a significantly greater search for sophisticated information on the part of many.

For pharmaceutical use, patients will continue to do various forms of self-care. In reviewing current consumer habits, the CBS consumer survey reports that nearly half of all households using prescription drugs borrow or use previously prescribed medication to self-treat similar illnesses or conditions when they reoccur. What is even more important is the finding that 14 million households report owning a copy of *Physician's Desk Reference* (or an equivalent) and 27 million report that they consult a *PDR* for information. FDA surveys show that probably more patients read the *Physician's Desk Reference* than do physicians. This aspect of the patient information market is large enough to have stimulated at least 13 *PDR*-type compendiums. In the years ahead the quality of this information will improve as will the devices for communicating it. Many of the books now in use will be replaced by electronic systems that speed access and that can incorporate automatic searching for side effects most relevant to the individual consumer.

The next decade will also see the emergence of consumer groups which evaluate health care providers. Consumer groups will have their members provide information with adequate privacy guarantees to local and national information networks to compare the outcomes of providers and treatment. Current examples include the evaluation of physicians and HMOs by the *Washington Consumer Checkbook* (Washington DC area) and the People's Medical Society (national). These will be tied to the dramatically improved medical record keeping procedures that group members use on a routine basis.

There will probably be several different consumer monitoring groups, giving consumers a range of choices about health care philosophy and approach.

Powerful home information systems in widespread use 10 to 15 years from now will be able to handle very sophisticated medical monitoring, record keeping, and diagnosis, as well as communicate with the information system of the consumer's health care provider and the consumer groups to which they belong.

These developments will be reinforced by the continued pressure on the part of large health care purchasers, namely employers, for more cost-effective care, including better monitoring of outcomes.

The current 13 or more *PDR*-type compendiums will be available in electronic form, continuously updated, benefiting from the enhanced consumer and provider drug use monitoring. Yet local consumer groups will be able to offer comparisons of products and weekly prices for local pharmacies and other outlets.

Eventually consumer groups will evaluate potential R & D directions and expenditures of pharmaceutical firms. Consumer groups will give awards and various other reinforcements to companies seeking the strategies most consistent with consumer values.

Much of what is described above will be used by the informed consumer. While this influential group could improve the market significantly by its monitoring, and the market will get "smarter" in the years ahead, there will always be the need for some "information minimums" of the type the FDA has been considering with the patient package insert (PPI).

CONCLUSION

The nature and quality of pharmaceuticals available for use will improve significantly over the next 20 years. Consumers can help shape that improvement by monitoring their health-care practices and by supporting consumer groups that follow pharmaceutical R & D prospects. Additionally, they can reinforce efforts in appropriate directions by pharmaceutical companies.

There are other trends that will shape the future of pharmaceuticals, such as the aging of the population, AIDS, FDA regulation, and Federal R & D and drug reimbursement expenditures, to name only a few. The basic points, however, are that the trends identified here—better health information systems, the focus on the biochemical uniqueness of each of us, truly significant pharmaceutical breakthroughs, equally significant advances in "soft technologies" that each of us control, changes in health-care provider incentives, and consumer monitoring of health care—will make the future of pharmaceuticals similar to that described in John's trip to the pharmacy at the beginning of this article.

28 CAN HEALTH PROMOTION ENABLE PEOPLE TO LIVE HEALTHIER LIVES INTO LATER LIFE?

James F. Fries, M.D., is associated professor of medicine at Stanford University and chief of the arthritis clinic there. He is also director of ARAMIS (The American Rheumatism Association Medical Information System), a national computer databank of patients with rheumatic disease. Dr. Fries is an avid runner, an expedition mountain climber, and author of 97 articles and several books, including *Take Care of Yourself, Taking Care of Your Child, Prognosis, Arthritis,* and *Vitality and Aging.*

Most people assume that the ills and afflictions of old age are unavoidable and that living robustly until we die is the exception, not the rule. It is also assumed that good health in later years results chiefly from good medical care. Dr. Jim Fries argues that the habits we develop in our youth or middle age will affect our health when we are old. He believes that a healthy lifestyle may decrease the number of people who develop chronic diseases and delay the onset of symptoms in those who do. So the healthy period of life prior to the onset of a chronic problem may be increased by a careful diet, exercise, stress management, and avoidance of cigarettes and alcohol.∎

Imagine two scenarios for our aging population. In the first, life expectancy and life span grow ever longer, but people grow old at the same point in time as now. Thus, an ever longer proportion of each individual life is spent "old," infirm, possibly sick, possibly senile, probably dependent. The prolonging of life has resulted, in effect, in the prolongation of dying. Health care cost increases exceed the most alarmist estimates.

In the second scenario, life expectancy continues to increase, but the rate of increase gradually slows as it approaches the length of the natural average biological life span in humans of approximately 85 years. In contrast to the first scenario, the age at which individuals pass certain milestones of infirmity grows ever later. Aging itself is postponed. Thus, heart attacks occur later, as do strokes. Emphysema and the various cancers begin later in life. Clinical problems from chronic disease decrease. Morbidity at the end of life is preceded by an ever lengthening period of vigor and vitality. The percentage of an individual's life spent infirm decreases. This is the compression of morbidity. This chapter will explore the evidence behind development of the compression of morbidity thesis, the role of health promotion in the compression of morbidity, and the mounting evidence that these phenomena are beginning to occur.

THE EXCHANGE OF CHRONIC DISEASE FOR ACUTE DISEASE

At the beginning of this century, life expectancy was 47.5 years. The leading cause of death was tuberculosis, accounting for over one quarter of all deaths, and major mortality was accounted for by diseases such as typhoid fever, appendicitis, polio, syphilis, diptheria, tetanus, and other acute infectious diseases. As a class, the major specific infectious diseases have now decreased as causes of mortality by over 99% in this century.

In place of the acute diseases are now chronic problems such as atherosclerosis, emphysema, cirrhosis, cancer in its many forms, and, in terms of morbidity, osteoarthritis. These conditions now account for 90% of the mortality and 90% of the morbidity in the United States.

In social terms, much of the turmoil of mounting medical care costs and need for increased numbers of hospital and nursing home beds traces to this "exchange" of chronic disease for acute. The individual now survives the acute illnesses to die at a more advanced age of a more chronic illness. As a result, the percentage of an individual life spent in a hospital, or infirm by other definitions, has steadily increased. Now, however, the exchange of chronic disease for acute is essentially complete since there is little serious acute disease remaining. With the completion of this exchange, this major force which has been increasing the morbidity burden of the country becomes much less prominent.

THE NATURE OF CHRONIC DISEASE

Our modern "medical model" of disease really traces to the "germ theory" in which illness was thought to be caused entirely by outside pathogens and medical treatment was devised in order to eradicate the external threat. Diseases such as tuberculosis and smallpox illustrate this principle. However, the currently prevalent diseases do not fit this model.

Rather, today's major diseases are chronic, degenerative, influenced by multiple risk factors, and not curable in the same sense as were the earlier infectious diseases. Perhaps the most differentiating characteristic, is that the present diseases are universal. People do not differ from each other as to whether they have the illness or not; they differ in how much of the particular illness they have. Atherosclerosis, for example, begins in the teens or twenties with the development of small fatty plaques on arteries which enlarge in size over the ensuing decades until clinical problems result. All individuals have these problems, but in some the rate of accumulation is minimal and ultimately inconsequential. In others it is rapid and leads to premature mortality.

The concept of diseases as having causes has given way to diseases having risk factors. Risk factors accelerate the development of a chronic disease. For atherosclerosis they include dietary fats, blood pressure, body weight, lack of exercise, cigarette smoking, and stress. For cancer, cigarette smoking, obesity, alcohol for certain cancers, and a variety of other environmental exposures lead to an increased risk of neoplastic change which increases with the amount of exposure to the risk factor. For emphysema, smoking is the primary risk factor, and for cirrhosis, alcohol. The most prevalent acute disease remaining is trauma, 50% due to automotive mishaps. The risk factors are impaired drivers, imprudence, and failure to utilize protective devices such as seat belts.

The emerging paradigm of chronic disease mandates an entirely different therapeutic approach involving preventive control of the rate of accumulation of the disease process rather than after-the-fact control of a complication. Health becomes much more dependent upon healthy lifestyles than upon the quality of the after-the-fact medical care.

Possibly the most important attribute of this new model, however, is the fact that changing the rate of development of chronic disease not only decreases the number of people who will

FIGURE 28-1.

THE INCREMENTAL MODEL OF CHRONIC DISEASE

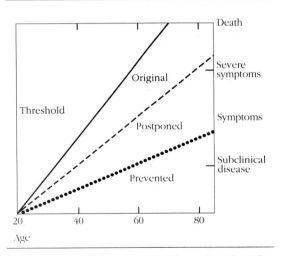

■ Note: (a) onset in early life, (b) different slopes for different folks, (c) the potential effects of life-style modification upon the slopes of the lines, and (d) the effect of changing the slope upon the time of life at which the symptom threshold is crossed. (Reprinted with permission from Vitality & Aging, W.H. Freeman & Co., San Francisco, CA 1981.)

develop clinical symptoms but also delays the onset of symptoms in those who do. Thus there is a prolongation of the healthy period of life prior to development of the first chronic disease symptomatology. Evidence that chronic disease may be postponed by lifestyle change is indisputable in the case of cigarette smoking and exercise, and it is almost certain with regard to other major risk factors described above. Thus the vital, vigorous, disease-free portion of life can be extended. Opportunity is great.

THE BIOLOGIC LIMITS TO LIFE

In contrast, the human life span is biologically fixed. Even after elimination of all disease and all accidents, people will die after living not much longer than at present. A full discussion of the evidence for the finite human life span and the calculations that estimate its magnitude is beyond the scope of this chapter. Several lines of evidence suggest, however, that the ultimate average human life span may approximate 85 years with a standard deviation of 4 to 5 years and that 95% of all deaths will ultimately occur in the period between 70 and 100 years of age.

It is initially surprising to many that the life span is, in fact, fixed and that life would not go on forever with the eradication of disease, because our medical model implicitly makes the assumption of potential immortality. On reflection, however, it is clear to farmer and scientist alike that the life span of all species is indeed fixed. Hamsters may live 3 years, horses 40, and Galapagos tortoises 150. This is not because Galapagos tortoises are healthier than human beings; it is because their species' life span is greater. In the United States, the oldest authenticated death was a woman dying in 1928 at the age of 113 years, 274 days. Anthropologic studies indicate that the human life span has been fixed for at least 100,000 years. The increasingly rectangular survival curves of our century demonstrate the failure of maximum age to increase. Physiologists document a linear decline in organ reserve beginning around age 20 or 30 which is independent of disease and must logically result in death without disease at the point when organ functions are insufficient to sustain life. An actu-

FIGURE 28-2.

THE INCREASINGLY RECTANGULAR SURVIVAL CURVES
OF THIS CENTURY

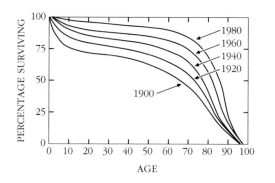

■ Note (a) the currently small level of death prior to age
50, (b) the steady improvement over each score of years, and
(c) and constant point of insertion at the end of the curve.
(Reprinted with permission from *Vitality & Aging*, W.H. Freeman & Co., San Francisco, CA 1981.)

arial law discovered in 1824 by Benjamin Gom-
pertz notes that mortality rates double every 8
years after the age of 30 and that this exponential
decline in survival is a constant characteristics of
all populations. A finite death for all must result.
Moreover, the *a priori* phenomenon of frailty is
increasingly evident as our population ages; frailty
refers not to illness but to a decrease in the adaptive powers of the organism. Decreased hearing,
eyesight, reflexes, strength, and reserve functions
of the vital organs cumulate in a decrease in the
ability of the organisms to survive even minor
challenge.

THE COMPRESSION OF MORBIDITY

Average life expectancy is anticipated to continue rising slowly. Increasing improvement will
become more difficult with time as the average
life expectancy begins to push against the biologic
limit to life. Advances in life expectancy in the
past have resulted from decreasing the number of
cases of infant mortality, tuberculosis, premature
heart attacks, and other diseases of middle age.
Chronic diseases are becoming less prevalent. As
premature death occurs less frequently, the natural life span remains, and further improvement

would require modification of the genetic characteristics of the race, not an immediately likely
prospect.

Postponement of the onset of chronic disease,
and postponement of the loss of adult vigor, can
increase at a much more rapid rate. Postponement
of morbidity results in its compression and its
diminution. Similarly, with the declines in vitality
that represent what we term aging, postponement
of loss of vigor results in a decrease in the period
of impaired function.

A STRATEGY FOR POSTPONEMENT
OF THE ONSET OF MORBIDITY

Lifestyle factors are the obvious target, since
the consequences of unhealthy lifestyles are extremely large. Cross-cultural comparisons, such
as with the Japanese, indicate that atherosclerotic
complications might be reduced by 70% to 90% as
a result of dietary and other lifestyle modifications.
The National Cancer Institute estimates that at
least 70% of all cancers could be prevented by
individual lifestyle-related actions. In terms of
postponement, such changes would postpone
death only by about 3 years, but they would
postpone the onset of morbidity by probably 5 to
10 years.

EVIDENCE FOR THE COMPRESSION
OF MORBIDITY

The relationship of disease to lifestyle is incontrovertible. The causative role of the major risk
factors for cardiovascular disease and for cancer have been demonstrated in experimental
animals and documented in multiple epidemiologic studies. Large-scale intervention trials have
demonstrated the ability to improve survival by
lifestyle interventions. Less frequently remarked,
a great deal of very common nonfatal morbidity is also linked strongly to lifestyle factors. For
example, varicose veins, gall bladder disease, her-
nia, gastritis, ulcer, reflex esophagitis, and hemorrhoids are clearly related to lifestyle. Most elective
surgical procedures are designed to treat problems that result from unhealthy habits.

We have experienced a 15-year decline in
the United States in the consequences of atherosclerosis. Over this period, heart attacks and

strokes have significantly decreased; age-specific rates are down by over one third. For males, the average age for a first heart attack has risen 4 years over a period of time in which the average life expectancy from age 40 has increased more than 2 years. Thus, morbidity has been compressed.

The compression of morbidity thesis notes that men traditionally have suffered greater rates of premature death than women and thus have considerably lower life expectancies from birth. This model predicts that the biologic limit to life will be approached most rapidly by the longest living cohorts (white females in the United States) and that their relative rate of increase in longevity will slacken first. This has now happened in the United States, where the widening difference between male and female life expectancies, reaching 8.4 years from birth in 1982, has now declined to 7.9 years. In Japan, the country with the foremost worldwide health statistics, the gap between women and men has now narrowed to only 4.9 years.

Lung cancer onset ages are rising in men even as the prevalence of lung cancer in men reaches a plateau and begins to decline. For women, lung cancer rates will continue to rise for another 6 or 7 years.

Nursing home utilization also begins to show evidence for the beginning of the compression of morbidity. Over the last 10 years, life expectancy from age 85 has increased from 5.6 to 6.6 years. Over the same period of time, the percentage of individuals over 85 in nursing homes has increased only from 20.5% to 21%. In other words, the average 85-year-old spends less time in a nursing home environment than previously. Implicity, the age of admission to nursing home, a difficult statistic to come by, is increasing.

Evidence for the compression of morbidity is mounting from a number of different directions, including the bioscientific, the epidemiologic, and the demographic as noted above. Historically, it is a new phenomenon, beginning slowly 15 years ago with the change in cardiovascular mortality, and gradually gaining momentum and breadth as the years have progressed. It is now a strong force and will become much stronger.

CAVEATS

The compression of morbidity will affect the percentage of time that an individual, on average, spends infirm. But the compression of morbidity will not make the large problems of our aging population to go away. The national problems of care for elders depend on the number of individuals in particular age groups. The last of the "baby boomers" are now 23 years of age, so for the next 40 years we will be facing greatly increased number of individuals entering the sixth, seventh, and eighth decades. The "rectangular society" is one in which essentially everyone born reaches at least the age of 70. This unprecedented social phenomenon creates very real problems which have not been faced by previous civilizations, and have not been solved by this one.

The second caveat is that we face a period of national social choice. If we adapt health promotion and disease prevention approaches, we can compress morbidity. If we neglect these approaches and concentrate on heroic high technology measures after the fact to prolong life at all costs, we may continue to increase morbidity.

FIGURE 28-3.

THE IDEAL SURVIVAL CURVE AFTER ELIMINATION OF ALL DISEASE

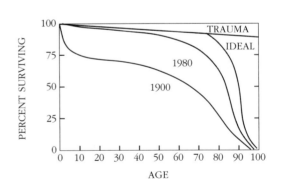

■ Note the large remaining role of trauma. (Reprinted with permission from *Vitality & Aging*, W.H. Freeman & Co., San Francisco, CA 1981.)

OPPORTUNITY

Thus there are two scenarios for the future; in one, morbidity is compressed and social, medical, and personal resources are mobilized in a primary effort to delay the onset of chronic illness, social isolation, and dependence. In the other scenario, the increasing number of elderly people requires ever more care and support. The opportunity is present for us to become the society that plans for healthy elders.

29 EXERCISE AND THE AGING PROCESS

Ralph S. Paffenbarger, Jr., M.D., is professor of epidemiology at Stanford University. He studies the determinants of disease in large population groups. Previously concerned with identifying the means by which poliomyelitis and other infectious diseases were transmitted, he now confines his research to chronic disease, including heart disease and cancer. He is particularly interested in identifying personal characteristics and lifestyle elements that affect life expectancy and reduce the risk of developing coronary heart disease.

Robert T. Hyde, M.A., is an epidemiologist with the Stanford University School of Medicine. He has been studying host and environmental influences on chronic diseases, seeking to identify trends, associations, and causal relationships of personal characteristics and lifestyles elements and their effect on health, aging, and longevity.

With the growth of modern populations that include an increasing percentage of elderly and aged persons, the term "senior citizens" has become a household word and the label for an extensive area of social responsibility. Great interest has developed in the activities and health requirements of these older individuals. In particular, new attention is being drawn to the importance of their habits and needs of exercise. There is widespread hope that a better understanding of exercise and aging can help to improve the quality of life and reduce the burdens of invalidism and expense associated with health care in the later years.■

Adequate exercise is a natural requirement of the body and is necessary to keep the vital systems of the body in good working order as long as possible: this may be called its maintenance function. Exercise also helps to avoid or delay chronic disease: this is often considered its protective function. Both of these functions can be regarded as capable of influencing the aging process, assuming it can be altered. Or, in another sense, aging may be considered as gradually altering the role of exercise in the maintenance of health as the body grows older.

There is much uncertainty in attempts to define the aging process itself. Some view aging as the running down of a biological clock. Others see it as deterioration of essential body systems. Or it is called the result of wear and tear, the effect of assaults by disease and environmental hazards. Many believe it is influenced by motivation, which is subject to psychological, social, physiological, and physical factors. In almost every line of thinking, however, aging is eventually assessed in terms of capacity for activity. Thus viewed, aging is seen to have a direct interrelationship with physical activity or exercise.

It is possible to look for signs of aging by applying batteries of tests to the body systems, i.e., measuring blood pressure, pulse, respiration, muscle strength, reflexes, audio visual acuity, balance, memory retention, and so on, but the overall aging process is best defined by capacity for the performance of external work while maintaining regulation of the internal environment necessary for survival. On this basis the successive stages in aging are usually defined as follows:

Middle age: The second half of a person's working career (age 40–65 years)

Old age: The immediate post-retirement period, when there is usually no gross impairment of function or homeostatis (65–75, sometimes called *young old age*)

Very old age: Usually some functional impairment, but the individual can still live a relatively independent life (75–85, sometimes called *middle old age*)

Extreme old age: Where institutional or nursing care is usually needed (85+, sometimes described as *old old age*)

Culturally and individually there are wide variations in the degree and rate of aging, so the above categories are only approximate and many departures from them occur. Physiological age, or the ability to be active, is the true criterion of aging status, not chronological age in years logged on a calendar. Thus, to some extent habitual exercise itself may be a good index of aging. Almost regardless of years, persons who are adequately active are likely to be physiologically younger than those who are less active. Here "adequate" physical activity may be defined as that necessary for the body to maintain its status quo, or at least minimize its rate of deterioration. The goal is to extend the vigorous middle years of life and so to postpone and abbreviate the ultimate decline that is the inevitable result of the natural aging process.

Most importantly, the interrelationship is a two-way street. If exercise is a bodily maintenance activity and an index of physiological age, the lack of sufficient exercise may either cause or hasten aging: "It is possible that a significant amount of age-based deterioration may arise from decreasing physical activity rather than advancing years," says a British Sports Council research paper. If that is true, persons who exercise little should become "aged" sooner than their more active cohorts, while physically active elderly persons should remain physiologically younger than their peers who have abandoned exercise. There are countless anecdotes that support these impressions, and perhaps almost as many refutations. In fact, only a large-scale, long-range epidemiological study of lifestyles could supply the data and analyses needed for scientific proof on any of these points. Complex patterns involving many variables would have to be examined. The findings of such investigations would be of great value, but in the meantime it is certainly possible to consider what kinds and amounts of exercise should be recommended for individuals in the advanced decades of life.

TYPES OF EXERCISE

In the course of daily living, however sedentary, everyone engages in several different kinds of exercise. At higher levels of exertion these have a variety of physiological effects. Some are good for the senior citizen, but others should be minimized.

Passive exercise occurs when the muscles and joints are set in motion or flexed by the application of power from an external source, as by a physiotherapist, a mechanical device, or forces of inertia in a moving vehicle. In an aged person such exercise could promote metabolic process, enhance blood flow, reduce stiffening of joints, and possibly avoid some wasting and edema, but it would do little to develop muscle strength or cardiovascular/respiratory fitness. Passive exercise does have further value in aiding recovery from injuries at any age.

Active exercise utilizes the power sources of the individual himself and involves many elements not required in passive exercise, e.g., motivation, feedback, balance, aerobic capacity, load bearing, and others. Normal load bearing, as occurs in sitting, standing, and physically active work, is essential to the healthy maintenance of bone and cartilage, especially in the support structures such as the legs and spine, hips, shoulders, arms, hands, and feet. The muscles and tissues that support these structures also require such exercise. These considerations are critical to the continued well-being of aged persons, but overload stresses should be avoided.

Isometric exercise is not recommended for the elderly because it involves putting a stress load on the muscles and joints without moving them. This also may severely overtax the cardiovascular system by constricting blood vessels and inducing a steep unrelieved increase in blood pressure. It is *static exercise* rather than *dynamic exercise*. Everyone has to do both kinds in order to get along, but if enough dynamic exercise is performed to benefit the cardiovascular/respiratory system as is needed, the musculoskeletal system will be trained sufficiently to serve the body's static or postural requirements without the need of an isometric exercise regimen.

Isotonic exercise flexes the muscles and joints in a reciprocal dynamic process such as working with cable weights, hydraulic machinery, or sculling or sailing a boat. A certain amount of this kind of exercise might be helpful for strengthening the muscles, but it should be as rhythmic as possible, and it should not be considered a substitute for the rhythmic and vigorous kinds of whole-body exercise that are undertaken to benefit the cardiovascular/respiratory system, described here under aerobics.

Aerobic exercise utilizes the oxygen supplied to the muscles by the cardiovascular/respiratory system. The oxygen transport capacity of an individual is established by the condition of his lungs, heart, blood vessels, blood, and muscles, influenced of course by all other systems of the body. Conditioning of the cardiovascular/respiratory and musculoskeletal system is affected by exercise, lack of exercise, aging, lifestyle, environment, and disease. Maintenance of good condition by adequate physical activity is always important, but it becomes especially important or even critical as aging progresses and the margins between health and disability are narrowed. Therefore, in popular usage, *aerobic exercise* has come to mean exerting oneself sufficiently to keep these essential systems in good shape, i.e., at or near their maximum capacity for doing work or physical activity. Some common measures of such exertion are working up a sweat, breathing deeply to take in more oxygen, and getting one's heart rate up to a count well above the resting pulse, so as to pump enough blood to meet the demands of the large muscles that are being urged into rhythmic motion as in walking, running, swimming, cycling, or in using a hoe, rake, broom, hammer, or handsaw.

Anaerobic exercise is required of the body when the cardiovascular/respiratory system does not supply enough oxygen for the work being demanded of the muscles. The necessary additional energy is provided from within by a different biochemical process, essentially a back-up or auxiliary system that is rather limited in capacity and difficult to enhance by training or other means. Perhaps because of their reduced activity, aged persons have less capacity for anaerobic exercise, yet probably tend to draw on that resource sooner if their aerobic capacities are diminished by aging or lack of exercise; either way, their maximum capacity for work is lowered as their years increase. According to some views the chief use of the anaerobic mechanism is to provide the muscles with an energy source that can be used immediately while the aerobic process is getting underway, which may take a minute or more, depending on the condition of the individual.

Physiological measurements have shown that although the elderly have a lowered maximum performance, they respond to training in much the same way as younger individuals. Often older persons seem to require less of a workout to achieve a given level of physiological benefit, although their response may be slower or more gradual. As do women, older men perform a particular physical task at a higher percentage of their maximum heart rate than younger men, unless the occupation permits slowing down on the job. The maximum rate itself is lowered with increasing age.

EXERCISE AND THE SYSTEMS OF THE BODY

It is convenient to assess the influences of exercise on aging and chronic disease in terms of the various physiological processes or vital systems of the body, though by interaction the effects on one biological mechanism sooner or later affect the rest. The processes and characteristics usually studied categorically are those of the cardiovascular/respiratory, musculoskeletal, gastrointestinal, genitourinary, neurosensory, metabolic, endocrine, and hematological systems. For brevity, some of these will be discussed below in groups, as will be noted. At least equally important, of course, is the system of the mind, whether assessed for its psychological and social manifestations, its psychosomatic symptoms, its electro-kinetic circuitry, or its cerebrovascular and biochemical requirements.

Thus far, with regard to aging there has been difficulty in establishing norms for any of the body systems. Experimental data are hard to obtain and subject to many biases and uncertainties, with wide variations among individuals of the same chronological age. Methods of study and measurement often are not standardized or are unsuitable for aged persons. These variations, plus others introduced by ethnic, geographic, secular, and temporal differences, tend to complicate the assessment of biological or physiological age and the effects of exercise on aging. While these limitations must be kept in mind, much information of value has been obtained in recent research.

The Cardiovascular/Respiratory System: Exercise and Heart Attack

Among the most emphatic results of epidemiological studies of physical activity have been the findings relative to risk of heart attack. These extensive investigations have not fully demonstrated cause-and-effect relationships between exercise and protection, or between inactivity and disruption, but their large-number statistical conclusions and the apparent sharpness of their circumstantial evidence have led to increasing acceptance that the studies do represent causes and effects. The results are consistent by age, time, place, and personal characteristics. They persist over time and show a dose/response pattern in which exercise is inversely associated with the risk of heart attack.

Some broad spectrum epidemiological surveys may reflect the real life situation more fully than detailed clinical studies. For example, the track records of college alumni relative to exercise and heart attack have been assessed in the presence and absence of other chronic disease, cigarette smoking habit, hereditary tendency, and other risk factors. The influence of exercise is substantially independent of the influence of any of those other characteristics. It appears as a protective effect in the positive sense or as an additional hazard in the negative sense. In other words, lack of sufficient exercise is a risk factor. This is important, since inactivity is considered to be one of the more common ways of hastening the aging process. Conversely, habitual adequate exercise is regarded as a healthful means of deferring such developments.

Potential evidence of self-selection, such as

student athleticism and varsity status, has been weighed against the reported exercise and health experiences of adult life and advancing age. Vigorous activity by alumni, not their student athletic prowess, determined their risk of heart attack. The college alumni studies have shown that even a relatively modest amount of currently habitual and recreational physical activity is significantly protective against fatal and nonfatal first heart attack and lowers risk of death from subsequent heart attack among survivors of prior heart attack. Since these alumni exercise data were assessed on a moderate scale where low and high levels of leisure-time physical activity were defined as below and above 2000 kilo-calories of energy expenditure per week, the findings should be relevant to exercise standards for older persons in general. Most elderly who are still in good health should be able to achieve the levels of exertion found effective among the alumni thus far. Further data on what levels and kinds of exercise the alumni themselves maintain as they get older would be worth studying, as current information about exercise in the later years of life is slender.

In San Francisco a 22-year study was conducted among 3,686 longshoremen aged 35–74, whose low and high levels of physical activity on the job were rated as being below and above 8500 kilo-calories per week. All of these men were required by union rules to spend at least an initial 5 years in the heavier duty jobs of cargohandling, and the average was 13 years. Some remained cargohandlers all their working life. Death rates, particularly from heart attack, were significantly lower among men in the high activity jobs than for those less active. Skill and work-gang politics may have enabled the older men to ease off a bit in their exertions, but certainly the aging process in these very active elderly individuals had not yet brought them to a delicate state of health.

The Musculoskeletal System: Exercise as Maintenance

Because of recent publicity, the relation of exercise to the well-being of the cardiovascular/respiratory system has appeared to be of central importance. But, among the elderly and the aged, conditions of the musculoskeletal system can become even more obvious matters of concern. Aches, pains, cramps, twinges, stiffness, and cranky, unstable joints are symptoms of structural and mechanical difficulties associated with aging, whether or not they are diagnosed as arthritis. Diminished connective tissues and support muscles lead to shortened stature and curvature and stiffness of the spine. Loss of knee articulation may hamper functional locking of the joint needed for stability. Cellular, molecular, biochemical, and physical changes that occur with aging in muscles and connective tissues produce losses of strength, power, elasticity, reflex, bracing, and control.

Wasting or deterioration of bone occurs rapidly when the body is reclined instead of standing up; also, cushioning and nutrient fluids are withdrawn or withheld from the synovial joints. Some of these effects can be reversed if erect posture and activity are restored, as during convalescence after confinement to bed. The ability to renew or revitalize tissues is slowed with age, so recovery may be difficult where injury has occured or proportions have become altered and strength has been lost.

Since loss of function may be impossible to restore, habitual and appropriate exercise of the musculoskeletal system is important for maintenance of ability. Reduction of mobility is one of the more consistent indices of physiological age. Furthermore, muscular activity is important to the proper functioning of metabolic, endocrine, and cardiovascular systems as well as to posture and movement. Exercise for the aging musculoskeletal system should be gentle and rhythmic rather than sudden or stressful. Flexing and stretching movements such as those used in warming up are especially beneficial and can reduce chances of damage from sudden stresses such as might occur in tripping, stumbling, or even more vigorous actions. Training that lengthens muscles can increase joint flexibility, while regular dynamic action of the joints increases flow of nutrient fluids to the cartilage.

Isometric exercises are not recommended, nor are other straining efforts, as harmful local over loading and injury can result. If cardiovascular status permits, judicious work with weights can help strengthen muscles, but like obesity a heavy musculature is not a recommended burden for a weak heart. The aerobic exercises required for cardiovascular fitness can also benefit the musculoskeletal system if care is taken to do adequate stretching and flexing exercises before and after the more vigorous whole-body workout.

The Assimilative Systems: Exercise, Diet, and Utilization

For brevity it is convenient to group here the gastrointestinal, metabolic, endocrine, and hematological systems as representing assimilative processes related to other factors such as diet and environment, as well as to exercise. There are significant interrelationships between diet and exercise, as in the control of obesity. It is routine knowledge that reduction of fat is best achieved by combining lowered caloric intake (diet) with increased caloric output (exercise), so that output will exceed input as is necessary to lose weight. If only one means or the other were to be chosen, it would be better to choose exercise, so as not to risk lack of needed nutrients. Many individuals who regularly engage in vigorous exercise testify that their appetite have not increased and may even be decreased by their activity but that they can eat whatever they please without getting fat. Studies in England and Iowa have shown that vigorously active men consumed more calories yet weighed less than men who had lower caloric intake but were not sufficiently active to achieve weight balance or weight loss. Weight alone is not as important an index of health as body composition, or the ratio of fat to muscle, and exercise promotes muscle whereas inactivity promotes fat. Diet and exercise experiments with primates have demonstrated that inactivity also promotes unfavorable cholesterol levels and atherosclerosis.

The healthy, active body tends to demand whatever it needs, i.e., a well balanced diet of fat, carbohydrate, protein, vitamins, and minerals. An individual who takes up exercise after having been sedentary for some time may actually gain weight with training, but the increase is muscle instead

of fat and the figure becomes trim. A paradox of aging is that after middle-age gains of fat, the elderly tend to lose weight, but the loss may be of muscle rather than of fat, especially if inactivity is a feature of lifestyle.

Some have observed that exercise may improve the ability of the body to utilize nutrients and rid itself of wastes more efficiently, promoting regularity and minimizing constipation. Physiological measurements of the effect of habitual exercise on the gastrointestinal tract are lacking, however. Exercise is known to increase glucose tolerance, probably by increased blood flow to the more active muscles, thus reducing risk of adult-onset diabetes, especially that associated with obesity.

Recently much attention has been directed to the effects of physical activity on blood cholesterol. Total cholesterol is unchanged, but high-density lipoprotein (HDL) cholesterol is favored and low-density lipoprotein (LDL) cholesterol is suppressed, while very-low-density lipoproteins are halved. These changes are associated with improved cardiovascular health and lower risk of heart attack, apparently by reduction or inhibition of atherogenesis. HDL-cholesterol has the strongest influence of all the lipids and lipoproteins on risk of coronary heart disease in old age, showing a significant negative association in both men and women up to age 80, according to a report of the Framingham Heart Study. Recent studies elsewhere have concluded that a prudent diet has more influence on cholesterol makeup or blood lipid profile than exercise as such, but those findings do not negate the important relationships of diet and exercise described above.

Exercise enhances fibrinolytic activity, and thus it may reduce risk of thrombosis. Vigorous rhythmic habitual exercise, especially of the large musculoskeletal structures such as the legs in walking, stair climbing, jogging, snowshoeing, cross-country skiing, or cycling, enhances the activity of red blood cells and oxygen transport throughout the body. Enzymatic activity, processing of nutrients, uptake, utilization, and scavenging functions are improved or maintained.

In general, there is no reason to suppose that

beneficial effects of exercise noted in younger subjects are not also applicable to elderly and aged individuals, even though some systemic changes are ascribed to aging. Although data for establishment of norms have been too uncertain to define what is normal, especially for the elderly, various physiological trends with age have been observed. An older person is different from a younger person both in structure and in functioning. Such changes can affect matters of immunity, capacity, adaptation, and maintenance, and may or may not be amenable to control by medication. As age increases, the margin for resistance or recovery is narrowed and the systemic costs of inactivity can become more critical. Exercise programs for the elderly may differ from those of youth, but their importance for the maintenance of vitally essential performance in all systems of the body is, if anything, increased as time goes by.

The Neurosensory and Cerebral System: Exercise and the Mind

Research differs on whether physical activity can have salutary effects on cerebral function. Certainly, motor training is one thing and mental agility another. Elderly individuals often function more slowly than younger adults, either because of slowed responses or from greater caution established by experience. Verbal and other tests administered to young and old may be confounded by elements in the background of the older person, or audiovisual or other localized deficiencies that can affect coordination, emotional control, speed, and accuracy. It is often difficult to tell whether an age-related decline in performance has been caused by neurosensory deterioration, losses in audiovisual perception, central information processing trouble, or atherosclerotic disease in the cerebrovascular system. Delay could be anywhere in the circuit of receptors, central processing, and muscular response, but it is believed by many to reflect loss of efficiency in the central processing system of the brain. Since brain cells are not self-replacing, channel capacity, signal strength, memory service, and response time would be adversely affected if the number of active cells is diminished by deterioration or blocking.

The elderly have better long-term than short-term memories, perhaps because these differ in their structural or electro-chemical principles. Learning difficulties in the elderly appear to reflect problems with short-term memory and with selective and integrative functions. The gradual deterioration of cerebral function with aging is a complex and sensitive area of human experience and study. If exercise tends to delay atherogenesis or thrombosis and loss of active neurons by cell anoxia, it might be shown beneficial to mental processes, at least from the standpoint of good maintenance. Exercise is a well-known adjunct of psychotherapy for mental patients and for social and personal adjustment, but this application in the aged could require a special set of values or maintenance objectives. It may well be that, where the maintenance of cerebral function is concerned, mental exercise of the brain is as important therein as physical exercise is to the other body systems. Also, many interactions are likely: not a few devotees of regular aerobic exercise often claim to have swept away mental cobwebs while endurance running.

Much is said about the importance of motivation in the elderly, the necessity of keeping up the will to stay alive and remain active and healthy. A similar motivation is needed to keep up the habit of ample vigorous exercise, but there is an element of feedback in the process: exercise is reported to promote favorable attitudes by enhancing the sense of well-being and love of life. This interaction of mind and body is elemental to most philosophies and is a chief principle of psychosomatic medicine. The individual incentive so often demonstrated in exercise patterns may have broader application to the process of aging. Dr. James Fries says, "Personal choice is important— one can choose not to age rapidly in certain faculties, within broad biologic limits." At this point the state of the mind, whether maintained by physical exercise or other essentials of upkeep, emerges as a psychosocial instrument on which, along with physical mobility, the caliber and success of most programs for senior citizens will depend.

EXERCISE AND CHRONIC DISEASE: PROTECTION AND THERAPY

Thus far we have discussed interrelationships of exercise and aging in vital systems of the body with or without reference to chronic disease. Inasmuch as various chronic diseases involve particular body systems, physiological and other considerations already mentioned will not be repeated here. The rationale for including a brief section on chronic diseases is that, as already mentioned, much confusion exists as to what is chronic disease and what is aging. Dr. Franklin Williams, director of the National Institute on Aging, has said, "Aging is not a disease. I think we need to make that distinction all the time. We need to look for explanations and causes whenever someone has a deviation from a healthy state and not to accept anything as just aging. That's been a bad myth."

If aging is taken to be an inherited, genetically determined process, the newest biomedical science of genetic engineering raises the question of whether modifications might become possible. Even without such speculation, those who seek to define aging are uncertain whether the aging process itself may be deemed naturally capable of adjustments along the way, or whether many observed variations in degeneration of tissues and faculties are effects of long-term and insidious chronic diseases that might be treated or avoided. By the same token, it may be difficult to determine whether exercise had avoided or arrested a disease or slowed down the process of aging. Some regard disease as hastening aging and countermoves as fending off disease. Or, disease can be thought of as an intrusion that alters the functioning of one or more key body systems and so disturbs the vital balancing of homeostasis. In this sense a chronic disease could be regarded as an overlay of additional hazard above and beyond the life-limiting influence of the aging process itself.

Whatever view is taken, much of the research on exercise in relation to chronic disease can also be considered applicable or transferable to aging, and vice versa. Thus, studies of the effects of exercise on the cardiovascular/respiratory system are often directed to heart attack or coronary heart

disease risk rather than to some calculated stage of aging of the elements of the system. Yet, even after the data have been adjusted for chronological age or analyzed on a birth-cohort basis, it could be postulated that a cardiovascular/respiratory system in good working order may be regarded technically as "younger" or less aged than one in poor condition. This would be valid whether the difference was thought to be due to heredity, cigarette smoking, exercise level, environment, diet, or some other cause. To the extent that physical exercise has maintained the health of a vital body system it has helped to keep that system "young." In conditioning the cardiovascular/respiratory system, exercise has reduced the risks of heart attack, hypertension, atherogenesis, thrombosis, edema, dyspnea, anoxia, and stroke.

The suggestion has been made that if a condition responds to treatment, it was due to disease; otherwise it is due to aging. Such a definition may be convenient for some purposes, but it will remain open-ended as long as there is still room for medical progress. On that sliding scale it is an attempt to assume that the true aging process is not subject to modification. Then we are expected to define stiffness of the joints as some form of arthritis and say it has been avoided or relieved by recommended exercise.

Lewis Thomas has rated present knowledge of cancer as being in the nontechnical or semitechnical state and concerned more with treatment of symptoms than with causes and prevention. Hypotheses of cancer etiology may relate it to heredity, cigarette smoking, sunlight, environmental toxicity, diet, viral assault, autoimmune deficiency, trauma, stress, worry, or aging, and confound attempts to distinguish an association with exercise aspects of lifestyle. If running discourages cigarette smoking it may tend to reduce lung cancer, but outdoor sports might help to promote skin cancer by increasing exposure to sunlight. If leanness in youth predicts one kind of cancer and obesity another, there may be implications for exercise as well as for diet, heredity, and lifestyle. Long-range epidemiologic studies of many chronic diseases are still in the exploratory stage. As chronic disease research continues, the topics of exercise and aging should be taken into account at every opportunity.

EXERCISE AND LONGEVITY

When considering the interrelationships of exercise, disease, and aging, the bottom line may be to ask whether physical activity extends longevity, i.e., by deferring all causes of mortality. Recent studies of data on college alumni have shown that habitual leisure-time exercise is related inversely to total mortality, though most strongly to cardiovascular disease death rate. In a 16-year follow-up among 16,936 Harvard alumni aged 35 to 79, all causes of death rates were one-third lower for men expending 2000 or more kilocalories per week than for those less active. Longevity estimates showed that in all 5-year age groups up to 65, at least 10% more active than inactive men would survive to age 80. The difference remained sharp above age 65 although narrowed a bit in the shorter follow-up time left before reaching 80. Between the ages of 35 and 80 the estimated additional life gained by adequate exercise as contrasted with sedentariness averaged upward of 1 to 2 years. This significant difference was independent of other characteristics such as cigarette smoking, obesity, hypertension, or heredity.

For any individual alumnus the gain in longevity might be well above the average cited. Also, considering the beneficial effects of adequate exercise on the various body systems, discussed earlier, it is logical to suggest that the years of life gained would be likely to occur in the middle as added active years, rather than at the end as years of extended disability. Another calculation, derived from the time required for sufficient exercise versus the estimated average gain in longevity by physically active alumni, is that the exerciser would in effect have each hour of exercise to live over again plus an additional hour besides.

LIMITATIONS AND OPTIONS FOR EXERCISE BY THE AGED

Lately much attention has been directed to aerobic exercise and endurance training. But aside from anecdotal reports on a few elderly and even aged athletes, the data have been chiefly on middle-aged and younger individuals. Recommendations as to jogging beyond age 65 have ranged all the way from "not recommended" to "go ahead." The commonsense view is probably somewhere between these extremes.

Once a training effect is achieved, a maintenance effect is desired. The aerobic response or training effect should be considered an index of exercise value rather than an objective in itself. Heart rates, blood pressures, vital capacity, oxygen transport, stamina, strength, and endurance are only part of the total body picture at any age and especially at advanced ages. The effects of stress and activity on all systems must be considered, even though the results of natural exercise for any system should be expected to be beneficial as contrasted with the consequences of inactivity. Jogging, for example, may not be recommended for a certain individual because of his musculoskeletal state; swimming may be proposed instead.

Injuries to cartilage and tendons are a common hazard to athletes of all ages, and the effects of aging make the elderly even more susceptible to these problems. The road to safety, however, is not necessarily to quit jogging or walking, but to be more careful about warming up and warming down before and after the main exercise, stretching and flexing the muscles and tendons and joints to make them loose and limber before subjecting them to stress and after they have done their hard work in training. "Start slowly and taper off" is the motto of a San Francisco runners club. These before-and-after regimens also influence blood flow and lactic acid concentration, both of which become of increased concern in older individuals.

Where for one reason or another a jogging or walking program is not feasible, swimming or bicycling or a good home stationary cycle may be a good substitute. The advantage of walking is that it can be done almost anywhere and requires no special equipment except good shoes and perhaps a favorite stick. The training benefits of walking depend on the pace and distance, or intensity and duration, and the fitness of the walker. Hills and stairways provide extra work that can enhance the results per mile, but they invite accidents and local-stress hazards for an aged person. In some surveys walking has ranked second only to gardening as a physical activity most favored by the elderly.

There is no need to take risks, but also no favor is done by steering anyone away from adequate exercise who could have benefited by engaging in it. In fact, the elderly and the aged are a select class of persons who by their survival have already proved their durability. Within reason, they should feel free to engage in whatever exercise or physical activities they see fit. Even a handicap is not necessarily a stop sign. People run marathons without eyes or feet, ski with one leg or no arms, and play basketball in wheelchairs. So, too, an aged amputee might feel better pushing his wheelchair around and doing the dishes than merely sitting still. Calisthenics are not the only way to limber up aging joints. Other rhythmical activities such as playing the piano, weaving or whittling, or furniture polishing may be as effective and more enjoyable.

Extra attention to posture and precision of movement can minimize the likelihood of accidental strains or injuries due to distraction, imbalance, poor reflex, or reduced vision or hearing. Taking the time and patience to be thoughtful about it can increase the enjoyment of any exercise and help avoid the risks of environmental hazards, uneven surfaces, soft or slippery spots, poor lighting, bad weather, and inadequate dress or equipment. Motivation and self-motivation are important: how much can be done depends on the individual, and if properly heeded, his own responses may be the best guide to what that is.

The ideals of an optimum training regimen for the elderly have been listed as safety, effectiveness, motivation, and low cost. Vigorous physical exercise is not recommended for individuals with certain adverse conditions: congestive heart failure, dissection aneurysm, recent embolism, thrombophlebitis, acute infectious disease, ventricular tachycardia, severe aortic stenosis, active myocarditis, acute myocardial infarction. Special precautions are recommended for people experiencing conditions such as deforming arthritis, marked obesity, severe hypertension, neural

and metabolic problems, electrolyte disturbance, reliance on heart pace or medications, and the like. Diabetics need to know how their insulin requirements are altered by exercise. The goal of exercise by aged persons is not primarily to extend life but to improve the quality of life while it lasts. However, if survival is considered to be optimal in healthy individuals and reduced in those with disease, adequacy of exercise may indeed increase longevity as well as quality of life.

DISCUSSION

Many of the research observations described earlier have centered on one body system or another—for example, the study of heart attack risk in the San Francisco longshoremen. But those elderly men who continued to work hard must have avoided not only heart attack but other disabling afflictions. Not just their cardiovascular/respiratory systems but their other vital systems had to keep on functioning effectively. It is very likely that their exercise pattern helped to maintain those as well. If the ability to remain highly active is evidence of deferred aging, these elderly longshoremen would seem to have remained physiologically younger than less active individuals of their chronological age.

Hard workers who become sedentary after retirement are likely to fare worse than those who continue to be energetic in their leisure years. The college alumni health studies showed that alumnus exercise habits influenced continuing health status, not student athleticism. Workers who retire from either physically demanding or sedentary occupations will improve their lot if they devote some of their new leisure time to vigorous activity. Both clinical and epidemiological studies of the kinds and amounts of exercise needed for best health maintenance and longevity are underway or proposed in a number of populations. The knowledge obtained from these will become clearer and firmer as follow-up of aging goes on and morbidity and mortality curves become more pronounced. Along the way, assessments should include attention to other elements of lifestyle and to matters of motivation, self-determination, and choice.

SUMMARY

Definitions of the aging process are uncertain. There is a lack of specific information on the "normal" physiological characteristics, activities, and health trends of individuals as their chronological age advances, especially in their later decades of life. Most observations to date have been derived from small-number studies, extrapolations from younger experience, or inferences from research not originally designed to assess aging. Current information on exercise, however, does strongly indicate that it plays an important role in health maintenance and the extension of longevity.

The wide variations encountered in physiological and sociocultural data suggest that much can be done to preserve or adjust lifestyles of the elderly so as to maintain capacity for activity and physical independence, fend off disease and deterioration, and enhance the quality of life in the later decades while the power and will to survive remain. The effort will be more than repaid in dividends of human satisfaction and intellectual and social progress. In particular, the predicted heavy burdens of invalidism and expensive but hopeless bed care may be reduced. With a rapidly increasing percentage of senior citizens in the total population, the sociomedical field faces equally great responsibilities to develop new knowledge and intervention programs to achieve these goals. Because physical activity influences the health of every individual, research and programs on exercise are of prime importance.

Programs and Prescriptions of Exercise for the Elderly

To the extent that adequate physical exercise is a requirement for health maintenance and a bulwark against chronic disease, programs and prescriptions should be designed to help keep the elderly motivated to elect and continue effective exercise, so individuals will not drift away from it and lose its benefits. Recognition of this as a wise policy has already led to the organization of regular exercise groups and of senior citizen activity programs, such as walking tours of museums, shopping malls, historic sites, and nature areas, with provision of the transporta-

tion necessary to bring a group together. Popular television programs on exercise bring guidance and participation to many individuals at home and can be designed to help elderly as well as younger viewers. Educational and social agencies have instituted courses in aerobic dancing, rhythmic exercise to jazz or ballet music, yoga, and swimming. There are senior marching bands, and a team of elderly cheerleaders received national attention. Group interest in exercise is very helpful, but athletic competition is not recommended for the aged because it may provoke overexertion and risks of injury.

Considerable progress has been made recently in developing guidance information for physicians as to prescription and surveillance of exercise for their patients. The very active personal interest of many physicians themselves in habitual exercise is a most promising and significant trend in contemporary professional thought and lifestyle.

A corollary is the importance of instilling good habits of exercise into the young, so they will be inclined to continue sufficient physical activity to maintain fitness throughout their middle years and on into old age. This view has led to the promotion of "life sports" such as skiing and swimming, in preference to team sports such as football or soccer, since the number of persons who may participate in team sports is limited by access and facilities, while there is no limit to participation in individual exercise alone or in club-oriented groups. In England a national program, "Sport for All—Come Alive!" has been launched to distribute information and promote appreciation of vigorous exercise, including moderate workouts for the elderly. Despite possible hazards, the international growth of Masters and Seniors categories in foot races, swimming meets, golf, bowling, tennis, and other sports activities is hailed as evidence that these programs have no intention of excluding the elderly and that the elderly have no intention of being excluded.

The recent upsurge in popular attention to sports and health is impressive, but there is reason to believe that hardly one third of the U.S. adult population habitually get enough vigorous exercise to quality as adequate in physical activity.

Attitude tests have shown that the elderly often fail to assess their own physical activity status realistically, usually overestimating it. This suggests the need of continuing public education on the subject, plus added support for activity programs.

Needs for Further Research on Exercise and Aging

With specific reference to exercise and aging, as well as to chronic disease, more accurate information is needed on both the physiology and the lifestyle of senior citizens, decade by decade into the later years of life. Better knowledge is needed of the scope, goals, types, standards, effectiveness, and results of exercise programs, including their significance to the individual and to the community. Information should be updated on the extent of facilities, utilization, encouragement, costs, and participation. Studies should attempt to determine what modifications of experience are being achieved, by what means, and with what effect on health and longevity.

Anecdotal and clinical data on the physiology of aging as affected by exercise will continue to be sought. There is a great lack, however, of more massive pertinent information on the lifestyles and health experiences of the elderly as they grow older. This deficiency hampers interpretation of much other data concerning them, as well as attempts to define and assess the aging process. The National Health Survey on Health and Nutrition has compiled a random sample of health data on Americans of all ages, but it includes little information on physical activity. A U.S. general population survey of physical activity and fitness has been proposed by the National Center for Health Statistics and is in the planning stage.

In view of difficulties encountered in obtaining reliable actuarial and clinical information on aged persons, more research is needed on better ways of gathering and processing data and interpreting the results. The complexities of aging, coupled with the complexities of lifestyle and other influences, present a formidable challenge to even the latest methods of analysis. Adequate design and evaluation of studies may often require use of several different approaches to a given problem, even on a seemingly familiar subject such as exercise.

Utilization of Findings

It is already clear that exercise or physical activity is a positive and pervasive element of health maintenance for everyone and especially for elderly and aged persons. Knowledge developed on this subject will be quickly applicable at all levels, from individual regimen to community program to national health policy. Because exercise and aging are so closely interrelated, improved activity programs may be expected to have an early and continuing favorable effect on the well-being of many senior citizens at a time in history when that is more needed than ever. The results of further studies in this field are likely to have important social and economic impact in the years ahead.

30 SOME MYTHS AND REALITIES ABOUT AGING

Ruth G. Newman, Ph.D., is a clinical psychologist practicing in Washington, D.C. For many years she specialized in working with disturbed children, their parents, teachers, and schools. Her books include *Psychological Consultation in the School* (Basic Books, 1967) and *Groups in Schools* (Simon and Schuster, 1974). She is vice president of the American Orthopsychiatry Association and a fellow of the A. K. Rice Institute for the Study of Group Relations.

What others believe about us frequently influences the way we picture ourselves, and self-esteem greatly affects our health. Therefore, the myths that we develop about ourselves and others intimately affects our lifestyles. The elderly are probably most affected by these myths. The way in which society views old age and what an older person actually experiences often contrast sharply. But the result may be the isolation of the elderly population, which leads to them being increasingly misunderstood. Dr. Newman has dealt with this vicious cycle professionally. Her work both with children and with the elderly brings a unique viewpoint to this discussion.■

One of the greatest ironies of our western culture is that although we have focused much attention on health care, preventive medicine, and living longer, healthier, and happier lives, we have not come close to wanting to deal head-on with the issues of those who *do* live longer. It is sometimes difficult to understand what it is that we want as a culture. In other words, if indeed we do wish that people were able to live longer, healthier lives, then why is it that once these people have attained an old age, we wish to have very little to do with them, if anything at all? The answers to this irony are far beyond the scope of this chapter, but it is clear that our isolation of the elderly may be one of the most important factors in their not being able to attain the longevity that they might otherwise have before them. Nor are our older members of society able to enjoy the fruits of their wisdom by virtue of their years and experience, and therefore their years are spent in a less than healthy fashion. It is not growing old that matters to most, but growing old healthy and growing old happy.

It has become evident to researchers of longevity that there is no magic potion that allows some people to become centenarians while others die at a much younger age. It seems clear now that a mixture of factors are at play: genetic, nutritional, alcohol consumption, physical activity, sexual activity, psychosocial involvement, and environmental factors. Even though all these play an important role in a person's ability to achieve longevity with happiness, when centenarians are asked what their secret has been, they often respond that sexual activity and community involvement have been most important. Now, this is not to say that the answer to a long life has been making love (though it may be!). But it is clear than an individual who feels a part of life and of the community is a person who feels needed.

There is solid evidence that a relatively low caloric intake (1500–1800 calories a day) and a diet high in fibers and low in fats contributes to a longer, healthier life. There is also evidence that biological propensities play a role in possible longevity. There is information to indicate that moderate drinking habits over heavy drinking patterns play a role in longevity. There is increasing information to show that exercise on a daily basis plays an important role in living healthy longer. And there is clear evidence that environmental factors that involve high pollution levels of all sorts (i.e., noise pollution, toxic waste seepage, air pollution, water contamination, etc.) unquestionably reduce the chances of long, healthy living. But the information regarding social involvement or social isolation is far less apparent. Nevertheless, it is becoming quite clear that this is a major factor in the health of the elderly and their increasing longevity.

Loneliness is everyone's next door neighbor. It touches people at different times in each life. It can come at night, it can come during broad daylight. It happens when we are alone and while we are in a crowd. It is there with the 8-year-old, the 18-year-old, the 38-year-old, and the 88-year-old. And it undoubtedly affects each intensely. However, at 8 and 18 and 38, there is far more likelihood that someone in the social environment will respond to the lonely. At 88, few may care.

The isolation and loneliness of the elderly is partly a result of the separations that have developed over the past century within the social stratas and family structure and community systems. Today, more than ever before, a person can live in the middle of any city or town and not know one single neighbor, nor the people who travel by the door each day (the postman, the electric meter reader, the gas man, and the telephone man). It is easy to be no one in the midst of a bustling city. Families are separated and isolated from one another, communities are apparently less and less dependent upon the elderly for any service (although this is a community's great loss). Western civilization seems to have created little need for the older person. And through all of this, the elderly have less contact available to them, contact by which the myths and realities of the elderly can be discarded.

Any approach to enhancing the health of elders should start with a clear understanding of the aging process.

First some basic facts:

- Americans over age 65 represent one out of every five U.S. households.
- As they age, women increasingly outnumber men. There are 16 million women over age 65, compared to only 11.5 million men.
- Like the general population, the largest concentrations of elderly are found in the most populous states. However, the proportion of people over age 65 varies greatly from state to state, with a high of 17.3% in Florida and a low of 2.9% in Alaska.
- Seventy percent of the population over age 65 are home owners and nearly 80% have paid off their residences. However, an estimated one third of the elderly live in substandard housing.
- Only 5% of the population over age 65 reside in nursing homes, hospitals, or other institutions. Family members and friends provide more than 80% of the care for older persons.

Beyond these fundamentals, many myths abound. Worse yet, even the elders frequently believe them. And in believing these myths, older people can and often do compromise their own health and well-being. Feeling helpless or senile, incapable, used or victimized is hardly a healthy attitude.

In 1975 the National Council on Aging commissioned Lewis Harris and Associates to survey Americans under 65 about their attitudes toward those over 65. After completing this survey, the Harris organization reported that most young Americans believed that older people were friendly at their best, but basically poor, sexless, physically impaired, and intellectually failed or incompetent. Some of the specific findings show what a dim view many of us have about the "old." Only 41% of those polled thought elders were physically active; only 35% believed them to be effectual; a slim 29% thought elders alert; just 21% thought them adaptable; and only 5% believed elders to be sexually active. These answers are far from true.

To further illustrate the schism between myth and reality, a poll was conducted in 1973 by Ben-

nett and Eckman which posed these four questions to people of all ages:

1. In general, old people need _____

   _____

2. One of the greatest fears of many old people is _____

   _____

3. Old people tend to resent _____

   _____

4. One of the greatest pleasures of old people is _____

   _____

Before relating what Bennett and Eckman found, fill in the answers yourself. How do your answers compare to their findings stated below?

1. Younger people most often names assistance as the major need of old people. Older people cited their dominant need as wanting to be liked and valued by others.
2. Younger people said that death and dying were great fears, while older people most often stressed financial insecurity. Death is not the primary fear of older people. Their fears are more immediate, reflecting realistic insecurity in regard to the opportunities available.
3. Younger people guessed that the object of older people's resentments was younger people! The older people, specifically referring to their treatment by others, said they most resented rejection.
4. Younger people judged that the greatest pleasure was in family, while older people more frequently chose companionship and love.

To see how deep some of these myths are embedded, try another test. Answer the following true and false questions.

1. Most older people who live into their eighties or beyond become senile before they die.   T F
2. Aged persons tend to regress and become more like they were as children.   T F

3. Women are more likely to live into their later years than men.   T F
4. All people start becoming more forgetful after the age of 20; older people cannot learn well.   T F
5. Fewer than 10% of all older people are college graduates.   T F
6. The majority of older people no longer have sexual desires.   T F
7. As people age, they almost inevitably become more withdrawn and disengaged from life.   T F
8. The majority of older people are in poor health by the age of 60.   T F
9. The suicide rate is higher for the elderly than for any other age group.   T F
10. As people become older, they tend to become more suspicious, complaining, and irritable.   T F
11. Older people worry much more and are much more suspicious, complaining, and irritable.   T F
12. Older people can no longer produce on a job or be very active socially.   T F
13. Senile behavior is always caused by brain damage.   T F
14. Alcoholic beverages are more hazardous for the elderly than for other adult age groups.   T F

How many "true" answers did you mark? If you checked more than three, you checked too many. Only statements 3, 5 and 9 are true!

Unfortunately, many myths die hard. One of the most persisting ones is that older workers are less productive than younger ones. In fact, our public policy on aging, and in particular retirement policy, reflects this belief. The truth is otherwise. The Andrus Gerontology Center at University of Southern California has studied this issue extensively. They not only found that older workers were as productive, they frequently found that they were more productive. Some of their findings are striking:

- In 1977, 4% of the workforce employed by Bankers Trust and Casualty Company were over 65. The majority of these workers were concentrated in clerical jobs. Approximately 30% were managers or supervisors. According to management, older workers were more dependable, had much better attendance records, stayed on the job longer, and did as much work as younger employees.
- Employees aged 60 and over comprise 20% of the sales force of the Texas Refining Corporation, a manufacturer and distributor of roofing materials and wall coverings. These older employees have the highest sales averages, according to management. In addition, their older workers were more dependable, inclined to stay on the job, and easier to work with.
- The Department of Labor in 1956, 1957, and 1960 did a series of studies on factory workers in two light manufacturing industries and clerical workers in government and private offices to investigate age differences in performance. The Department's findings show that clerical workers aged 65 and over had the highest performance record.
- In the early 1950s, the Bureau of Business Management at the University of Illinois examined the effectiveness of over 3000 retail, industrial, office, and managerial workers who were aged 60 or older. They found that in terms of absenteeism, interpersonal relationships, and quality and quantity of work, the majority of these older workers performed as well as or even better than younger workers.

The research done on elders and their capacities shows that:

1. Intelligence is relatively stable throughout life, unless the person is suffering from a health condition affecting cognitive abilities. Sometimes heart or circulatory problems or even advanced cancer can reduce awareness or diminish mental activity. Most important, learning is possible at any age.
2. Physical activity can continue throughout a person's life. Certain kinds of activities can remain relatively constant. Lifestyle and environmental/cultural factors, rather than

age, are primarily related to the amount of activity in a person's life.

3. Creativity can occur at any age.

4. Individuals with more education have better health and appear able to adapt more successfully.

5. Personality does not normally change drastically with aging: people show a consistency throughout life. When personality does change, the change is not directly the result of aging.

6. The sex drive and related behavior continue at any age.

7. Age is a poor index of the differences between people in their abilities to find pleasure in living and to experience happiness.

In order to an individual to maintain a healthy outlook on life, he or she must have the self-confidence to go beyond the myths and believe in the realities. The same can be said for communities and cultures. It is, by and large, the way in which each of us imagines aging and the elderly that most affects their outlook on life. In such a youth-oriented culture as our own, aging and the elderly are avoided. Sadness, loss, helplessness, and a lonely lifestyle describe our fears of the elderly. This obviously has to change in order for the elderly to function happily and healthily in our society.

31

SOCIAL NETWORKS AND SOCIAL ISOLATION AMONG THE ELDERLY

Meredith Minkler, Ph.D., is associate professor of public health education at the University of California at Berkeley. She also is director of the Center on Aging at Berkeley. With Carroll Estes, she edited *Readings in the Political Economy of Aging* (Farmingdale, NY: Baywood, 1984), and she has written numerous articles, book chapters, and monographs on aging and related topics.

"Social isolation of the elderly is for the most part a problem that is socially created and maintained," writes Dr. Meredith Minkler. "As such, it is a problem that will not be solved without a serious societal commitment to policies and programs that reflect a basic belief in the dignity, autonomy, and social worth of all individuals, regardless of age." In this chapter, Dr. Minkler describes the protection and support to be found in social networks and she suggests ways in which individuals and communities can intervene to prevent the social isolation of the elderly that often follows the death of a spouse, mandatory retirement, or the onset of health problems.∎

The losses associated with old age often are mistakenly believed to involve primarily declines in physical or mental capacities. What is often forgotten is that for many of the elderly, a far more serious loss is the sense of place in the social milieu. Widowhood, retirement, sudden geographic moves—these and other life changes often involve disruptions in an older person's support network. When these disruptions are particularly harsh—as, for example, with the sudden death of a spouse, unwelcomed mandatory retirement, or the move to a nursing home— the consequences for physical, mental, and emotional health may be profound. Network breakdown and social isolation are among several key risk factors which help explain why some older people become ill while others remain in good health. Put more positively, older persons who are immersed in strong support networks appear more likely to maintain their health and to resist disease than those without strong supportive ties.

In this chapter we will look at social networks and social isolation among the elderly. Following a general discussion of this topic, we will consider several different contributors to social isolation in this age group. Finally we will examine a number of promising avenues for intervention that may help prevent or remedy social isolation in the elderly.

For the purposes of this discussion, *social networks* will refer to the web of interpersonal connections in which people live and function. *Social support* will be used to describe the resources, both tangible and intangible, that people receive through their networks and that they give to others. *Social isolation* will refer to a process through which people may lose their sense of personal integrity or their ties to people and other social resources.

THE SOCIAL NETWORKS OF OLDER PEOPLE

When we think about social networks, it is helpful to use Kahn's metaphor of the convoy. It suggests the movement of each individual through life, surrounded by a set of people to whom he or she is related through the giving and receiving of social support.

As individuals age, people are added to or subtracted from their convoys through death, changes in job and family life, and geographic moves. With these changes, the potential of the social network for providing social support also varies over time.

The networks of older people are smaller than those of younger people, with major losses often recurring around age 70. But despite a contracting social world as a consequence of the death of friends and relatives, geographic moves, and other changes, most of the elderly have the basic ingredients for social support. Over half are married, for example, and four out of five have at least one surviving child. Contrary to the popular myth about America abandoning its elderly, all but 5% of older people live outside of institutions and three fourths of those who have children see them on a weekly basis.

While these statistics suggest a high degree of social contact for many of the elderly, however, other facts should not be overlooked. Of today's population aged 65 and above, for example, greater proportions are women, widowed and very old, than in previous times. In fact, the death rate of people aged 85 and over dropped 20% over the last decade, suggesting a greater number of frail elderly living alone and whose children often are themselves in their sixties or even seventies.

The network characteristics of older people vary widely by sex, socioeconomic status, and other factors. Contacts with relatives, for example, tend to be more common among older people in higher socioeconomic groups, while contact with children is highest among working class elders. The latter are also far more likely to live with their children than are elderly persons from upper- and middle-income backgrounds.

As in other age groups, the social networks of elderly men are considerably smaller than those of older women. For many aged men, the wife is in fact the only close friend or confidante and the one who connects him to the larger social world.

The friendship networks of older persons also vary along several dimensions. Friendship contacts are more frequent among persons of higher socioeconomic classes and among elders in good health than among those who are poor or less healthy. Studies by Lowenthal and her colleagues at the University of California, San Francisco, also provide some evidence that career women may have more restricted social networks later in life than those women who played a more traditional wife and mother role and who accordingly spent more time fulfilling the role of social facilitator.

It has been said of older people that "they are who they were, only more so." This statement holds true particularly with respect to the involvement of elders in voluntary associations and other groups outside of their immediate family and friendship circles. The extent of participation in voluntary groups earlier in life thus tends to be a better predictor of late life group activity than does gender, race, or social class.

In discussing the social networks of older people, it is important to recognize the role of other factors that may work to influence their degree of social activity. Transportation problems, sensory losses, and declining health thus may prevent even the most sociable of the elderly from interacting as much as they would like with family, friends, or members of a church or voluntary association.

Such factors, which work to inhibit the opportunities for elders to engage in social interaction, have been referred to as "social isolators." In reality, a whole host of potential isolators from the biological to the sociostructural levels have been identified.

Social Isolation Among the Aged

In their book *Isolated Elders*, St. Louis professors Eloise Rathbone-McCuan and Joan Hashimi provide a holistic framework for understanding social isolation in later life. While critical of the myth that the majority of America's elderly are lonely and isolated, they nevertheless identify a variety of economic, physical, social, and other factors that may "predispose" older people to isolation.

Isolators may include such obvious factors as the death of a spouse or serious physical or mental illness, as well as more subtle factors. Age discrim-

ination, myths about the asexuality of the elderly, and a conservative political climate which restricts funds for senior centers, meals on wheels, and other health and social programs thus also may serve to contribute to the social isolation of older people. In the remainder of this section, we will look at several examples of different types of social isolators and how they may create or exacerbate the isolation of certain groups of elders in our society.

Bereavement. Studies dating back to the turn of the century have shown that people who are recently bereaved are at elevated risk for disease and even death during the 2 years, and especially the first 6 months, following the death of a spouse. In one of the best known of these studies, Parkes and his colleagues conducted a 9-year follow-up of close to 5000 elderly widowers in the late 1960s. These investigators found a death rate that was 40% higher than expected in the first 6 months after the death of the spouse, with close to half of the deaths attributable to heart disease. Dubbed the "broken heart study," Parkes' research brought increasing attention to bear on the medical consequences of loneliness.

Subsequent studies tended to confirm the overall finding of increased rates of death and disease in the months following bereavement. But they also suggested that this elevated risk for death and disease was far more likely to older men than it was for older women. As noted earlier, one likely explanation for this finding is that men are far more likely to name their spouse, and only their spouse, as a source of social support. Women, in contrast, frequently have a number of close friends and confidantes from whom they continue to derive support during and after the bereavement process.

Given these differences in sociability by gender, it is perhaps not surprising that the risk of dying is significantly decreased for widowers if they remarry, while there is a much smaller decrease for women upon remarriage. While other factors can't be ruled out—for example, the possibility that healthier men are more likely to remarry in the first place—it seems likely that widowed males reestablish supportive networks through remarriage, and that this in turn protects them to some degree from the adverse health consequences of bereavement.

Limitations on Mobility. Frequently overlooked in discussions of social isolation and the elderly are problems with mobility which may sharply curtail an elderly person's contact with family, friends, and the outside world. Such limitations may be of a physical nature, where difficulty seeing, walking, or climbing stairs may prevent older persons from maintaining valued social contacts or participating in routine social activities. But mobility problems may also be rooted in the social and economic environment. Elderly persons living in high crime, inner city neighborhoods frequently are afraid to venture outdoors and may face social isolation as a consequence. Inadequate income also prevents some elderly persons from attending social and recreational events or in other ways participating in social activities. Finally, for the rural elderly, lack of access to transportation has been found to be a key contributor to social isolation and loneliness.

Over the past several years, a variety of programs such as senior escort services in high crime neighborhoods and adult day health centers featuring transportation to and from an elder's place of residence have begun to emerge as a means of overcoming the limitations on mobility faced by some elders in the community. Yet as important as these programs are, they don't begin to meet the critical need for safe, low-cost transportation and other forms of assistance with mobility among America's rapidly growing elderly population.

Ageism. While at first glance age discrimination may seem an unlikely cause of social isolation, the pervasiveness of age prejudice in our society and the ways in which it shapes our definition and treatment of the "problem" of old age implicate it as an important root cause of alienation and isolation among the elderly.

A classic manifestation of ageism, for example, is mandatory retirement, a practice widely used in the United States, beginning in the late 1800s, as a means of helping employers rid themselves of their most expensive workers. While the mandatory retirement age in the United States

recently was raised from 65 to 70 for most occupations, many older workers continue to experience strong *de facto* mandatory retirement pressures at earlier ages, and many continue to report that they leave work against their will.

Mandatory or forced retirement may contribute to social isolation in two key respects. First, and particularly for blue collar workers, the loss of work-based social ties may represent a major loss in social support. While the literature is controversial, some investigators have hypothesized that physical and mental health problems which sometimes follow retirement may be strongly associated with the loss of these important social contacts.

Retirement may also increase one's chances of becoming socially isolated through its effects on income and standard of living. An estimated one third of the elderly poor in the United States, for example, become poor upon reaching retirement age. For such individuals, significant loss of income at retirement may necessitate sharp declines in social activities and may in other ways limit opportunities for social interaction.

While forced retirement is among the most overt expressions of ageism that may contribute to social isolation, it is by no means the only one. Negative portrayals of the elderly in the mass media and prevalent societal myths and stereotypes of the aged as useless, decrepit, and asexual work for many elders to reinforce their own negative self-images and in turn may contribute to an unwillingness to identify with other people in their age group. The cultural dread of aging in American society—aptly termed "gerontophobia"—thus not only works to alienate older people from their society but also from one another.

Chronic Brain Disorders. Among the greatest fears about growing old in American society is the fear of losing one's mental abilities. "Chronic brain disorders" is one of several terms now used to refer to a host of diseases most frequently characterized by impairments of memory, intellectual functioning, judgment, and orientation. Long neglected by the medical community and the general public, these disorders are a focus of increasing research and societal attention. In the process, their isolating influence, both on afflicted individuals and on their loved ones and caregivers, has begun to be recognized.

Alzheimer's disease is the most frequent cause of irreversible dementia in adults and is a disease responsible for some 120,000 deaths per year. Recently termed the "disease of the century," Alzheimer's is a devastating condition in which the individual progresses—often agonizingly slowly—from forgetfulness to total disability and death. The causes of Alzheimer's disease are still unknown and there is as yet no cure. While only 6% of the total population aged 65 and above suffer from Alzheimer's disease, its prevalence increases with age, so that an estimated 15% of persons aged 80 and older have the condition.

Patients with Alzheimer's disease and related disorders frequently experience social isolation as a consequence of the fear associated with their diminishing intellectual functioning. Patients frequently attempt to conceal their illness from others—a practice that itself may engender considerable isolation. For other victims, personality changes may alienate friends and relatives, and cognitive impairments may also work to decrease the individual's ability to maintain social relationships.

As noted earlier, the social isolation associated with Alzheimer's disease and other chronic brain disorders is not limited to the individual patient but frequently extends as well to family members, and particularly to those in a caregiving role. The social isolation for family members may stem in part from the losses experienced when a beloved victim of the disease becomes almost a stranger as a consequence of personality changes and/or diminished mental and physical capacities. For the family caregiver, social isolation also may result from the toll that caring for an ill parent or spouse may have on one's other social relationships. The spouse or daughter-in-law putting in a "36 hour day" caring for a loved one with Alzheimer's thus may have little emotional or physical reserve—let alone the time necessary—to nourish and enjoy other relationships. As caregiver, she may herself become socially isolated, and this isolation, coupled with the stress of caring for an ill spouse or

relative, may lead to health breakdown. A recent study by Fengler and Goodrich of the wives of elderly disabled men indeed found that over half of the women suffered significant illnesses of their own and were thus "hidden patients."

While the great majority of elderly people in the United States are mentally healthy and alert, dramatic increases in the size of the "old old" population, aged 75 and above, suggest that chronic brain disorders, and the social isolation they frequently entail, may well become more common in the years ahead. Programs, policies, and research which address the social needs of patients and their families should be placed high on the social agenda if we are to help alleviate the social isolation commonly connected with these disorders.

Intervention Strategies

The social isolators described above illustrate the range of possible factors which may cause or exacerbate social isolation among the elderly. These isolating factors were seen to occur at all levels from the individual (as in the case of Alzheimer's disease) up through the broad societal level (ageism, mandatory retirement policies). Just as these social isolators operate on multiple levels, so may interventions be designed on a number of planes to help prevent or alleviate social isolation in the elderly. The examples provided below are suggestive of the range and diversity of approaches that have been employed or might usefully be developed to help prevent or reduce social isolation among the elderly.

Individual Level Interventions

Support Groups. Intention networks or social support groups have come into vogue, particularly in the last 15 years, as a means of (1) helping individuals develop and maintain new interpersonal ties and (2) providing social resources to help people experiencing similar types of problems and stressors to better cope with these problems.

In the latter category, support groups for individuals adjusting to bereavement, mastectomy, or to a family member's diagnosis of Alzheimer's disease have had encouraging results. Raphael thus followed 200 recently bereaved widows at elevated risk for morbidity and mortality, randomly allocating them to treatment and control groups. The treatment group received specific support for grief and encouragement of mourning over a 3-year period and demonstrated a significant lowering of morbidity over the subsequent 13 months. In contrast, no decreased morbidity was seen in the control group which had received no supportive intervention.

The impact of intentional support groups for the elderly appears to be greatest among those who are the most socially isolated. The Tenderloin Senior Outreach Project (TSOP) in San Francisco, California, is illustrative of the role that intentional network building may play in improving the health and quality of life of isolated residents of the nation's low-income Single Room Occupancy hotels (SROs). Through the TSOP, weekly support groups facilitated by university graduate students are held in eight hotel lobbies. Elderly residents are encouraged to identify common problems and concerns and to collectively seek solutions to these problems. Through their joint efforts, hotel-based minimarkets have been established to reduce problems of inadequate food access; a network of 48 "safehouses" or places of refuge has been set up in the neighborhood to help prevent crime; and a Health Promotion Resource Center has been opened for and by the low-income elderly. TSOP's visible effects on individual health and morale thus have been accompanied by improvements on the broader community level as residents, empowered through newfound supportive ties, work together to change their lives and the life of their community.

COMMUNITY-BASED HEALTH AND SOCIAL SERVICES

While the majority of America's elders enjoy good health, approximately one third of the community-based elderly require some degree of long-term health and/or social services. While most such long-term service is provided by family members, effective community-based supports are needed, both to assist families in their caregiving role

and to provide autonomy and social support for those elders lacking families and/or other social resources. A comprehensive continuum of community-based health and social services for the elderly is needed that would include at one end a variety of services for the ambulatory independent elderly, those who are socially well integrated and in need only of minimal assistance (e.g., transportation, outpatient medical facilities, congregate dining, or multipurpose senior centers). Toward the middle of the continuum would be the more substantial services, such as adult day health care and sheltered housing, which can help the frail elderly remain in the community. Skilled nursing homes, hospice services, and community hospital care would comprise the far end of the continuum and would focus on those with the most severe mobility restrictions and dependence on outside assistance. At each point along the continuum, the social as well as the more narrowly conceived health needs of elders would be addressed. A premium would be placed on maintaining elders in their communities and helping family members and others continue to provide the level of care and social support that they do best without overtaxing their personal strengths and resources.

Unfortunately, the heavy skewing of federal and private sector service dollars toward institutional long-term care and hospitalization has in reality meant that only this end of the continuum of services has been developed to any significant degree. Lack of attention to the social needs of the community-based elderly has been a key factor responsible for inappropriate nursing home placements and has contributed further to the social isolation of some community-based elders.

SUPPORTIVE SYSTEMS AT THE NATIONAL LEVEL

Closely related to the provision of adequate community-based health and social services is the need for supportive systems at the national level geared toward enhancing social integration and quality of life for the elderly. Included here would be a federal commitment to income maintenance and to federal financing for comprehensive community-based health and social services for the elderly, including respite care for family care-givers and major reforms in Medicare and Medicaid, making these programs more responsive to meeting the social and preventive health care needs of older persons.

Efforts also must be made on the broad societal level to end age discrimination and those policies (e.g., mandatory retirement) which may increase social isolation among the elderly. The Gray Panthers, the Older Women's League (OWL), and other groups working to combat myths and stereotypes about aging are making important contributions to the fight against ageism and hence to reducing some of the social isolation that stems directly or indirectly from this source.

In a time of fiscal conservatism and cutbacks in domestic spending, particular care must be taken to avoid hurting those services and programs vital to the autonomy and social integration of the elderly. Cost-saving measures that slash transportation and mobility assistance programs may in the long run increase costs by decreasing the capacity of frail elders for remaining outside of institutions and in the community. Yet even aside from these fiscal cost considerations, the human costs of such budget cuts in terms of quality of life and social integration of the elderly must not be overlooked.

The generation that "greened" America is now graying America. As our society ages, we would do well to heed Paul Berry's remark that "If we don't know we are a community, we can't know our losses." Social isolation of the elderly is for the most part a problem that is socially created and maintained. As such, it is a problem that will not be solved without a serious societal commitment to policies and programs that reflect a basic belief in the dignity, autonomy, and social worth of all individuals, regardless of age.

32

MOTIVATING THE ADOLESCENT: SPECIAL NEEDS AND APPROACHES

Dale C. Garell, M.D., is clinical professor of pediatrics and family medicine at the University of Southern California. He also serves as medical director of California Children Services in Los Angeles, regional media consultant to the Job Corps, and consultant to maternal and child health in the School of Public Health, University of Hawaii at Manoa. He has published several articles on adolescent health care.

Anyone who wakes up in the morning in the household of one or more adolescents knows that the day is frequently defined for the entire family by the way the adolescent feels that day. It's not unlike waking up next to a grenade. "O Lord, please let my teen be happy and pleasant and well-mannered and responsible this morning," is the prayer whispered every morning in millions of homes. "Why bother?" asked Dr. Dale Garell. Then he reminds us: we were all there once. And nobody lives through adolescence without some tragedy befalling them at least twice daily. This chapter will be a godsend to many who deal with adolescents on every level.∎

Anyone who has ever tried to tell an adolescent what to do "because it's good for them!" knows how difficult it is to get acknowledgement, much less respect. Adolescents are not noted for their cooperation or responsiveness to advice from any corner, whether from their parents, teacher, physician, or even peers— an understatement of the challenge to the health promotor anxious to improve adolescent behavior.

Still, there is evidence that with appropriate techniques and a basic understanding of adolescence, it may be possible to positively influence teenage health behavior. Effective approaches have been reported in the prevention of initial smoking in seventh graders in the Houston school systems (Evans), in reducing risk behavior in alcohol misuse (McAlister), using effective group techniques in weight control in obese teenagers (Mellin), in taking responsibility for their own family planning (Litt), and even in developing sound teenage child-rearing practices (Hardy). These investigators, working on high risk problem areas during the adolescent years, have found a surprising degree of success.

WHY BOTHER?

Despite these somewhat limited successes, the question remains, why bother? For the more than 42 million teenagers (ages 12–21), adolescence is really a healthy period of time, particularly when compared to older age segments of the population. And yet many adolescents worry about their health, see themselves as engaging in unhealthy behaviors, and believe they are less healthy than peers or adults.

Despite this relatively good health, *teenagers are the only population age group whose mortality rates are rising rather than falling!* Three quarters of all deaths during adolescence are violent—homicide, suicide, automobile collisions, and other accidents. Add to this more than 1 million teenage pregnancies yearly, the fact that over 50% of all sexually transmitted diseases occur between the ages of 12 and 21, and increased alcohol and drug abuse and you have a period of sig-

nificant high risk behavior and a group that is ill-prepared to handle much of it.

Other important reasons also justify intervention during adolescence. Many of the diseases of adult life result from behaviors originating in youth; these include obesity, elevated blood pressure, increased levels of cholesterol, smoking, alcohol and drug use, and early cervical cancer, to mention but a few. All of these conditions share one common dimension: they may be preventable if intervention strategies can be developed to alter adolescent behavior and assist them in choosing their health practices wisely.

And herein lies the challenge to those interested in changing their health behaviors. The opportunity exists for primary prevention of adult diseases and for the prevention of potentially destructive teenage behavior *before* it becomes incorporated into a permanent way of life.

This chapter explores the current knowledge of teenage motivation and how this knowledge might be applied to working with adolescents in groups or individually.

STATE OF KNOWLEDGE REGARDING THE MOTIVATION OF ADOLESCENTS
Adolescent Development

Adolescent growth is part of a lifelong continuum in which certain tasks are essential preparation for becoming a functional adult. Establishing one's own identity and achieving independence requires by its very nature a certain amount of experimentation in order to arrive at acceptable values, beliefs, and practices to incorporate into adult lifestyles. Therefore, approaches to changing adolescents need to be directed not toward elimination of these activities, but to how adolescents can experience them and derive their own standards of behavior.

A very good illustration of this point is in the area of sexual development. The goal for adult life is not absence of sex but meaningful sexual activity. Effective programs that encourage healthy attitudes and beliefs about sexuality are geared toward readiness and timing as the individual passes through various stages of adolescent development.

Where To Begin?

Adolescence has been described as a transitional period between childhood and adulthood, having its onset with puberty and ending with the assumption of adult roles and responsibilities. Using the age range from 12 to 21 as a rough guideline, there can be considerable variation in completing the tasks of adolescence. For some, adolescence is a short-lived period in which the exigencies of adult life quickly come to play— social, economic, education, and work pressures during the teenage years are major determinants of early progression to adult responsibilities. Other teenagers extend their adolescence well into their 20s, continuing many of the challenges of the adolescent period of development. Because of this diversity, every adolescent needs to be seen as an individual rather than as a collective average—something that society has great difficulty in doing.

Early, Middle, and Late Adolescence

It helps to divide the adolescent period into three age periods. During *early* adolescence, most healthy young people experience major physical changes with the onset of puberty. They are more like children than adults. They focus on issues of identity, establishing peer relationships and daily tasks of living. During this early period, guidance from parents and values learned immediately preceding the adolescent period are usually not challenged. However, during the *middle* period of adolescence, teenagers experience most of their physical changes in growth and develop independent thinking, frequently in conflict with parents and other adult values and characterized by experimentation and testing. The ability to use abstract thinking—to consider the future— becomes part of the adolescent's skills. The *late* adolescent period is characterized by behavior more like adults than children, with identity formation almost completed, an awareness of their own sexual identity, and movement toward separation from family to function independently on their own as effective adults.

The movement toward adulthood, therefore, can be seen for most adolescents as a series of developmental periods, involving establishment of an identity (Erikson); the capacity for abstract thought (Piaget); a positive sense of one's self, and a potential for establishing intimate relationships with others.

Adolescent Health Behavior

Positive health behavior is based upon the skills acquired and the behaviors practiced that can help teenagers function in adult society. Yet many behaviors are based upon a perception by adolescents of their own excellent health, strength, and sense of relative "invincibility." Adolescence is a time when experimentation with drugs and alcohol, smoking, variable eating habits, and sexual experimentation may have no perceived negative consequences. Motivation to change or even to initiate "healthy" behaviors is really an antithesis to the normal experimentation of adolescence. In fact, some researchers have shown that the adolescent's view of his personal vulnerability to illness and of the severity of various health-risking conditions becomes fixed by age 12 and remains fixed through age 18, suggesting that effective intervention should focus on the preadolescent age group or upon the young adult (Radius).

THEORIES OF ADOLESCENT HEALTH BEHAVIOR
Basic Studies

A number of basic studies can provide the foundation for understanding theories of adolescent health behavior. The Health Belief Model (HBM), developed by Lewin in 1944, postulates that health behavior is a function of susceptibility to the particular illness as perceived by individuals, the degree of illness or the consequences that might result from contracting the condition, the benefits or efficacy in preventing or reducing susceptibility if health action is taken, and the physical, psychological, economic, or other costs related to a particular behavior. The Social Learning Theory described by Bandura in 1976 emphasizes the role played by the interaction between self-generated and environmental determinants; in other words, behavior is governed by awareness, motivation, and incorporation into belief systems and the reproduction of that behavior.

Other health behavior theories have been on the ability of the individual to communicate and the effective persuasion of that communication. If the communicator wants the message to be accepted and acted upon, individuals exposed to the message must pay attention before communication can begin. Comprehension of the message is equally important; agreeing with the message is vital if the communication is to have an effect in the desired direction. Holding onto the beliefs is essential when the individual is challenged by messages contrary to the accepted belief (communication theory). Finally, attitudes and behaviors have been found to be strengthened by "innoculating" individuals against arguments to which they may be exposed.

Research on Adolescent Behavior Theory

"Problem behavior proneness" implies that the adolescent is moving away from conventional attitudes, values and traditional expectations about normative behavior. Kellerman and his associates described the importance of self-esteem and self-worth upon subsequent adolescent behavior. While other researchers have tended to minimize the importance of the adolescent's perception of themselves, how adolescents feel about themselves has been found to vary directly with their attitudes and beliefs.

Adolescent health behavior can also be viewed from a cultural and societal vantage point. Environmental factors may play a key role in understanding motivation. Structuring an environment in which health is a norm, developing alternative models and skills training can be used to create core groups of adolescents who can rebel against "unhealthy" behaviors and help their peers to do the same. This is an alternative to the pressure from peers, the media, and negative adult role behavior.

In 1980, Perry surveyed 362 high schools in California and rated these schools on positive as well as unhealthy environments for adolescents. She studied absenteeism, annual student suspension rates, and the number of daily office referrals. She found that adolescent involvement in making rules and planning for environmental redesign significantly reduced negative behaviors. Developing clearer organizational rules and smaller units, seeking parental support, and involving the adolescent in problem solving also positively affected outcomes of adolescent behavior.

APPROACHES TO SPECIFIC ADOLESCENT HEALTH PROBLEMS

For the most part, health promotion programs for adolescents have been targeted to specific behaviors or health problems. Efforts to change behaviors during adolescence have focused on such specific projects as reducing smoking, increasing physical fitness, and preventing unwanted pregnancies, alcohol and substance abuse. Since it is not possible to detail all of the research concerning the adolescent period, a few programs are described by way of illustration.

Obesity

Perhaps no problem is of greater significance to adolescents and their parents than that of being overweight. It involves a complex series of factors—genetic, familial, environmental, emotional, and physical activity—that affect the individual adolescent's weight and body image. Shapedown is a program developed at the University of California, Division of Adolescent Medicine, in San Francisco which has been very successful in helping adolescents to lose weight. Using a group format and an interdisciplinary approach, Shapedown employs the use of a moderate diet in which types of food, quantity of food consumed, and frequency of eating are regularly discussed. A daily aerobic exercise program is recommended, and adolescents learn to monitor their own heart rate to ensure they are not exercising beyond their cardiovascular fitness level. A wide range of behavioral techniques are also used, from monitoring to goals setting. Cognitive restructuring is used in a simplified form.

Shapedown focuses on the many behaviors associated with obesity and weight gain: hyper-emotional eating, internal cue responsivity, compulsive eating, eating style, eating environment, assertiveness, idleness, and peer interaction. Depression, self-esteem, and locus of control are monitored. Parents meet to discuss supportive measures, weight management principles, role definition, and communication patterns. Over a 15-month period, the experimental group had an average weight loss of 10 pounds as compared to a control group that showed little or no change over the same period. The key elements in the program—team work, parental support, and information about weight, stress-management, and alternative behavior—have made this program a continuing success. Plans are underway to repeat Shapedown in other parts of the country.

Smoking

It is generally agreed that the most effective way to attack the problem of smoking is to persuade the adolescent not to begin smoking in the first place. It is encouraging to note that over the last several years teenage smoking has decreased. One study has shown that smoking among high school seniors dropped from 29% in 1977 to 21% in 1982. Significant decreases have occurred among boys of all ages and among girls ages 12 to 16. But older teenage girls continue to smoke at increasing rates. These findings should be somewhat qualified, since there may not be an actual increase. Perhaps increased social acceptance of smoking by young women has resulted in more self-reporting.

It is also true that when both parents smoke, there is an increased incidence in smoking among both teenage boys and girls. This may be due to role modeling by parents or the availability of cigarettes in the home. Virtually all investigators report that adolescent smokers and non-smokers alike really believe that smoking is po-

tentially dangerous to one's health. Obviously, this fear is not enough to deter the onset of smoking or to motivate smokers to stop.

Among the many factors associated with cigarette smoking, social factors appear to be most important. Smokers have friends who smoke; it is also likely that the modeling of smoking behavior by teachers, television and media personalities, and cigarette advertising plays a significant role in encouraging early experimentation with tobacco and providing social support for ongoing smoking.

Individual characteristics associated with cigarette smoking include high impulsivity, rebelliousness, an impatience to assume more adult roles, and a strong orientation to peers. Smoking may also play an important role for some teenagers in establishing a sense of identity and for still others to compensate for low self-esteem.

The Life Skills Training Program, sponsored by the American Health Foundation in New York, uses a social learning model with emphasis on social and psychological factors motivating cigarette use. Again, the use of the group process is an effective method for influencing behavior changes. The program attempts to increase the participant's awareness of direct social pressures to smoke and to decrease susceptibility to indirect social pressures. It also strives to increase participants' ability to cope with anxiety, particularly in social situations, and to become more aware of both immediate and long-term effects of smoking. The group discusses smoking beliefs, biofeedback, decision making, anxiety, communication skills, assertiveness, and peer pressure. Classes are led the first year by outside specialists and the following year by teenage leaders. In a subsequent study carried out in the New York schools, results have shown that only 8% of students who received this intervention had begun to smoke, whereas 19% in a comparable control group had started smoking. Of particular interest is the positive effect of the program on the initiation of smoking by girls, a previously mentioned high risk group.

Alcohol

There is little question about the importance of alcohol as a major vehicle for adolescent acting out behavior. Studies document that virtually *all* adolescents experiment with drinking at one time or another, and a sizable group of adolescents between the seventh and twelfth grades (22% of females and 34% of males) are reported to drink on a weekly basis. Other surveys report that more than one third of high school seniors may get drunk on a weekly basis.

As with most adolescent health behaviors, the causes of alcohol abuse are a complex set of factors: age of onset, with an increasing percentage of regular drinkers during later adolescence; variations in alcohol use by the sexes, although females are rapidly catching up with males; relative lack of involvement by family and interest in school activities; peer pressures; the media; the image of what constitutes a mature adult; parental histories of alcohol abuse; and genetic as well as personality-based determinants.

A number of programs have used a factual approach to alcohol education by providing information regarding the hazards of drinking. These programs do not take into account the variety of emotional contributions to adolescent drinking behaviors, and as a result they are limited in their effectiveness. Intervention programs can increase their effectiveness by considering a variety of emotional determinants—the use of alcohol for pleasure, curiosity, escape, or to increase social interaction, and to prove oneself.

Other programs have attempted to emphasize the importance of the adolescent choosing to behave responsibly, emphasizing the relationship between alcohol use and lifestyle values. Programs that are designed to improve self-esteem, reduce anxiety, promote responsible decision making and problem solving, and teach assertive responses to the environment thus offer alternatives to using alcohol to solve life's problems.

A teenager with severe alcohol problems, as with adults, cannot be helped unless he or she becomes fully involved in the process and accepts the serious consequences of alcohol abuse. Alcoholics Anonymous can be an effective intervention resource. It emphasizes self-help, self-awareness, positive group interaction, reality testing based upon the experiences of others, and a no-nonsense view of the world, emphasizing the underlying responsibility of the individual to accept and change his or her own behavior.

For many, alcohol is but one of a multitude of other chemical substances used simultaneously. Mixtures of alcohol and other drugs only compound the problem of developing responsive interactive programs. Once physiological dependence occurs, medical intervention with detoxification is the only alternative. Once the teenager is substance-free, other behavioral and psychological programs can be effective.

Compliance

Compliance is related to the ability of the person to comply with a prescribed course of treatment, including taking medication, adhering to a diet, or making changes in lifestyle. Studies in the general population suggest that noncompliance (not following a prescribed course of medical action) ranged in the adult from 30% to 70%! Studies of noncompliance among adolescents are relatively few in number. Litt and her associates at Stanford University have been studying teenagers who are undergoing medical treatment for juvenile rheumatoid arthritis. Their studies show that the adolescents who comply with their prescribed medical treatment are those who have high self-esteem and are allowed more autonomy. A critical factor appears to be the duration of the teenager's illness and the multiplicity of disease symptoms. These findings are also supported by studies by Korsch and her colleagues in Southern California. Korsch has discovered that children and adolescents with chronic renal disease who are noncompliant are usually perceived to have poor self-esteem and social adaptation. Litt found in 1985 that adolescents' own self-assessment of past compliance may be an important factor in determining whether or not an adolescent complies with a current treatment program. While studying more than 100 teenage females beginning an oral contraceptive program, Litt found that patterns of compliance established during adolescence or even earlier, when perceived by the adolescents themselves, are valuable predictors of whether or not they will continue to take oral contraceptives.

A brief review of what can be learned from these intervention programs is summarized in the following list.

- Group discussions.
- Use of peer leaders/understanding adults.
- Provision of information about specific condition with rationale for why teenagers should change their behavior. Clear instructions on what to change and positive reinforcement.
- Incorporation of the following in the design and planning:
  - Psychological determinants: understanding of adolescent's development stage, identity, and independence.
  - Social determinants: understanding of peer behaviors, parental behavior, other positive and negative role models.
  - Environmental determinants: school setting, socioeconomic level, governmental programs and services, laws, recreation, and workplace.
- Use of approaches that seek to increase:
  - Communication skills.
  - Assertiveness.
  - Problem-solving capability.
  - Ability to cope with stress and anxiety.
  - Self-esteem and self-worth.
- Involves the adolescent in own or other adolescent's care: self-help, peer support, reality testing and feedback. Respects confidentiality and builds trust.

WORKING WITH THE INDIVIDUAL ADOLESCENT

So far, this chapter has focused on the work of special programs dealing with specific health problems of the adolescent. Inherent in all of these approaches is a plan, usually on a large scale, with a specific intervention strategy and a specific target goal. These programs are frequently done in conjunction with schools, health departments, specific medical or psychological study groups, or community-sponsored organizations. They represent a broad-based approach to groups of adolescents.

On the other hand, what is likely to work with the adolescent, who brings his or her own unique experiences, strengths and weaknesses, attitudes and values to a particular health problem? How can the clinician, counselor, parent, or interested adult work toward changes in behavior? To be sure, individual approaches are more subjective and are less likely to be supported by statistical validation. Nevertheless, it is ultimately the *individual* adolescent who determines the importance and value of healthy behavior.

UNDERSTANDING, ACKNOWLEDGING, AND EXPERIENCING A POTENTIAL HEALTH PROBLEM

Without the individual's acceptance that a problem exists, there is relatively little chance of effecting a significant change in behavior. This is true for adults and teenagers. The learning curve is a function of the acceptance by the adolescent of a need to change his or her behavior. Many parents have experienced the defiance of the teenager who seems bent on self-destructive behavior: "I told him so, but he wouldn't listen" or "He knew better, but just couldn't seem to stop himself" or "I don't know what got into him. He just continued to act as if he weren't thinking at all." Such adolescent resistance is expected and occasionally may be healthy behavior.

Many teenagers do not recognize that their behavior is potentially self-destructive. This may be due to denial, internal stresses, poor self-image, peer pressure, rebellion against parental behavior, or inappropriate adult role modeling. For whatever reasons, the adolescent may not be able to assess his or her own behavior objectively. Without an objective perception, change is unlikely to occur.

Approaching the Problem

Listening to the adolescent without questioning and interpreting value judgments may be the only effective approaches at first. Indeed, the reasons for seeking changes in behavior may not be motivated by the adolescent but may come from parents, teachers, or the courts.

Helping the resistant adolescent to understand and acknowledge the presence of a problem relies on providing another "pair of eyes." The individual counselor may say to the teenager, "This is what I see, these are my perceptions," then carefully label her interpretations as being her own rather than those of the teenager. Such interpretations may be the only possible approach unless there is further insight by the teenager and the development of a nonjudgmental trust in the counselor.

Perceiving Value and Return for Changing Behavior

Why change? Why alter behavior that may be pleasurable and may fulfill some need? For many adolescents, there may appear to be no logical reason to change behavior, particularly in the face of peer pressure and current stresses.

After a teenager has recognized a particular problem, however, the counselor may help by encouraging him to observe his current behavior. From that perspective, he may be able to see the particular benefits or disadvantages of such behavior within themselves, discover that he has ambivalent feelings, and decide that the outcome of such behavior may not be as fully controlled as he would like.

Recognizing Whose Choice It Is To Change

The adolescent does indeed have some choices when he can recognize the various alternatives and positive or negative consequences of his actions. Whether or not we personally like that choice, little change is likely to occur unless the adolescent recognizes that he must make the decision—not the counselor, his parents, or his peers.

Interestingly enough, once an ongoing relationship has been established and trust is developing, the adolescent frequently seeks ways to involve the counselor in the decision-making process. This may take the form of acting out in seemingly negative fashion or describing the actions of the proverbial "friend" who may have a similar problem, or asking the counselor directly for advice. Again, it is important to avoid premature intervention. Offering advice and taking charge will undermine the adolescent's future decision-making capabilities. The goal of the counselor is to encourage the adolescent to make knowledgeable, independent decisions in a given situation. In this way the adolescent will learn to take responsibility for the outcome of that decision.

When the counselor is asked directly by the teenager for advice, and when it appears to be in the best interest of the adolescent to give advice, the counselor's viewpoint should be clearly identified as one belonging to the counselor and *not* necessarily the same as the teenager: "If you are asking for my opinion, this is what I would do in that particular situation. However, the choice is still yours to make."

Decision Making and Support

Once the teenager has made a choice, the counselor's role becomes one of helping the teenager to strategize, developing possible scenarios, supporting the teenager's decision, continuing to be available to deal with periods of added stress and/or possible failure, and not undermining the decision that has been made.

A teenager's first choices may not be the most beneficial or necessarily have the most likely positive outcome. What is important here is not the fact that the teenager made the *right* choice but that he made a choice at all. By continuing to be available to the teenager, even when the first choice may not be optimal, the counselor continues to support the teenager's search for a positive outcome. Such a supportive role assists the adolescent in learning to make decisions by himself.

When the choices appear to be self-destructive, direct intervention may be needed, helping the adolescent to reexamine various alternatives and pointing out unforeseen consequences. While there may be concern for harm or risk to the teenager, the very fact that the issue arose in the first place and can be openly discussed implies that the teenager may be unable to prevent these behaviors on his own. This should be seen as a request for help. The counselor need not fear losing the developing relationship if forced to directly intervene; on the contrary, not intervening not only may lead to problems for the teenager but may also destroy the counselor's future effectiveness.

When used appropriately, role playing, behavioral contracts, journal writing, psychotherapy (either individual, group, or family), experiential activities, self-help groups, and structured experiences can be effective tools. But there is no simple set of interventions that is invariable successful. Each adolescent requires a specific approach tailored to individual needs. "Successful" intervention designed to alter adolescent health behavior is not so much a function of technique, as it is a function of the counselor's attitudes and authenticity. Understanding adolescent behavior, having a basic trust in the adolescent, supporting individually determined choices, emphasizing involvement in the decision-making process, and developing the adolescent's self-esteem and patience are key elements in the counselor's work.

A FEW FINAL WORDS OF ADVICE

1. **Avoid becoming pals, becoming a contemporary of the adolescent in an effort to influence health behavior.** Most adolescents are very suspicious of "adolescent adults" — those individuals who try to dress or speak the language of the adolescent. Adolescents are quick to pick up on insincerity and the underlying manipulation of such interventions and to reject them. When adults or parents speak comfortably and honestly about their beliefs, the adolescent will be much more willing to respond. The goal is not to manipulate the adolescent, but to listen, inform, and be honest.

2. **Bribery is a form of manipulation that will get you nowhere.** Careful thought must go into behavioral rewards for positive behavior. If the adolescent perceives that he is being manipulated by the offer of a reward, he will reject that out of

hand. Emphasis on joint decision making about future health behavior, done in collaboration with shared goal setting, is the most effective way of reinforcing a desired behavior.

3. **Avoid the use and abuse of authority and power.** To be sure, appropriate limits need to be set for most adolescents. However, pulling rank on the adolescent because of parenthood or positions of power often provokes rebellion and noncompliance. Adults frequently fail to recognize that the adolescent may already know the potential benefits or harm of any given action. Asserting power assumes that the adolescent is not aware of the consequences. On the contrary, the adolescent may be fully aware of the expected result, and may be unable to alter this behavior by himself. Adults should support the adolescent rather than force him into a response.

4. **Patience is critical.** It is critical to recognize that it may take time for the adolescent to respond in the desired way. By seeing behavior as a set of small steps moving toward behavioral change, the counselor can deal with his own frustrations at what must at times appear to be little or no progress. Reinforcing the small steps and acknowledging that progress, however gradual, is being made may be as effective for the counselor as it is for the teenager.

Future Directions

Considerable progress has been made in the last decade to understand adolescent behavior and to improve the outcome of health behavior programs. Despite these efforts, relatively little is known about what motivates adolescents to change health behavior. Most research has been descriptive; in other words, it has identified those teenagers who have the best chance of changing, relying upon specific factors that make change possible. We still do not understand how these factors work, particularly in interaction. Jessor has shown that "problem" behaviors do spark other behaviors; that is to say, there appears to be a strong relationship between drinking and smoking marijuana; with cigarette smoking and deviant behavior, as well as correlating negatively with such positive behaviors as regular attendance in school, leadership activities, and perceptions of self-worth and self-esteem.

Five- and ten-year follow-up studies are needed to discover what really works over a longer period of time. It is not enough to report that interventions work during the adolescent years. Permanent change in behavior remains the goal.

Consumer research is still another area that needs to be explored. We should investigate the ways in which the mass media—including television, music videos, and magazine articles—can affect health behavior.

Perhaps the greatest need is for the development of effective programs to address issues of violence—the number one cause of teenage mortality. We need to understand the relation-

ships between alcohol and other substance abuse and automobile fatalities. Mothers Against Drunk Driving (MADD) and Students Against Drunk Driving (SADD) are attempting to offer effective intervention programs. Further work is needed to understand the "epidemics" of teenage suicide and gang violence. Whenever health promotion programs tire of traditional prevention activities, the broader social context offers an unlimited source of high priority problems needing practical solutions.

Finally, studying the variety of influences, both internal and external, that affect health behavior remains one of the endeavors showing the greatest promise. Simply said, adolescents do not all behave alike. They are complex beings with conflicting motivations. Theories and treatments that help one adolescent today may be useless in helping him tomorrow. Understanding these interrelationships represents the challenge for future investigators.

33 CRISIS IN ADOLESCENCE: AN UNEXPECTED OPPORTUNITY FOR GROWTH

James S. Gordon, M.D. teaches in the Department of Psychiatry and Community and Family Medicine at Georgetown University. For 10 years he was a research psychiatrist at the National Institute of Mental Health. His latest book is *The Dancer and the Dance: Bhagwan Shree Rajneesh and His Disciples* (Viking Press, 1987). He is co-author of *The Healing Partnership, New Directions in Medicine*, and *Mind, Body and Health*. He practices psychiatry in Washington, D.C.

Jim Gordon is a pioneering psychiatrist who has worked with troubled teenagers since 1967. He was one of the first physicians to study the effectiveness of teen hotlines and runaway shelters. And when physicians were reluctantly beginning to admit that medicine's focus on the body alone might be too restricted, Jim had already written extensively about mind/body relationships in health and healing. In this chapter, Jim explains his use of psychotherapy to treat physical symptoms and his use of the very characteristics of adolescence—energy, imagination, loyalty, and independence—to resolve emotional crises. He reminds us that "crisis is an opportunity as well as a danger." ▪

Adolescence begins with the biological changes of puberty and culminates in the assumption of an adult's role and status. In the West, for more than 200 years, it has been regarded as a distinct and stressful stage of life. In the early years of this century, the pioneering psychologist G. Stanley Hall wrote that this time of life was uniquely fraught with "storm and stress."

This perspective, which has been reinforced subsequently by many psychoanalysts and a general consensus of parents, has come under some scrutiny in the last 20 years. Margaret Mead, Daniel Offer, and others have suggested that adolescence is in fact no more inherently stressful or stormy than other developmental periods (infancy, middle age, or old age).

Still there are profound biological, psychological, and social changes which mark adolescence and set it apart from earlier and later developmental stages. Adolescence begins with sexual and intellectual maturation. It is characterized by the development of secondary sex characteristics (pubic hair, breasts, a deeper voice), the enlargement and maturation of genitalia, and the ability to procreate. At the same time, there is an increase in young teenagers' cognitive flexibility and their capacity for abstract reasoning.

As the adolescent begins to develop an identity as a student and worker, he seeks to differentiate himself from his parents. Although adolescents may embrace some parental attitudes, hopes, and expectations, they rebel against or rework others. Meanwhile they are identifying with peers at a similar stage of life and developing a world view which acknowledges that they are a part of a larger "we," a generation with similar concerns.

During the last 40 years in the United States the changes of adolescence have taken place in a social and economic climate which itself has shifted and changed at an ever increasing rate. Teenagers in America in the 1950s and early 1960s lived securely in a vessel framed by social, conservative, and economic growth and by individual and national self-confidence. In the late 1960s and early 1970s this vessel was challenged and shattered by the profound social and cultural upheavals of the civil rights movement and the Vietnam war, by widespread use of drugs, and by an unprecedented and pervasive sexual freedom. Young people swam joyously (if erratically) in the rolling waters of change. Now, in the mid-1980s, large numbers of adolescents are behaving like survivors. They are clinging to spars of personal success and social and economic security.

Contemporary middle- and upper-middle-class young people grow anxious about their future in an uncertain economy at an early age. From junior high school on, they anxiously scramble to win places in the prestigious colleges and graduate schools that may help them to achieve the same economic level as their parents. Other youngsters, particularly in our inner cities, are disillusioned by those schools that bore them and poorly prepare them for life as adults. In increasing numbers, they become high school dropouts and teenage mothers, sealing their membership in a permanent underclass.

Over these struggles hangs the threat that maturity itself will elude the young. The shadow of nuclear war and ecological destruction is a continuous if not always apprehended presence. It makes many adolescents wary of bringing children into the world. AIDS threatens to turn the very flag of adolescence—its burgeoning sexuality—into a means of destruction. Apprehension about potential hazards is making many teenagers less idealistic, more practical, more cautious about their relationships and more limited in their aspirations.

Still, amidst all these pressure to conform, all these threats to their well-being, young people continue to be enormously resilient, and adolescence remains a time of experimentation and exploration. In times of personal crisis, the adolescents' experience in adapting to continual and profound change in and around them can in fact become an extraordinary virtue, a source of immediate strength and enduring optimism.

During the last 20 years I have worked as a psychiatrist and physician with thousands of troubled and troubling young people. Some have run away from homes where they did not feel welcome. Others have used alcohol and drugs to wall themselves off from challenges and conflicts they did not know how to meet. Some became incapacitated with anxiety; others descended into bewildered and infantile psychotic states or deep depressions. Many came to me with physical illnesses that developed during or were exacerbated by the stresses of adolescence: asthma, arthritis, epilepsy, colitis, and juvenile diabetes. Others exhibited physical symptoms like anorexia, obesity, and bulimia.

Although these delinquencies and disorders and these crises of social, physical, and emotional life are in many ways different, they share certain common features and often evoke similar responses. Something has gone wrong, out of control, in the body, mind, or behavior (and often enough in all three) of a young person. Parents feel a need to define the problem and treat it, to exert a controlling force that will restore the adolescent to that previous state in which he or she was, or appeared to be, normal. We feel a desire to bring the adolescent home to the family, to end the drug use, to feed the anorexic, to quell the asthma attack.

In life-threatening situations there is a need to act and to control. The diabetic's insulin must be carefully regulated to avoid a coma that could cause death; a starving anorexic must be fed; and a desperately depressed suicidal teenager must be restrained. Still, it has seemed to me over the years that the emphasis, particularly in situations that are not immediately life-threatening, must be aimed in another direction. As its Chinese ideogram suggests, crisis is an opportunity as well as a danger.

If we rush to return the runaway teenager to his home, or treat the symptoms of a physical disease, or suppress, through medicine or psychotherapy, the rebellion that psychiatric symptoms may reflect, we may be doing the young person a lasting disservice. We need to see the disease, disorder, or delinquency as a symptom in itself. We need to regard it as an opportunity for the young person to discover, explore, and heal the deeper disharmony that the symptom reflects. If we are willing to look at a problem and to help them to look at a problem in this way, the crisis can indeed be an opportunity. It can become

the vehicle for resolving developmental difficulties that might otherwise have been ignored, and for achieving an intelligence, indeed a wholeness, which might not have been possible.

We, as adults, can help young people in the process of exploring the origins of the crisis and coming to its resolution. We can help them make creative use of the very characteristics of adolescence which often seem so problematic: their enormous physical energy; their need for independence and for independently defining themselves; their restless, questing minds and vivid imaginations; their refusal to accept on faith the words of their elders; their sometimes desperate need for mutuality and their intense attachment to their peers.

Here are two examples of rather different kinds of adolescent crises and some ways I have dealt with them.

THE RUNAWAY

When I first began to work with adolescents in 1967, perhaps as many as a million were running away from their homes each year. Their departure was defined by police as a crime, punishable by incarceration. The medical profession viewed it as a disease. The Psychiatric Diagnostic Manual (DSM II) listed the "runaway reaction of adolescence" as a mental disorder alongside depression, anxiety, and schizophrenia.

In the free clinics, hotlines, and runaway houses with which I consulted we redefined running away. We accepted, at least provisionally, the runaway's definition of his or her situation. Leaving home was a legitimate, if poorly understood, response to a difficult if not untenable situation. In the programs we created, we responded not to the parents' panic or the society's disapproval but to the needs of the young people. We created situations in which they could receive the food and shelter they needed without stigmatizing themselves as patients or delinquents. We provided them with counselors who would be responsive to their points of view and responsible not to the parents or society but to the young people themselves.

We did not see our job as forcing—or even necessarily helping—young people to return home. We were there to provide them with some material and emotional security in a time of insecurity and uncertainty, to encourage them to understand themselves and the situation they had fled. Instead of viewing them as irresponsible, we assumed they were responsible: they had made a *decision* to leave home. Now they could look at the options that were available to them—going to school or work, living on their own or returning home. Then, perhaps with our help, they could make a decision about what to do next.

In the runaway house we created, we encouraged the young people to be active participants, not passive victims. We expected them to cook and clean alongside their counselors, to actively investigate the options available to them, to make phone calls and set up interviews with parents and potential employers, counselors and probation officers. We invited them to participate in daily group discussions in the house, to share their plight and their insights—about parents and schools, themselves and one another—with other young people in similar situations.

Often in the course of a few days, many of the young people changed. Away from the pressures of the disturbing home situation, in a climate of respectful though not uncritical acceptance, they seemed less disturbed and impulsive, more thoughtful and responsible. If they were no longer forced to see themselves as the sole problem, the delinquent or disturbed one, they could relax and look at the whole problematic situation. Many young people, who had refused to speak to the therapists whom their parents chosen, now actively sought out counselors who seemed to understand them. With our encouragement they learned to redefine the situation: it wasn't just their problem or their parents' problem, but a family problem. Most contacted their parents and invited them into a family counseling program designed to explore and resolve the situation that had precipitated their flight.

Redefined, dealt with in this way, the crisis of running away became an opportunity for the young person and, indeed, the entire family to look at the dysfunctional patterns that had induced the child to run. In many families the runaway's "delinquent" or "disturbed" behavior provided the catalyst for changes that otherwise might not have occurred. For many runaways the experience of living cooperatively with other young people, of looking thoughtfully at and taking responsibility for their behavior, was a significant step toward greater independence and respectful mutuality.

It is interesting to note that in time our efforts to respond to the needs of runaway young people contributed in a significant way to a societal redefinition of running away. In many states, it is no longer a crime for a juvenile to run away from home. The American Psychiatric Association in its latest Diagnostic Manual no longer defines running away as a disease. The approach we developed has now become a model for those in the mental health and juvenile justice establishment who work with runaways and other troubled adolescents who cannot stay at home.

PHYSICAL ILLNESS

During adolescence bodies change in profound, sometimes distressing, sometimes gratifying ways. Sudden growth is accompanied by awkwardness; sexual changes which bring pleasure may be attended by physical discomfort–menstrual cramps and premenstrual tension—and emotional distress. Easy intimacy between the sexes is complicated as well as enriched by sexual and romantic feelings. Adolescents often regard their bodies as uncertain or out of control. They tend to feel they are on display and they have mixed feelings about the visual, verbal, and physical attention which others pay to them.

When the ordinary physical and emotional transformations of adolescence are compounded by serious physical illness, the effect can be quite disturbing. The already questionable reliability of the adolescent's body is further compromised by a crippling injury or a medical illness that may flare up without warning. The injury or illness may have serious behavioral consequences: restrictions in diet, exercise, or movement. These alter interpersonal relationships and patterns of group participation and may produce more self-consciousness. A teenager with asthma may be unable or afraid to participate in sports or dancing. A juvenile diabetic cannot safely eat the food which often provides a focus for peer activities.

The need for medical management of an illness disturbs the delicate balance between freedom and restraint which adolescents and their parents are trying to maintain. Stringent therapeutic regimens often provoke childlike rage, frustration, and rebellion in the adolescent whose health seems to depend on an orderliness and compliance against which he is straining. Why do I have to watch my diet or carry an inhaler or test my urine, the adolescent asks. Why do I have to be sick and different, a teenager angrily demands of herself, her parents, and an unkind Providence. It's embarrassing to inject insulin or reach for your inhaler when you're sleeping over at a friend's house.

Often the illness (and its management) becomes a weapon in intergenerational conflict. The rebellious diabetic binges on junk food, terrifies his parents with his elevated blood sugar, and is rushed to the hospital. As the pressure escalates to do schoolwork or to conform to the rules at home, the asthmatic has an attack. Meanwhile parents may become frantic, then controlling and punitive: if you don't stick to your diet you can't go out.

When I work with physically ill young people and their families, I try to see the illness as an opportunity. Young people can use their growing powers of observation, their capacity for introspection, and their interest in the changes in their bodies to turn the illness into a tool for self-awareness. If one gradually helps the young person to view it that way, this can be a catalyst in the ongoing process of maturation.

I begin by asking my adolescent patients why they are ill now or, if it is a chronic illness like asthma or diabetes, why it has become worse. What has happened recently at home, in school, with their friends? Have they changed their diet or their intake of alcohol or drugs? Do they now feel differently about themselves or their bodies? Do acute attacks or exacerbations occur more often at home or school? Are they related to changes in diet or mood? Are there times in the menstrual cycle when the illness is more severe? Can

they anticipate when they will feel worse or better? How do their relationships with other people affect their symptoms?

The way these questions are posed sends a message that transcends the gathering of information. They indicate my respect for the adolescent's growing capacity for introspection and problem solving. My questions imply: "You can understand what is going on and why it is happening to you. In fact, you already know a good deal about your illness, though at first you may not be aware that you know. The answers you give are not only clues for me as a clinician but for you as a patient." They also lay the groundwork for making the adolescent an active partner in his own treatment. "If you understand, you can have a hand in making it better. I am an expert on your illness but treatment, like understanding, is collaborative. You are not a victim of a disease but a student of it and a participant in its treatment. We are engaged in an experiment in which you are both experimenter and experimental laboratory."

In both history taking and treatment I often use the adolescent's self-consciousness, self-concern, and imagination (which to many seem like liabilities) as therapeutic tools. I question the young person very closely. I may say, "Try to figure out exactly what precipitated an asthma or anxiety attack. Were you anticipating a stressful situation? Did a disturbing thought come to mind? How did you feel about the people you were with and how do you think they felt about you?" To amplify the process of self-observation and make it ongoing and prophylactic, I use other techniques. I advise some young people to keep a journal of how they feel emotionally and physically; sometimes I suggest they use drawings, clay, or poetry to record their changing state of mind and illustrate the way their body feels.

I often follow this kind of inquiry with a psychotherapeutic approach, treating the physical symptoms very much as if they were psychological ones. With adolescents I find that the expressive techniques of bioenergetics and gestalt therapy are particularly helpful in dealing with the emotions that precipitate or accompany their illness: I may say, "Talk to your fractured leg or your diabetes, and express your anger at the restrictions the limb or the disease places on you. Imagine you are your irritable colon or your wheezing lungs, and experience the emotions that come up."

I teach adolescents a variety of techniques to help them relax and thereby remove the physiological stress that may precipitate or exacerbate their illness. Depending on the illness and the adolescent's personality, I may focus on deep breathing, progressive muscular relaxation (tensing and relaxing muscle groups), or autogenic training (feeling and visualizing parts of one's body as warm and heavy). Later, when they are able to relax a little, I may show the adolescents pictures of the afflicted organs or the necessary healing process. I encourage them to use their imaginations to affect their bodies. I may say, "Visualize a warm light playing softly on the pain of your arthritic joint; imagine your fracture healing efficiently, the callus forming on the bones, reaching out to bridge the broken area; close your eyes, breathe slowly, and picture your bronchial tree expanding, opening up when you begin to wheeze."

Instead of simply telling a young people what to eat and what to avoid to improve their health, I treat them as collaborators. I may ask a young woman who is anxious or has difficulty sleeping or is plagued by acne to observe the effects of diet on her symptoms. "What happens when you eat a great many sweets? Does it make any difference when you cut down?" If she continues to eat candy and drink Cokes, I won't push her to stop or make her feel guilty for continuing. The distressing symptoms are, after all, hers. "Try for a few days not to eat sweets," I may say. "See if it makes a difference in your restlessness, in your acne, then *you* decide."

I also teach some young people about massage and acupressure. I show them points to work on to reduce stress, relieve symptoms, or improve functioning. At each visit I ask about their success. Most young people enjoy the sense of mastery that comes from taking care of their own bodies, from using their minds and breath and hands to help themselves.

I use a variety of other techniques to break the habitual, self-defeating patterns that often precipitate or accompany physical illness. Many of them are identical to the strategies I use for young people who exhibit emotional problems. Sometimes I prescribe the very symptoms that are most troublesome to young people and their parents. If the adolescent can experience the symptoms fully, often he can leave them behind like old shoes he has worn out.

Instead of demanding that the fearful, dependent, regressed teenager perform well and grow up, I may suggest that she spend more time with the dolls she has abandoned under parental pressure. For my part, I understand that they provide an anchor, a source of easily manipulable gratification and security in times of rapid change and uncertainty. I am giving her permission to seek the comfort that her regression offers her. The girl in turn feels that she is understood and approved, not condemned or hurried by me. When *she* is ready to grow up, she will give up her regression.

Similarly, I may tell an angry or hyperactive boy to be more active. I may suggest running or calisthenics or swimming, pounding pillows or kicking and screaming in a temper tantrum. Sometimes, particularly with some of the most aggressive and violent young people, I suggest karate or kung fu lessons. The physical exercise is formidable, indeed exhausting. Moreover, the discipline of a wise and skillful teacher can help adolescents transform an anger that rules them into an assertiveness of which they are securely the master.

I try to be flexible in my choice of approaches. I improvise experiments that seem to arise out of the unique situation of each adolescent, and I quickly change them if they don't work. Often, as with the kung fu or karate, they combine physiological utility with psychological exploration. Usually they offer young people a challenge, an opportunity to discover sides of their personality they had consciously suppressed or unconsciously repressed.

For example, I have told some overweight teenagers who were terribly embarrassed about their bodies to dance naked in front of a mirror.

Sometimes they are initially horrified at the suggestion. But if they do it—and virtually all of them do—something happens. It breaks down their denial and forces them to accept their bodies as they are. This acceptance is a precondition for change. Sometimes they wind up laughing at their self-consciousness, and sometimes they begin to lose it. And fast exuberant dancing usually improves their mood, energizes them, and helps them to lose weight.

Without violating the adolescent's confidence and privacy, I try to work with the parents, sometimes in family sessions with the adolescent, sometimes separately. If their support seems crucial to a frightened and dependent adolescent, I ask parents to participate actively. I may ask a mother to do a relaxation technique with her child or to massage the young person's back or feet. If the adolescent is struggling to achieve greater independence, I may suggest that the parents leave the monitoring and treatment of the illness to the young person and me. I reassure them that their child is being cared for and reduce the anxiety they feel—and communicate—to their son or daughter.

CONCLUSION

The examples I have given only hint at some ways of dealing with adolescent crisis. They do not, of course, cover the wide range of potential crises. I have not talked at all about the impending death of an adolescent, the loss of a parent by death or divorce, problems of long-term addiction to alcohol or drugs, or psychosis in adolescence. But I believe the principles I have outlined and the perspective I have described can also be helpful in these and other situations.

Those who work with adolescents—including their parents—can help young people to gain confidence in their ability to deal with and grow through crisis. In this process we can value and make use of the adolescent's capacity for introspection and self-observation, for intelligent analysis and responsible decision making, even though these may be limited by lack of experience and impulsiveness. As adult family members, friends, or professionals, we can offer adolescents an opportunity for respectful and collaborative action. We can teach them and we can learn with them rather than merely treat them.

As we try to help, we need to remember that the excess pressure which young people feel from parents, teachers, or themselves to find or resist an immediate solution to their problem needs to be relieved. We need to be patient and encourage them to be patient as well as persistent and firm. Many avenues may have to be explored. Failure to negotiate one or another of them need not be regarded as a defeat. Something can be learned from it. And when yet another crisis arises, just when we felt things were going so well, we have to take a deep breath and relax.

We must remember that the adolescent *does* have time. Decisions about school or work or a living situation or the choice of a therapeutic regimen are almost never final. They are moments in development, not end points. Dropouts and runaways can and will return when they are ready. Teenagers do stop drug use and delinquent behavior and they do outgrow many emotional and physical illnesses if they are encouraged and helped to grow through them. If all of us—professionals, parents and adolescents—can remember this, we will discover the many opportunities that it brings.

34 VARIETIES OF INTEGRAL CANCER THERAPIES

Michael Lerner, Ph.D., is a MacArthur Prize fellow at the Institute for Health Policy Studies at the University of California at San Francisco. He is president and founder of Commonweal, a center for services and research in health and human ecology in Bolinas, California. His article, "A Report on Complementary Cancer Therapies," appeared in *Advances* (Winter 1985).

According to Reiser and Rosen, "There is a vast difference between curing and healing. A patient can be cured but not healed. There are also times when a physician can help a patient to heal, even though he cannot cure him." Dr. Michael Lerner describes the principles of integral cancer therapies, which focus on healing the whole person with cancer rather than on the treatment of the cancer alone. Integral therapy combines established moods and experimental regimens to treat the patient at the physical, emotional, and spiritual levels. Dr. Lerner explains his support of therapies for which the quality of life and functional ability are as important a goal as life extension and disease-free intervals.∎

There is an intense and growing interest among physicians and patients in cancer therapies that address the whole person, not only in the search for a cure but also in the attempt to enhance and perhaps extend a life worth living. In different times and cultures, medicine offered systems of care that patients felt failed to address their needs as whole people. Alternative systems have emerged from outside the reigning medical perspectives to redress the imbalance. This is happening in cancer care in the United States today.

The American cancer treatment and cancer care systems include established cancer therapies, such as chemotherapy, surgery, and radiotherapy; adjunctive cancer therapies, such as psychological therapy, relaxation, and therapeutic touch; and alternative cancer therapies, including nutritional, psychological, spiritual, and alternative "immune" therapies. What we are witnessing is an increase in the use by patients of adjunctive *and* alternative therapies, which I group together as complementary cancer therapies. But along with this development, comparable changes are occurring within the domain of established cancer therapy: an increased interest in considering the needs of whole people for humanitarian as well as therapeutic reasons, a feeling that the present established therapies have their limits, and an increased interest in exploring the best elements in the complementary cancer therapies.

I have titled this chapter "Varieties of Integral Cancer Therapies" to emphasize the fact that different patients and therapists experience enormously divergent therapies as integral. Thus integral cancer therapies, as I refer to them, can consist of any possible combination of established, adjunctive, and alternative therapies. To avoid any misunderstanding, I perhaps should add that most ethical therapists and intelligent patients attracted to complementary cancer therapies include established treatments of known efficacy in their efforts to create integral cancer therapies.

PRINCIPLES OF INTEGRAL CANCER THERAPIES

Integral cancer therapies may be drawn from any or all of the schools of cancer therapy as long as informed patients experience them as addressing their needs as whole people. The choice of therapies will differ according to the training, beliefs, and resources of the patient and the physician. In this section, I describe nine principles or characteristics of integral cancer therapies. Many of these principles arise from some of the deepest perennial philosophies of medicine, and numerous authorities have cited them in different forms.

1. Integral cancer therapy focuses on the whole person with cancer, rather than on the treatment of the cancer alone. Integral cancer therapies include but are not limited to technical treatment of the cancer. The primary Hippocratic injunction to the physician to "Be of benefit, and do no harm" is an explicit instruction to consider the whole patient. A therapy that is technically successful in preserving physical life, but leaves the person within the body in a condition that he or she considers excessively compromised, does not satisfy this injunction. The principle of benefiting the whole person has become a theme of contemporary established medicine.

2. Integral cancer therapy places a major emphasis on the autonomy of the cancer patient and his or her legal right to choose or exclude therapies. The principle of autonomy in at least one leading text on medical ethics holds second place only the Hippocratic principle of benevolence, and is based on one of the most profound principles in English and American ethics and jurisprudence.

There are in medical ethics various principles that impinge on individual autonomy. Under certain conditions "medical paternalism" impinges on patient sovereignty, and sometimes concerns for family and society introduce the limiting principle of "utilitarianism." Yet, even granting these qualifications, integral cancer therapy would propose a fairly substantive reevaluation of the current practice of patient autonomy to allow a patient a wider range of sanctioned choices among both established and complementary cancer therapies. The conditions under which patient autonomy is currently abridged often do not meet the dictates of clear scientific reasoning or common sense.

Full participation in the choice of therapies engages the self-healing capacities of patients who thereby are encouraged to pursue therapies that make sense to them, enhancing the feeling that life is not completely out of their control. The value of granting the patient genuine autonomy in decision making is also widely supported by ethicists and physicians concerned with humanizing medicine. I perhaps should add that the principle of patient autonomy in no way compromises the physician's responsibility to advise the patient about established therapies whose effectiveness in treating some cancers is scientifically supported, or to warn of the real perils of some alternative cancer therapies.

3. Integral cancer therapy explicitly acknowledges that healing can take place at many levels, including physical, emotional, mental, and (for those who assign meaning to the term) religious or spiritual levels. In their valuable study, *Medicine as a Human Experience*, Reiser and Rosen state, "There is a vast difference between curing and healing. A patient can be cured but not healed. There are also times when a physician can help a patient to heal, even though he cannot cure him. Sometimes the latter opportunities can offer the highest joys and privileges a physician can hope to know." To cure, Reiser and Rosen point out, comes from the Latin word *curare*, meaning "to take care or charge of" and denotes successful medical treatment, while to heal comes from the old English word *haelen* and means "to make or become whole," being closely related to the word *holy* from the same root.

That healing can take place at many levels is one of the most profound principles of integral cancer therapy. Thus the therapist pays close attention to the level of healing that the patient (or the patient's family) is experiencing at any point in the cancer process and also to the particular levels of healing that the patient regards as the most significant.

4. Integral cancer therapy recognizes that knowing, like healing, also takes place on many levels for human beings, and that scientific knowing is not the only kind of knowing that is important to whole people. The concept of different kinds of knowing has important implications for a wide range of areas in integral cancer therapy. Does a patient *feel* that the chemotherapy is beneficial? Does a patient *think* she will do well with the proposed surgery? Does a patient *believe* his retirement contributed to the cancer? While such feelings, thoughts, and beliefs may not determine the course of therapy, or be susceptible to verification, they can profoundly affect several levels on which healing occurs.

5. Integral cancer therapy presumes that diagnostically similar cancers may have significantly different etiologies and develop in different internal biological milieus in different people. Further, whether or not similar cancers have different biomedical etiologies, patients may be cured or find relief in different therapies even when they have the same cancer at the same stage. As a result, integral cancer therapy does not presume either in clinical practice or research that there always will be a single therapy that is "best" for a specific cancer at a specific stage. When there is clear scientific evidence of the efficacy of a specific therapy for a specific cancer at a given stage, this evidence is welcome. But for many of the most common cancers, which are among the most resistant to treatment, there is no presumption that a single package of integral therapies will be optimal for all people with the same cancer. Different people have different belief structures, different life histories and situations, and they often manifest distinctive forms of "biochemical individuality," any or all of which may affect the outcome of integral cancer therapies.

Reiser and Rosen write: "Imagine 100

patients, 100 identical men with identical cancers of an identical organ (as though such were possible!). . . . Histopathologically, perhaps, they are all nearly the same, but the essence of their struggles, defeats, triumphs, and setbacks is not found here. It is found in the intangibles. For each, the experience of life is unique. . . . Clearly, modern medicine has tended to ignore these matters, though they are usually what is most on our patients' minds." This principle of difference gives concrete meaning to Sir William Osler's dictum that "It is more important to know what kind of patient has the disease than what kind of disease the patient has." To know the kind of patient who has the disease is to be able to consider the ways that will assist this particular human nature in creating the conditions that allow healing to take place.

6. Integral cancer therapy assumes that if an adjunctive therapy is not likely to do any harm, it may benefit the patient by promoting general health, by actively engaging the patient in the therapeutic process, and by promoting activities that increase positive placebo effects because of the patient's sense of self-control and self-care. Integral cancer therapy does *not* hold that, in the absence of data regarding life extension or cure, complementary cancer therapies should be considered *without* value for cancer patients (a misuse of the null hypothesis). While ethical complementary therapies may or may not have any effect on the progress of the cancer itself, they can have the beneficial effects just described and therefore a patient and therapist, with all appropriate safeguards, can legitimately consider their use.

7. Physicians prescribing integral cancer therapy believe strongly that "in the absence of certainty, there is nothing wrong with hope." Hope can take place on different levels for different patients and mean different things. Norman Cousins speaks of cancer patients who accept the diagnosis but not the verdict.

Unexplained remissions occur with even the most severe cancers, even when they are at an advanced stage. For many cancers that are only slightly less severe, there are statistically demonstrable groups who survive, and these groups can be the focus of hope for a patient. One can hope that one's life after a cancer diagnosis will be filled with positive and intense experiences of living, growth in the face of a life-threatening disease, healing of relationships within one's family, and the accomplishment of goals heretofore set aside.

8. Integral cancer therapy places a strong emphasis on the quality of direct personal attention received by a cancer patient, and on the aesthetic and emotional qualities of the environment in which this care takes place. Thus, the nursing staff, family members, and friends are of the utmost importance and are treated as capable of making a great difference not only with respect to relief and comfort but also in contributing both directly and indirectly to the energies that the patient has available to focus on the healing process. This principle reemphasizes for our time another great maxim of medical ethics, the fifteenth century injunction for physicians, "To cure occasionally, relieve sometimes, and comfort always."

9. Integral cancer therapy is predisposed to believe in the overwhelming significance of love in many forms. "The main reason for healing is love," said Paracelsus. David McClelland, Ph.D., of Harvard recently showed Harvard students a film of Mother Teresa taking care of dying patients and measured immunoglobulin A in the students' saliva before and after they watched this act of love. Immunoglobulin A is, among other things, a defense against colds. Half the students considered Mother Teresa "too religious" or a fake, yet despite their views the immunoglobulin A level of many students increased significantly. The implication is that exposure to selfless love may

have an immunosupportive effect independent of conscious beliefs. The cancer patient can certainly make good use of faith and hope—faith in the competence of the doctor and hope for any authentic goal. But above faith and hope, the cancer patient can make good use of love. Throughout history, love, if only as in tender loving care, has been regarded as a strong element in healing at the physical, mental, and emotional levels relevant to an individual's passage.

THE HISTORICAL AND CULTURAL CONTEXT OF INTEGRAL CANCER THERAPIES

Reviewing the history of cancer therapy is essential to understanding the changing character and interplay of the therapies we label "established" and "complementary" and placing them within the context of a legitimate medical pluralism. Historians of cancer in antiquity report that some cancer patients did surprisingly well with gentle therapies analogous to many of the complementary therapies today. On the other hand, the great early physicians in the West did not know of any nutritional or herbal "cure" for cancer or it surely would have been passed down to us in the historical texts.

An Overview of the History of Cancer Therapy

Malignant neoplasms were present in Egyptians mummified 5000 years ago, but the reported incidence was very low among the tens of thousands of early Egyptian bodies that have been examined, although the limits of the methodology suggest caution in interpretation. From the Egyptian medial papyruses, to Hippocrates (the "father of medicine") in 400 B.C., to the first-century Roman physician Celsus, to the Islamic physician Abul Quasim in 1000 A.D., the early physicians spoke with surprisingly consistent voices about cancer. Said Hippocrates: "It is better not to apply any treatment in cases of occult cancer for, if treated, the patients die quickly, but if not treated they hold out for a long time." Said Celsus: "Though no violent measures are applied in the attempt to

remove the tumor, but only mild applications in order to soothe it, [the majority of patients] attain to a ripe old age in spite of it." Said Abul Quasim: "The Ancients said that when a cancer is in a site where total eradication is possible . . . and especially when in an early stage or small, then surgery was to be tried. But when it is of long standing and large you should leave it alone. For I myself have never been able to cure any such, nor have I seen anyone else succeed before me." Herbal remedies reportedly were palliatives but not cures. The essence of quality cancer care for over 5000 years was to distinguish between the tumors that could be excised and the tumors that were better left alone or treated with palliative, gentle methods.

In seventeenth-century Europe, surgery before anesthesia and antisepsis was barbarous and dangerous to the extreme. In the eighteenth century, there was a new recognition that behavioral and environmental factors played a part in cancer, including breast cancer in nuns, lip cancer in pipe smokers, and cancer of the scrotum in chimney sweeps. The nineteenth century saw the founding of the first cancer hospitals; the development of the microscope, anaesthesia, antisepsis, and X-rays; and great advances in surgery and research. There was also an increase in the number of reports linking cancer incidence with personality factors and psychological states.

Cancer therapy in the twentieth century defies encapsulation, but there are some developments of special note for integral cancer therapy. Such supraradical procedures in surgery as hemiocorporectomy—cutting off the lower half of the body— reached their apogee in the 1950s, a point marked by the publication in 1955 of George Crile's *Cancer and Common Sense*, a plea for less drastic surgery. In the 1970s and 1980s, the use of both chemotherapy and radiotherapy may have its apogee, and a more moderate and discriminating use of these therapies may have begun. For all three of the major aggressive therapies—surgery, chemotherapy, and radiotherapy—the current period appears to be characterized by refinement of techniques, reassessment of achievements, and increasing acceptance of adjunctive supports to diminish side effects or enhance outcomes. Psychological therapies have gained greater acceptance. Both within and outside the medical community, there has been a strong movement toward recognizing complementary therapies and focusing on medicine for the whole person.

Complementary Cancer Therapies and American Medical History

What patients and therapists regard as integral cancer therapies differ with time and culture. Today, the virtually universal tendency toward medical pluralism in the health systems of complex industrial cultures expresses itself in the United States in a network of complementary cancer therapies of widely divergent origins and qualities, including some of the best and the worst in American health practices.

An excellent study documenting the nature and extent of patient and physician interest in unorthodox cancer therapies was conducted by Barrie Cassileth and her colleagues at the University of Pennsylvania Cancer Center. Cassileth sought to understand the reasons for "the sustained and apparently growing appeal of anti-medicine, non-medicinal, life-style-oriented alternatives during a period of technological advance in orthodox medical care." Cassileth's study involved 304 inpatients at the University of Pennsylvania Cancer Center and 356 patients under the care of unorthodox practitioners. She found that the patients using unorthodox therapies believed their cancer could have been prevented by diet, stress reduction, or environmental change, but those treated exclusively with conventional therapies did not. Metabolic therapies, diet therapies, mental imagery applied for antitumor effect, spiritual approaches, and alternative "immune" therapies were among the most common alternative therapies used by the patients engaged in unorthodox therapies. Cassileth writes:

41% expected the therapy to achieve a cure or remission; 18% anticipated prevention or halt of metastatic growth. These expectations were less than fully realized: 22% of patients on imagery, 43% on megavitamins, 53% on immune therapies, and 61% on metabolic regimens believed these therapies were effective (in bringing about cure or remission, augmenting other treatments, or preventing spread). Chemotherapy was judged similarly efficacious by 56% of patients, radiation by 59%, and surgery by 72%.

Most important, Cassileth found that 30% of the patients' conventional physicians supported the use of alternative treatments, that only 8% of the patients using these therapies refused any conventional treatment, and that 60% of patients using the unorthodox therapies continued to use conventional therapies as well. She concludes:

This study shows that many patients receiving alternative care do not conform to the traditional stereotype of poorly educated, terminally ill patients who have exhausted conventional treatment. Similarly, although some unorthodox practitioners may well fit the characteristic portrait of quacks and charlatans, many are well trained, few charge high fees, and most, on the basis of patients' views and our own observations, sincerely believe in the efficacy and rationality of their work.

In my research, I found no cure for cancer among the complementary therapies, little scientific evidence on which to evaluate them, strong anecdotal evidence that some patients did well while using them, a convergence of interest between ethical complementary cancer therapists and progressive established cancer therapists, and large numbers of intelligent patients seeking to integrate established and complementary therapies in their own packages of humanistic cancer therapy.

I found that many observers of complementary therapies agreed on a general model of patient response to these therapies, despite their great diversity: some patients are hurt or receive no benefit while using these therapies; most report subjective benefits of greatly varying duration; some had reasonably good prognoses on established therapies but used complementary therapies with a view to improving general health and reducing the probability of recurrence; and a small but important minority of patients with grave prognoses survived the cancer while using complementary therapies (often alongside established therapies).

I found that patients who used complementary therapies intelligently fit roughly into three groups: "exceptional cancer patients," who undertook to face their cancer and work actively with it, whether their goal was cure, prolonged life expectancy, better quality of life, or a better death; "healthy cancer patients," namely those exceptional cancer patients who had the time and made the choice to pursue vigorous health-promotion therapies and became physically healthier in many respects, reporting many benefits in the quality of their lives, in pain reduction, and in resilience, under a variety of therapies; and "cancer survivors," including a small number of cancer patients who survived grave prognoses and a much larger number who used complementary therapies as "insurance" along with established therapies to treat cancers with much better prognoses.▪

The emergence of a new and more balanced perspective on complementary therapies is a profound turning point in the recent history of cancer medicine in the United States. The history of American medical attitudes toward cancer therapy reflects the struggles of the American medical profession over the last two centuries. As Paul Starr has shown, in the years 1760 to 1850 most American physicians had low social status and low incomes as they struggled to establish allopathic medicine in a democratic frontier society and an open medical market. From 1850 to 1930, there was a fierce battle for dominion in the medical market place, the stakes being control of licensing authority and control of medical education. Organized allopathic physicians finally won.

The last half-century has seen new challenges to physicians from corporations and the state, and more recently a renewed challenge from a

wide range of "other therapies" that practice at the boundaries (or beyond) of physician-dominated medicine.

Cancer medicine has a unique position in this history. During the last century, as cancer became the symbolic disease of our time, it naturally attracted intense attention from both established and alternative practitioners. Many of the fiercest territorial battles for control of the medical market pitted organized allopathic physicians against "quack" practitioners of alternative cancer therapies. Some of these quacks were, unquestionably, quacks. Others were "premature" exponents of complementary cancer therapies that are edging into the mainstream today.

As a result of this combative past, of the symbolic resonance of cancer, and indeed of the billions of dollars poured into biomedical cancer research, cancer medicine has until recently been far more vociferously defended against the introduction of complementary therapies than has any other area of American medicine. Thus, it has been commonplace for holistic physicians to report that they can use alternative therapies for other health problems without attracting legal attention, but that applying the same therapies to cancer has frequently resulted in loss of licensure or other sanctions.

Today, the war over cancer therapies continues in the trenches, but the social membrane that for decades largely succeeded in insulating cancer medicine from the complementary therapies that were widely used in other medical areas appears to have become more permeable. This change is in part due to the emergence in established medicine of a more adaptive mechanism to sort out useful and acceptable complementary developments from those that still do not meet current standards.

The interest of society as a whole in health promotion, self-care, and personal growth coincided with the extension of complementary therapies into areas ever closer to cancer, until a blanket exclusionary principle no longer held credibility. The mechanism for debarring alternative cancer practitioners is wielded as vigorously as ever, but

▪ As Dan Ullman, M.P.H., points out, this classification does not include desperate cancer patients who are in highly anxious emotional states and often make irrational use of these therapies.

the progressive wing of the cancer care community is fully engaged with behavioral researchers, nutritionists, and others in exploring the substance of the most promising approaches that alternative and adjunctive therapists have been utilizing for decades.

THE INFLUENCE OF ADVANCES IN NUTRITIONAL RESEARCH ON INTEGRAL CANCER THERAPY

The confluence between established and complementary positions in cancer therapy is clearly visible in the area of nutrition, which plays an important role in many integral cancer therapies.

The publication in 1982 of the *Diet, Nutrition and Cancer* report by the National Research Council of the National Academy of Sciences marked a turning point in the development of patient and physician perspectives on integral cancer therapy. The Research Council Committee, chaired by Clifford Grobstein, M.D., made an extraordinarily extensive and coherent review of the relationship between diet and the onset of cancer. It issued interim dietary guidelines for reducing fat, increasing whole grains, fruits, and vegetables (especially citrus fruits and carotene-rich and cruciferous vegetables), minimizing carcinogens both from natural sources and from inadvertent or intentional additives, and minimizing alcohol intake (especially when combined with cigarette smoking). Perhaps most important, the report summarized the vital epidemiological significance of high animal fat diets in many of the major cancers for which effective therapies have not been developed.

While the report was primarily concerned with prevention, it raised a question that remains in the minds of many physicians and patients considering nutritional approaches to cancer control: If some cancers are demonstrably associated with poor nutritional patterns, may not the dietary habits that are known to decrease their incidence also decrease the incidence of cancer recurrence, extend disease-free intervals, or even slow or reverse the progress of an existing cancer? There are strong theoretical arguments on both

sides of the question. Clinical research on this subject is in its infancy. It is not known whether different results might be achieved by nutritional interventions, based upon the degree to which different people with the same cancer may have different metabolic constitutions (and different belief structures).

In any event, those who were aware that nutritional-metabolic cancer therapists commonly advocated a primarily vegetarian wholefoods diet and nutritional supplements saw a striking parallel between such a regimen and the diet and individual nutrients that the Committee's study found prevented some cancers. Cassileth's data add a suggestive finding on this point. While 22% of the patients using imagery believed the therapy was helpful in controlling their cancer, 43% taking megavitamins and 61% in nutritional-metabolic programs believed that their therapy had some effect. There are several possible explanations that would attribute no particular significance to this finding. Was this last percent purely a result of different belief structures and placebo effects varying with the different therapies? But there is at least a possibility that the nutritional-metabolic therapies may have contributed significantly—the numbers are powerfully different—to the benefits that patients experienced.

Perhaps the most intriguing recent example of convergence between established and complementary nutritional cancer therapies results from a study on diet and breast cancer. In an article in *Hospital Practice*, Ernest L. Wynder and David P. Rose, respectively president and chief of nutrition and endocrinology at the American Health Foundation, point to research showing that among postmenopausal breast cancer patients the 10-year survival rate at the Japan Center Institute was 60% and the survival rate at Vanderbilt University Hospital was only 31%. Among premenopausal patients, however, the 10-year survival rate was virtually the same—66% in Japan and 61% in the United States.

The authors cite studies in Hawaii showing that the average fat intake of white Hawaiian females was greater than that of Japanese Hawaiian females and increased with advancing age. They also discovered that although the incidence of *in situ* breast carcinoma was about the same for both groups, the rate at which the lesions progressed to clinical significance was significantly greater among postmenopausal white patients. "These and other findings suggest that it may be appropriate to conduct a randomized prospective clinical trial on the efficacy of a low-fat diet as adjunctive therapy in postmenopausal breast cancer. The diet used might be based on the Japanese model," which is generally lower in fat. Most of the alternative nutritional cancer therapies provide the low-fat diet that Wynder and Rose recommend. Macrobiotic practitioners, for example, sometimes report particularly good outcomes with breast, colon, and prostate cancer, all of which have a lower incidence in Japan than in the United States.

The alternative therapies have pioneered the use of nutrition for breast cancer; established cancer researchers have contributed the important observation that the efficacy of such a therapy should probably be far greater for postmenopausal then premenopausal patients. It is not difficult to imagine that when these two lines of cancer work converge, the result will be a nutritional adjuvant therapy for breast cancer.

One of the most fascinating sociological facts regarding the acceptance of different treatments proposed by complementary cancer therapists is that psychological therapies have moved into the modern mainstream far more rapidly than diet and nutritional therapies. On the face of it, one would expect a materially-oriented scientific paradigm to be receptive to the material orientation of diet and nutritional therapies, particularly given the incontrovertible epidemiological evidence on cancer prevention and the animal studies on both prevention and control. This has not been the case. How many people remember that in *Anatomy of an Illness*, Norman Cousins reported using not only laughter and psychological approaches but diet, supplements, and vitamin C to heal himself? Oddly, our cultural-medical filter preserves Cousin's "laughter thera-

py" but strains out his equally vigorous nutritional program.

THE INFLUENCE OF THE NEWLY ASSESSED LIMITS OF ESTABLISHED THERAPIES ON INTEGRAL CANCER THERAPIES

I noted earlier that the use of radical surgery probably reached its apogee in the 1950s and that chemotherapy and radiotherapy appear to be moving toward greater refinement of techniques and away from more extensive application. The general trend toward the less aggressive use of established therapies is not necessarily a uniform one. In regard to breast cancer, for example, some alternative cancer therapists are now suggesting that bilateral mastectomies may be more effective than lumpectomies in preventing the recurrence of some types of breast cancer. In their view, the factor exciting recurrence may be in the breast tissue itself. Similarly, at the highly regarded complementary cancer therapy center in Bonn, the Janker Clinic, the staff often uses high-dose chemotherapy and radiotherapy for brief periods of time with selected cancers to achieve what they consider superior outcomes. The fact remains that proposals for radical surgical techniques and for intensive chemotherapy and radiotherapy, although they may be effective and humane choices, are now generally being considered in a cultural and scientific atmosphere conscious of the limits of the established therapies.

The greatest contribution to this atmosphere is the widespread belief among the general public, shared by many scientists, that the 15-year-old, multibillion dollar war on cancer did not live up to the promises that were made at its inception. An emblematic example of this disappointment is found in the remarks of John Bailar, former editor of the *Journal of the National Cancer Institute*, who worked at the NCI for 25 years and is now a Harvard epidemiologist. As reported by the Associated press, Bailar told the American Association for the Advancement of Science:

My overall assessment is that the national cancer program must be judged a qualified failure. . . . It has not produced the results it was supposed to produce.... I have not said that the treatment of cancer is of no value.... The problem is that it is not getting better very fast.

Bailar also took issue with statistics that The National Cancer Institute used to suggest that substantial progress is being made in the treatment of cancer. The death rate from breast cancer is steady, he pointed out, and the survival rate in serious cases has not changed. Statistics that announce an increased survival rate result from the fact that more cases of mild and benign cancer are being found and "cured."

The growing consensus on the limits of established therapies even extends to the obviously exciting new research into the inner mechanisms of the cancer process. While it is recognized that the explication of these mechanisms may lead to clinical progress—the long-hunted "silver bullet" may yet be found—there is also an appreciation of the possibility that understanding the micromechanisms may not be equivalent to finding a cure. This cautiousness can be framed as a question: to what degree are the micromechanisms of cancer going to hold the answer to cancer control, and to what degree is the answer in prevention, health promotion and behavioral approaches, coupled with the humanistic use of selected established therapies for cancers for which they are clearly efficacious?

PIVOT POINTS IN INTEGRAL CANCER THERAPIES

From the point of view of the person with cancer, there are characteristic pivot points in the cancer experience that the medical literature often ignores, yet they can have a profound effect on the patient. As Naomi Remen has suggested, it is vital that the patient and the clinician recognize these pivot points so as to navigate them with the greatest possible skill and compassion. Any effort to develop an integral cancer therapy must consider them. Not all cancer patients go through all these pivot points, but all these points can be critical for cancer patients.

One can argue about whether disregarding the pivot points, or mishandling them, will influence

the course of disease. But the importance of pivot points does not depend on the conclusions of that argument. It is sufficient to note that insensitivity to the experience of the patient at these times often has a great effect on the morale, hopes, fears, self-esteem, and expectations of the patient. Whether or not these factors affect survival time, they deeply affect the lives of people living with cancer.

The Initial Visit and Diagnostic Procedures

The first pivot point in the cancer experience is the visit to a physician by a patient with undiagnosed symptoms that may signal cancer and the initiation of diagnostic procedures. If cancer is a possible diagnosis, how should the physician and the patient cope with the situation? If there is reason to use diagnostic procedures that carry any known or debated risk of spreading the cancer, clearly the patient should be informed of these risks. Beyond this, the physician should be aware that, for the patient, the period from the initial visit to the completion of the diagnostic process can be a time of great agony and uncertainty. The physician should openly acknowledge the possible difficulty of this period, inquire into what if anything he might do to help the patient through it, and prepare the patient for how and when they will discuss the diagnostic results.

The Diagnosis

How and when *should* a physician tell patients that they have cancer? There is certainly no single right answer. But there are skillful and compassionate approaches to the task of discussing the diagnosis.

Norman Cousins has suggested that there may be a sharp acceleration in the progress of cancer for many patients immediately following diagnosis. He acknowledges the possibility that this may reflect the natural history of the disease, but his concern is that the fear and panic resulting from the diagnosis may depress the patient's resistance and accelerate the cancer process. Cousins proposes that the physician emphasize the possibility of a positive outcome and his willingness to fight alongside the patient for survival. One of Cousins' suggestions is that when the physician delivers the initial diagnosis, a recovered patient with the same initial diagnosis be in the room so that the patient has visible proof of the possibility of recovery. The American Cancer Society has built a program around the obvious value for a newly diagnosed patient of seeing a recovered patient.

The concern of many thoughtful physicians about the biological and psychological effects of a badly presented cancer diagnosis may be related to the widespread custom in many countries of not telling patients of a cancer diagnosis at all. In Japan, according to Emiko Ohnuki-Tierney's beautiful anthropological account of health and illness in that country, cancer patients are almost never told their diagnosis. The family is told and usually decides not to tell the patient. Even professors of medicine at major medical schools are not told when they have cancer. A leading Japanese physician explained, "Human beings react very strongly to the notion of death. We should let the patients spend the rest of their short lives without anxiety." Even patients at the National Center for Cancer Research in Tokyo are not told they have cancer. "A doctor at the National Center for Circulatory Diseases told me that patients believe that, whereas all other people there may be cancer patients, 'I am somehow an exception.'"

It may be, of course, that without being told, most Japanese cancer patients consciously or unconsciously know that they have cancer. Bernard Siegel reports that in families where the children request that their mother be spared the diagnosis, the mother almost always knows what is wrong without being told. Bernard Fox has described to me studies in England and the United States showing that most cancer patients who are not told of their diagnosis still know that they have cancer. Fox points out that in such a circumstance, the failure to tell the patient of the cancer diagnosis may be worse than silence, for the patient may infer from the silence that the disease is completely hopeless and be struck by a feeling of helplessness.

In regard to informing patients, western Europe generally occupies a middle ground between American and Japanese practices. At the

Lukas Klinik in Switzerland, a spiritually-oriented center operated by followers of Rudolf Steiner (founder of Anthroposophy), director Rita LeRoi reports that many patients come to the clinic not knowing their diagnosis. The clinic practice is to give them the diagnosis for therapeutic and spiritual reasons. The staff believes that patients need to know the diagnosis to fight for life and to make the best use of the time remaining for the evolution of their souls.

While there are many different cultural and personal practices regarding the discussion of a cancer diagnosis, there is unfortunately no doubt that many common practices in the United States are unnecessarily hurtful to the patients. To take a typical example, it is not compassionate for a surgeon to come to the bedside of a patient emerging from anesthetic and surgery in the recovery room, deliver a brusque cancer diagnosis, and then leave the patient in an exquisitely vulnerable physical and psychological state to cope with this shattering disclosure alone. It is not compassionate to deliver a cancer diagnosis by a registered letter or over the telephone (appropriate on rare occasions). It is not compassionate to give a cancer diagnosis in a hurried office visit without judging its effects on the patients and family. As the saying goes, beginnings are important. Cancer patients will remember the moment of being informed of their diagnosis for the rest of their lives. For many patients, the real possibility of both death and suffering is suddenly placed before them. While much of the practice of cancer therapy is frustrating and unrewarding, the moment of presenting the diagnosis is a time when a skilled and compassionate physician can profoundly affect the lives of the patient and the patient's family.

Ernest Rosenbaum, a San Franciscan oncologist, has written at length on how he handles the discussions of cancer diagnoses. He often tape records the session because he has found that many patients go into shock after they hear the word *cancer*, and do not recall anything else from the interview. He wants them to be able to replay the interview later. Bernard Siegel has made a long study of how to give cancer patients a diagnosis and convey genuine hope both for what their remaining lives can be and for their possibilities of overcoming the cancer. "Our patients do not ask that we always cure them, but only that we respect them as human beings," he says.

Perhaps the key to effective communication of a cancer diagnosis is to make every effort to determine the kinds of hope that are most meaningful to the patient and to provide an assurance that the physician cares about these hopes and will be with the patient throughout the entire cancer process.

Physicians should be aware of all the forms that hope can take and how the focus of hope shifts through the course of illness as expectations change. In discussing the principles of integral cancer therapies, I noted some of the forms that hope can take. Precisely because cancer is understandably associated with so much dread, the list is worth repeating and expanding. There is the valid hope that one will experience a rare and extraordinary healing—medical literature substantiates such experiences, even with very advanced cancers. There is hope of being among those who experience the best possible outcome for the particular cancer from which the patient is suffering. There is hope for prolonged disease-free intervals of life. There is hope for time to attain a cherished goal. There is hope for freedom from physical pain and psychological suffering, hope that one will not experience side effects from treatment, hope of having a special period of time with family and friends. There is hope for personal growth, for time to live among Mexican ruins, for a new level of awareness to the beauty of life not achieved before the prospect of dying came so near. To understand, to admire, to support those hopes is the role of the physician and friends.

An Early Time to Assimilate and Heal

Virginia Veach, Ph.D., a psychotherapist in San Francisco, proposes that the next frequently ignored pivot in cancer is the need of the patient for a quiet and supportive setting in which to go through the shock of diagnosis (and often the shock of diagnostic surgery and sometimes of initiating treatment as well). In a comfortable setting with good, nourishing food and a caring friend, the cancer patient can take the time needed to assimilate this enormous life transition. Veach calls this an early opportunity for healing that is often missed. She believes it is very important during this period to protect the patient from a premature onslaught of advice about what to do. If this time is given to the patient, and the shock is assimilated, she believes the patient will usually emerge from the shock without prodding and will begin to ask questions about the available therapy choices.

Choosing a Course of Treatment versus the Rush to Treatment

Cancer authorities regularly urge that patients with serious cancer diagnoses get more than one opinion about treatment options and carefully explore the medical team and hospital to which they intend to entrust themselves. In practice, however, patients are often rushed into treatment immediately following diagnosis, and there is no suggestion that they should explore established alternatives, to say nothing of complementary therapy alternatives. The presumption, sometimes made explicitly, is that any delay will have grave consequences. This is another critical pivot point in the cancer experience. The rush to treatment ignores the good medical practice of informing the patient of the value of a second opinion. It ignores the need of many patients for time to assimilate the shock of diagnosis. It compromises the therapeutically valuable feeling of patients that they have made an informed personal choice after consultation with their physician and others, and that therefore they have some real control of events at a time and in a setting when much sense of control disappears. And medically, the rush to treatment is often based on questionable evidence regarding the immediate need to initiate therapy.

If time is taken to make an informed choice from among treatment options, the question arises as to how a lay person, often in a state of shock, can possibly understand the complexities of options among both established and complementary therapies. In fact, this question reemphasizes the importance of giving the patient time to assimilate the shock of cancer diagnosis. And of course the patient may make unwise choices. Virginia Veach simply encourages her patients to keep exploring options until they find a course of therapies that makes sense to them. The advice is deceptively simple and very useful. Sound and responsible information should greatly narrow the options, but Veach's advice is often the best guideline in choosing among the remaining options.

The Commitment to Live and the Purpose of Life

Naomi Remen finds that many patients embark on a course of therapy while they are still numb with the shock of diagnosis. But she often sees a turning point in the course of therapy when patients resolve an inner struggle over whether they dare to hope and fight for life. Making a commitment to live is the central pivot point in Lawrence LeShan's psychological therapy. LeShan believes that if a desire to live is based primarily on the fear of death, it does not stop the progress of cancer, and that a desire to return to life as it was before is at best a Band-aid. In LeShan's view, helping the patient to "find his own song," the deepest and most fundamental reason to live, activates the forces that can hold the cancer at bay.

Often, Remen reports, a commitment to live goes along with a decision to let go of what is not essential to a patient's newly reconsidered life. At this point, she reports, many patients embark on major health-promoting changes in their behavior.

LeShan reports similarly that his most successful patients are the people who engage themselves in an effort to heal on three levels: physical, psychological, and spiritual. The physical work may include established and complementary approaches to regaining health. The psychological work is the recovery of the deep purpose of life. The spiritual work, whether or not it is so labeled, is the dedication to something greater than oneself and one's immediate family. The dedication does not have to be to an endeavor normally defined as spiritual. It may be a commitment to devote oneself to a conservation cause, or to

being a Big Brother, or to something else with no apparent spiritual dimension.

Often, the emergence of a commitment to live and of a new sense of purpose in life is accompanied, gradually or suddenly, by deep and varying insights and by periods of expanded awareness that patients cherish. This expansion of awareness and the sense that life has been transformed leads some patients to report that, while they would not have chosen to get cancer, they nonetheless would go through the experience again rather than miss discovering what they have learned in the process.

The Recurrence of Cancer

Recurrence of cancer is a major pivot point for many patients. They may have suffered through rigorous courses of therapy, or made profound and sometimes arduous changes in their life, or carried out deep explorations of self-inquiry, or felt certain that they were successfully combating their illness, and then suddenly, often after a new psychological or physical shock, the cancer recurs. It can be an equally difficult point for compassionate physicians who believe that established therapies in the search for a cure are all they have to offer. At this point there may be a replay of many of the previous pivot points and a new fundamental question about whether one dares hope again to overcome the cancer. The key to this transition may be to explore fully the despair over recurrence so that the grieving can be completed. Often, new levels of awareness then emerge from this intense suffering, with potentially life-saving or simply life-enhancing consequences.

The Decision to Terminate a Therapy

Established physicians today will generally terminate a course of therapy only when there is absolutely no hope left for its effectiveness. But it is important for physicians and patients to recognize that patients have a right to call a halt to therapies that cease to make sense to them. A course of chemotherapy with a probably terminal cancer may be slowing the progress of the cancer, yet patients may decide that the treatment is depriving them of valuable time in which to live their lives. The same is true with complementary therapies: a macrobiotic diet is an arduous commitment for most people, and whether or not it appears to be improving health, patients may decide that life is too short, literally, to give up ice cream.

Choosing Life or Death

LeShan divides all cancer therapy and care into two periods: the time when one fights for life with every tool at one's disposal, and the time at which one prepares for death. Some therapists, he suggests, are more dedicated to the fight for life and may be insensitive or even psychologically brutal to the patient who has accepted death. Other therapists may be more skilled with the work of dying, and may urge patients to accept death before they are personally ready to do this. Anyone who spends a good deal of time with people who have cancer can see some people with very advanced cancers who wage the most extraordinary and beautiful fights for their lives and see others who choose with equal courage and beauty to accept death early in the cancer process. There is no right or wrong here, only recognition of the pivot points, which may occur more than once, at which people choose to fight for life or prepare for death, and the importance of supporting that choice, however wrong-headed it may seem to someone with a different proclivity.

The choice to prepare for death sets in motion a series of subsequent pivot points that I will not discuss at length here. They include the decision of whether to die in a hospital or at home, and the string of decisions concerning which naturally occuring opportunity to die will be allowed to run its course by the patient, family, and physician. This is an extraordinary and much overlooked subject. In the cancer process, there are often peaceful and painless ways to die that are regularly overlooked in hospital practice because the patient can be kept alive. For some people, the opportunity to die a natural death is an important goal. At present, these people must generally opt to die at home because hospital practices often prohibit the deliberate choice not to interrupt a natural process.

ENVISIONING AN INTEGRAL CANCER THERAPY NETWORK

In this section I propose one vision of how integral cancer therapy might be organized. I imagine a network of established and complementary cancer therapists who have decided to work together to enhance ethical treatment options for their patients, to improve the quality of life for patients and their families, to widen their own knowledge about interrelated approaches to cancer treatment and care, to facilitate important research, and to expand concepts of professional training.

Characteristics of the Network

The core group would consist of respected established and complementary practitioners who would only invite other practitioners to join by unanimous agreement. The group would inform the state medical board of its plans and shape its program around state legal requirements to safeguard network members and patients.

The practitioners would need to establish some common ground which might not include the principles outlined above of integral cancer therapy and the need for special care at the pivot points in the cancer process. All the members of the network would negotiate among themselves the basis for referring patients to one another. They would also provide descriptions of their treatment protocols to each other. All members would define the areas of cancer care in which they believed they were effective and the kinds of outcomes that referred patients might expect in working with them. These protocols and statements would form the basis of an informed consent form for patients entering treatment in the network.

Patients could enter the network through any member practitioner, but the group would also include a referral specialist who understood the resources in the network and had the clinical skills to diagnose, understand, and prescribe. Any group member could send a patient to this specialist to develop an overview of treatment options.

In many instances, the referring group member would act as the patient's "therapy coordinator"— the professional who would stay with the patient through the entire cancer process. But in all cases the patients would be encouraged to select their therapy coordinator for themselves, so that they would not experience the common feeling among cancer (and other) patients that their care is fragmented and that they are, in a sense, abandoned as whole people among the subspecialists.

Development of Research Priorities

Bernard Fox has emphasized the difficulties of conducting research on outcomes in the type of system that I am proposing. I am not a methodology specialist, but the following considerations might serve as a point of departure in determining research goals and methods.

One primary goal of initial research would be to inform group members and patients about sample patient responses to different combinations of therapies within the network. A second goal would be to assess patient and practitioner satisfaction with the network so that regular improvements could be made. A third goal would be to develop instruments for helping patients clarify their goals and select their treatment "packages" and for predicting patient satisfaction with different packages. A fourth goal would be to develop scales of general well-being, functional ability, and other quality-of-life measurements for cancer patients. A fifth goal would be to explore the difficult issue of assessing disease-free intervals or extension of life, and then to correlate these outcomes with quality-of-life and functional- status measures for different kinds of people with different cancers. A sixth goal would be to measure outcomes for the system as a whole against outcomes for established therapy practices with similar populations.

Throughout, the major aim would be to associate outcomes with different uses of the system, and the research would be guided by a logic of inquiry rather than a logic of proof. The researchers would not permit the ultimate scientific need for definitive research designs to divert them from the initial human need for approximate hypothesis-generating measurements that could lead to better outcomes and other improvements in the system.

A regular function of the system would be medical rounds for all practitioners to present and discuss cases. The system would place great value on developing and sustaining a clinical overview of the outcomes achieved by different practitioners with different kinds of patients. Collective efforts to assess clinically emerging patterns of outcomes would be encouraged as a basis for future research.

Humane Use of Established Therapies

For patients who did not have specific personal preferences, the network would provide a set of guidelines for health promotion and for using a mixture of established and complementary therapies. The idea behind this "package" would be to identify the combination of elements that worked best for most people. In general, a major emphasis of the network would be the integrated, supportive use of complementary therapies and the moderate and appropriate use of established therapies.

The guidelines would emphasize a commitment to the humane use of established therapies and the network's preference, in the absence of conclusive scientific evidence substantiating the clear effectiveness of toxic therapies, to use such therapies moderately rather than vigorously. To minimize distress over the likely possibility of receiving different recommendations from the oncologist, radiologist, and surgeon, patients would be advised to expect differences of opinion among established practitioners.

All established therapy practitioners would offer adjunctive complementary therapies for which there is scientific or suggestive evidence showing that they encourage positive outcomes.

Surgery patients would be walked through the surgery arrangements in advance of treatment and provided with whatever levels of information they wanted (some patients want to know everything, others nothing.) Operating-room teams would treat patients under anesthetic as though they were present in the room listening to the conversation. Patients would be encouraged to bring tape recordings of music into surgery with them and could also get tape recordings of operating room conversations afterward if they wished. The network would also encourage presurgical and postsurgical programs of enhanced nutrition and of visualization techniques to support good outcomes.

With both radiotherapy and chemotherapy, there would be a similarly strong emphasis on using nutritional and psychological techniques to support the treatments. The objectives of such support would be to decrease the negative side effects of the treatments and to enhance their anti-tumor effects.

Philosophy and Use of Complementary Therapies

The philosophy of the complementary therapies program would be to support patients in maximizing health-promoting physical, psychological, and spiritual initiatives consistent with their own beliefs and attitudes. The network would offer a standard program of such therapies, but patients would be encouraged to shape the program to their own needs.

The standard program would be one of diet, nutritional supplements, psychological counseling and support groups, stretching and aerobic exercise, progressive relaxation, visualization, breathing practices, meditation, and some form of direct healing work, such as therapeutic touch.

The network would also offer an education and recreational program consisting of inspiring and informative books, audio- and videotapes, and films. Art, music, movement, crafts, and nature appreciation would be encouraged for their direct therapeutic benefit.

One example of such a broad program can be found in the Bristol Cancer Help Center in England, where patients come for 1 or 2 weeks for a vegetarian diet, nutritional supplements, biofeedback training in progressive relaxation, and educational and philosophical orientation exploring the goals and spirit of the program, psychological counseling, and healing by the laying on

of hands. The patients return home with the diet regimen, the supplements, the knowledge of how to continue relaxation, meditation, and visualization, and the address of a nearby psychotherapist and a healer to continue their work should they want to. The Bristol Cancer Help Center program is effective in raising morale and teaching a sound, basic approach to physical, psychological, and spiritual healing.

CONCLUSION

This proposal that we integrate what is best in established and complementary cancer therapies comes at a time of forceful and continuing debate on the topic. I have emphasized throughout this chapter that most patients and physicians who engage in integral cancer therapy include in their programs the moderate use of clearly efficacious established therapies. I have also emphasized that among those who engage in integral cancer therapies, as among those who use only established therapies, the dramatic and complete reversal of serious cancers is the rare exception rather than the rule.

What I find in most patients and health professionals who are integrating established and complementary therapies is the profound conviction that this eclectic and personalized approach to cancer therapy is worthwhile. I regularly encounter patients engaged in these integrated therapies who, given their initial diagnosis, appear to be exceptionally well.

But what is most striking to me about many of these people with cancer has nothing to do with evidence of extended disease-free intervals or life expectancy. What amazes and touches me is that through this difficult life passage they have found inner resources of strength, wisdom, and insight that they often had not experienced before. They do not live with the certainty of clear victories. They live with the knowledge that the cancer process may worsen or return at any time, and with the personal conviction that how they live may affect when or whether it does so. But the kind of life they develop is also the one that they would want to follow even if their efforts had no impact on the course of the disease. The great cancer therapists I know seem to come to share these qualities of being. But it is never clear who is teaching whom.

Someday, if we are fortunate, the National Cancer Institute and the private foundations supporting cancer research will see fit to fund the new kinds of clinical research that will answer the scientific questions about the effects of integral cancer therapies on different cancers in different people. This research, if it is done well, will make quality of life and functional ability as important as life extension and disease-free intervals.

But even this research will not tell us the whole story that is being written in cancer medicine by patients and physicians engaged in integral cancer therapies. That larger story involves the struggle for the humanization of medicine being played out with the great symbolic disease of our time. The humanization of medicine is good in itself. It does not have to be justified in terms of life extension for patients. The act of treating sick people with compassion and sensitivity to their own unique healing patterns entirely justifies itself. And the struggle for the humanization of medicine, in turn, is one of the major forms of the struggle for planetary healing that mankind is waging with itself.

35 WHAT YOU SHOULD KNOW ABOUT SMOKING

Tom Ferguson, M.D., is co-author (with Gail Schmidt, R.N.) of *The Smoker's Book of Health* (G. P. Putnam's Sons, 1986). He founded the journal *Medical Self-Care*, and he is a regular contributor to *American Health* and a contributing editor of *Prevention*.

According to Dr. Tom Ferguson, at least 80% of smokers want to quit, and two thirds of them seriously attempt to do so. But for many, quitting cold turkey is impossible. Dr. Ferguson explains why smoking is so addictive and suggests ways for smokers to improve their physical health and protect themselves from disease without necessarily kicking the nicotine habit completely. Good nutrition, vigorous exercise, and social support can help even the heaviest smoker to control his smoking, writes Dr. Ferguson, and he explains how these factors can aid a 3-pack-a-day smoker in freeing himself from an expensive and dangerous habit.■

Researcher Gail Schmidt, R.M., and I interviewed 200 smokers, asking them about their health concerns. We were struck by the high level of guilt that these smokers were experiencing. We were prepared to find them blasé; we found instead a great deal of suffering and torment.

"Sometimes I just sit there in front of my mirror with a cigarette in my mouth and watching myself inhaling that poison gas," one smoker lamented. "I know that if I was in a concentration camp and someone tried to make me do that, I'd want to kill them."

We had expected denial of the health effects of smoking. Instead, we found that these smokers *over*estimated the negative effects of cigarettes on their health. We were astounded at the number of additional years of life they believed they would gain from quitting. Estimates ranges as high as 20 years. "If I could quit today, I know I'd see my daughter have children," one smoker said. "If I don't, I'll be lucky to see her married."

We expected resentment toward nonsmokers. But we found that smokers have become *extremely* sensitive to the effects of their smoking on nonsmokers. They are much more likely to refrain from smoking while in the presence of nonsmokers than they were 5 years ago.

They told us that they felt confused about the role that smoking plays in their lives. They no longer view smoking as a pleasant, relaxing, and helpful personal ritual. But at the same time they feel that it *does* provide them with undeniable benefits. As one woman smoker put it, "It's like being in love with a man who's no good. You *know* you're a fool. But you just can't help it."

In addition to their own feelings of confusion and guilt, smokers must deal with an increasing number of antismoking messages and a much more open display of antismoking sentiment: antismoking advocates in some cities have used spray cans to "zap" smokers. A Los Angeles man was stabbed when he refused to put out his cigarette. Another smoker was shot by a New York transit policeman in a dispute over smoking.

Among many groups, especially the more affluent and better educated, smoking has become something of a social stigma. This widespread change in attitude toward smoking has made many smokers feel part of a persecuted minority.

With few exceptions, smokers say that they'd like to take more control of their smoking. About 80% to 95% of smokers say they'd like to quit, and about two thirds of present smokers have made serious attempts to do so.

These smokers feel terrible because they have been unable to quit. One smoker explained: "After I go to bed at night, when I'm in that dreamy place just before sleep, I always think, 'I'm *not* going to smoke tomorrow. I'm *not* going to do this to myself any more. I think of how bad it is for me, how bad it is for my daughter. And I feel this big burst of resolve. But then, first thing in the morning, I grind that coffee and pour myself a fresh cup, and the second I take the first sip, I reach for a cigarette."

Those who have children at home feel guiltiest of all: "Ever since my daughter started to talk, she's told me she wished I didn't smoke," one smoker told us. "'That smoke stinks' she'll say. 'Your smoke really bothers me. It makes me want to throw up. I can't breathe when you're blowing all that smoke around.' And even though I *know* it's hurting her, I'll sit there in the house and smoke anyway. I *really* hate myself for that."

When we asked them what kinds of information they would find helpful in their efforts to take control of their smoking, they listed the following topics:

1. Why smoking is so addictive.
2. How to cut your smoking risk by adopting a healthy lifestyle.
3. Strategies for cutting down.
4. Tools to help you quit.
5. Dealing with weight gain after you quit.

In our recent book, *The Smoker's Book of Health*, we have attempted to provide health-conscious smokers with extensive information on these and other topics. The sections that follow provide brief summaries of the topics that our subjects rated as "most needed."

1. Why Smoking Is So Addictive

Smokers obtain many benefits from smoking. They use cigarettes to relax, to keep alert, and to concentrate on difficult tasks. Smoking serves as an effective anaesthetic for both physical and psychological pain. It provides the smoker with a comfortable and familiar ritual. In addition, withdrawal from nicotine results in unpleasant physical symptoms. But to understand the nature of tobacco addiction, we must understand the pharmacology of nicotine.

Nicotine is an extremely powerful and versatile drug which can produce an astonishing array of effects on the human nervous system. Smokers can generate different effects by employing different puffing patterns. Thus smokers can—and do—use nicotine to regulate their nervous and endocrine systems to achieve the mood they desire.

A pack-a-day smoker inhales smoke about 200 times each day. Every inhalation delivers a tiny dose of nicotine directly to the brain within 7 seconds—faster than heroin injected into a vein. (The heroin must pass through a good part of your body's circulatory system before reaching the brain, while the nicotine-rich blood from the lungs passes directly to the brain.)

Nicotine addiction is a stool with four legs: one is the environmental stimuli—finishing a good dinner, having a cup of coffee, driving a car, stress at work (*The Environmental Factor*). The second is moods and feelings (*The Mood Factor*). When you are depressed, tired, or hungry, or you feel bad, needy, lonely, abandoned, or betrayed, you reach for a cigarette (*The Friendship Factor*). And if you stop smoking, you will experience physical and psychological signs of withdrawal (*The Addiction Factor*).

For those who see themselves as more vulnerable or sensitive than others—as many smokers do—smoking can serve as an important psychological support. In extreme cases, individuals may undergo profound personality disorganization as the result of a voluntary or involuntary smoking cessation. It should come as no surprise that smokers in many studies have repeatedly described smoking as "their best friend," and expressed their feeling that their cigarettes are one of their few psychological resources in a stressful life.

The lesson from all this is that any effort to control one's smoking must deal with all of these factors.

2. How To Cut Your Smoking Risk: Building a Healthier Lifestyle

Eating. Some researchers believe that nutrition plays an even greater role than tobacco in cancer prevention. According to current estimates, smoking contributes to approximately 120,000 premature deaths per year, while poor nutrition plays a key role in about 133,000.

There is substantial evidence to suggest that a healthy diet can cut one's risk of cancer. A Japanese study found that those who frequently ate green vegetables had one-third less risk of getting cancer as those who did not. The author, Dr. Takeshi Hirayama of the National Cancer Research Center in Tokyo, concluded that "even heavy smokers can reduce their chances of dying from cancer by eating more vegetables." Dr. Hirayama speculates that beta carotene, vitamin C, and fiber are the principal factors in this decreased cancer risk.

There is substantial evidence supporting the role of beta carotene, one form of vitamin A, in preventing cancer. Beta carotene is found in dark yellow, orange, and green fruits and vegetables. Fruits and vegetables especially high in beta carotene include asparagus, broccoli, carrots, apricots, cantaloupe, and leaf lettuce. The American Cancer Society recommends eating high levels of vitamin A to help prevent cancer.

Michael B. Sporn, M.D., chief of the lung cancer branch of the National Cancer Institute, warns, "No human population at risk for the development of cancer—and this specifically includes cigarette smokers—should allow themselves to remain deficient in vitamin A."

There is some suggestion that vitamin C, vitamin E, selenium, and indoles may also help prevent cancer.

Exercise. Some experts, including running guru and cardiologist George Sheenan, believe that the best thing a health-concerned smoker can do is to start a regular exercise program. "I've never told any of my patients to stop smoking,"

Sheenan says. "I've even, on occasion, advised people to *return* to smoking because they had gained 15 or 20 pounds and were beating up on their kids and their lives were completely miserable. But when smokers start exercising, many of them find themselves cutting down or quitting without any special effort at all. The body has a mind of its own, and if you start exercising regularly, it will either quit or will cut down to a relatively low-risk level."

Exercising regularly may be especially useful for those who use smoking to deal with tension. Instead of "taking 10" to have a smoke, instead of "counting to 10," the new exerciser realizes that he can almost as easily go out and "*run* 10."

Even if smokers who begin exercising *do* continue to smoke, studies suggest that their health risks are cut substantially, but the great majority of smokers who establish a regular exercise routine find themselves dropping the habit.

According to Dr. Peter Wood, Director of the Stanford University Heart Disease Prevention Program, "Smokers who begin exercising regularly generally find themselves tapering off and quitting without giving the matter much thought. They find it much easier, because they're not just giving something up, [but] replacing their unhealthy old habit with healthy new one—working out."

For those who smoke *and* exercise, death rates are lower than for nonexercising smokers:

EXERCISE LEVEL	NEVER SMOKED	PACK OR MORE/DAY
None	834*	1416
Slight	579	1347
Moderate	486	1065
Heavy	474	998

Environmental Factors. Cigarette smoking multiplies the risk of those exposed to toxic substances in the workplace. The most dramatic of such substances is asbestos. One study showed that smokers who worked in the asbestos industry were 53 times as likely to develop lung cancer as nonsmokers who were not asbestos workers. Asbestos workers who are *heavy* smokers are up

*Deaths per 1,000,000 man-years. Source: Hammond, E., *Journal of the National Cancer Institute*, 1964, 32: 1161.

to 87 times more likely to die of lung cancer.

Exposure to radon gas among uranium miners and to carbon monoxide among parking garage attendants, traffic police, and others are also high risk factors. Other toxic substances that may interact symbiotically with smoke include vinyl chloride, nickel, 2-napthylamine, sulfur dioxide, cotton dust, and silica dust.

Social Support. Social factors are extremely important in determining who smokes and who is able to quit.

Most people begin smoking in their teens. During this time, they are working to disentangle their identity from the influence of their parents. They are establishing an identity and stronger links with their friends.

Teenagers are much more likely to start smoking if their closest friends do so. Nearly 90% of teens who smoke say that one of their four best friends smoke. But only 33% of nonsmoking teens have a smoker among *their* four best friends. Teens are also more likely to smoke if one or both parents or one or more siblings smoke.

Starting to smoke can serve as a rite of passage into early adulthood. The beginning of teenage smoking often stems from a transitional life change, such as graduation from high school or college, moving, or the loss or absence of a parent.

Conversely, for a person trying to quit, having the wholehearted support of family and friends is one of the best predictors of success.

3. Strategies for Cutting Down

Not all health-concerned smokers will choose to quit. It may not make sense, at least at the present time, to try to quit, because their chances of success are extremely slim. For some people, at least in the short term, the chosen path will be to reduce their dose and add health-supportive measures.

Smoking filtered cigarettes substantially reduces the risk of lung cancer, but apparently does *not* reduce your risk of heart disease, presumably because it is the carbon monoxide, not the tar, that increases heart disease risk. Other strategies for cutting down include:

- Switch to chewing tobacco.
- Switch to such "cigarette substitutes" as a carrot, licorice stick, toothpick, shower, or walk around the block.
- Switch to a pipe or cigar (this works only if you don't inhale).
- Smoke only half of each cigarette (but *don't* cut them in half—use red felt tip pen to mark them).
- Change your routine: stop carrying cigarettes, no smoking at your desk, etc.
- Take fewer puffs on each cigarette.
- Don't inhale as deeply—or at all.
- Avoid situations in which other people are smoking.
- Start a smoking journal in which you identify each urge to smoke, then list how you responded.
- Be aware of your stress danger zones: remember that the way to HALT smoking is to keep yourself from situations in which you are **H**ungry, **A**ngry, **L**onely, or **T**ired.

4. Tools to Help You Quit

The big one here is nicotine gum. The same nicotine that keeps you addicted can help you kick the habit. You can kick one leg out from under the four-legged addiction stool by getting your drug hit from nicotine gum rather than cigarettes.

"It's like being given the key to your jail cell," one successful ex-smoker told us. You can continue to get your nicotine "fix" while avoiding the cancer-causing chemicals, the carbon monoxide, and other irritating gases in cigarette smoke.

A piece of nicotine gum contains less nicotine than a cigarette. And the effective blood level that results from chewing it is much less than that from smoking. Overdose doesn't seem to be a problem. If the gum is swallowed, the nicotine is broken down in the liver before it reaches the brain. And if you try to chew too much, the nicotine will make you nauseous long before you reach toxic levels. This automatically limits the quantity used.

Studies show that nicotine gum (brand name: Nicorette) is the most successful tool for quitting ever devised. They suggest that you can increase

your chances of successfully quitting by 50% to 100% by chewing the gum in addition to taking other steps. Smokers who quit using Nicorette experience little or no difficulty going cold turkey. And Nicorette is most effective with smokers who are most heavily addicted to nicotine.

The secret of success with the gums seems to be to keep using it. Most physicians recommend using the gum no longer than 6 months, although most quitters discontinue it much earlier. Many ex-smokers choose to carry a supply around with them for years afterward to serve as a "security blanket" in case they should be faced with an overwhelming urge to smoke.

Nicorette *is* expensive in the early stages— about $20 for a 10-day supply. (About the cost of a two-pack-a-day habit). But most smokers quickly cut down to much less gum.

Potential quitters should remember that millions have quit successfully without the gum. Still, many health-concerned smokers may wish to try it. This is the only drug which has been proven to help smokers quit.

Once you have decided to quit, set a date. Tell all your friends and ask for their help. Make a public commitment. If you have decided to use nicotine gum as part of your program, visit your doctor to discuss your plans and get a prescription.

Pick a time as free from stress as possible. If you can, arrange for a vacation or time off. Set up supportive activities with friends and support people during the first months. Occupy your time. Avoid situations in which you will feel pressure to smoke.

You may wish to make a ceremony of smoking your last cigarette. Invite your friends to watch. If your friends ask what they can do to help, ask them to throw you a quitting party.

Throw out all your ash trays. Have your teeth cleaned. Put a "No Smoking" sign by your front door. Ask visitors who wish to smoke to do so outside. Congratulations! You're a nonsmoker!

If you use Nicorette, chew it slowly until you taste the flavor or feel a tingling sensation in your mouth. As soon as you do, *stop chewing*. Park the gum in your cheek.

When the taste or tingling is gone, begin chewing again—slowly—until you taste the gum again. Continue this stop-and-start method. Continue for about half an hour or until the taste disappears.

The reason for this stop-and-start process is to provide yourself with an effective dose without feeling nauseous. If you do begin to feel a bit sick to your stomach, stop chewing until the feeling goes away.

Your goal is to chew in such a way as to provide yourself with enough nicotine to prevent withdrawal symptoms, but not enough to produce such side effects as dizziness, light-headedness, nausea, irritation of the mouth and throat, hiccups, or an upset stomach. Other possible side effects include excessive salivation and palpitations of the heart. These typically occur during the first 2 or 3 days, and can usually be controlled by slower chewing.

People with extensive dental work may find that the gum sticks to their dentures or bridges. If this occurs, ask your dentist for advice. If you have heart disease or other chronic illness, you should use the gum only under close supervision of a physician.

Don't expect the gum to give you the same "hit" that smoking did. Your goal is to maintain a steady, moderate blood level sufficient to prevent withdrawal symptoms.

You'll soon find the pattern of chewing that works best for you. Most people find six to twelve pieces of gum a day adequate to control the urge to smoke. But in any case, don't chew more than 30 pieces per day.

As the days and weeks pass, you'll find yourself gradually cutting back. After 2 to 3 months, you should find that the amount of gum you are chewing is substantially reduced. You will find the urge to smoke becoming less frequent and less intense. Feel free to chew as frequently as you wish. Most physicians advise that you continue chewing the gum until your urge to smoke is controlled by one or two pieces of gum per day. Almost all smokers who use this method find themselves discontinuing the gum within 6 months.

Nicorette should not be used by pregnant women or by nursing mothers. If you become pregnant while using the gum, see your doctor.

And remember that the gum is only *one part* of your smoking control program.

5. Dealing with Weight Gain

The smokers we spoke with listed fear of weight gain as a major barrier to quitting. Weight gain is also one of the main reasons that people attempting to quit are unsuccessful.

Many of those who quit *do* gain weight. The average weight gain is 5 to 7 pounds. Those who smoke two or more packs a day may experience an even greater gain.

Weight gain after quitting is the result of two factors—an increased sugar craving and a change in the body's appetite setpoint.

To understand the increased sugar craving that quitters experience, we must look at yet another effect of nicotine. Nicotine causes an increased release of glycogen, a stored form of sugar in the liver. Thus each puff produces a quick burst of energy to the brain. This is very pleasurable and helps to increase the smoker's sensation of alertness. After quitting, smokers may feel less alert, and they may attempt to duplicate their accustomed "glycogen fix" by snacking on high sugar junk foods. This can contribute to weight gain.

Messages from your brain keep your weight fairly stable by increasing or decreasing your appetite. Scientists call this mechanism your appetite setpoint. Nicotine seems to be able to re-calibrate the body's setpoint upward.

The good news for quitters is that regular exercise can lower your body's setpoint. Nonsmokers who exercise regularly tend to weigh about the same as smokers. All the more reason to start a regular session of daily exercise before—or immediately after—quitting.

The best strategy for dealing with increased sugar craving seems to be simply not to have high-sugar snacks available. The key to this part of weight control lies in the hand that pushes the shopping cart. In a nutshell, you need to throw all the sweets out of the house and cross them off your shopping list. Good substitutes include carrots, celery, apples, oranges, unbuttered popcorn, unsweetened yogurt, and dry-roasted sunflower seeds and peanuts.

What Nonsmokers Need to Know About Helping Smokers Take Better Care of Themselves

Help nonsmokers by being supportive, not critical and angry. Make it clear that you care for the person and fear that their smoking will do them harm. Here are some messages that smokers say they would find helpful and supportive in their efforts to control their smoking:

"I love you. Please quit smoking."

"I want you to quit smoking because I couldn't stand to lose you. I want you to be around for a long, long time to be my friend."

"I accept your need for a cigarette, but please don't force me to breathe your smoke."

"If you ever want to start a smoking control program, I'll be glad to help in any way you'd like."

"I'll give you 100 dollars (or other sum or gift) if you can stay off cigarettes for 90 days."

"I would be delighted to handle all the organization, food, and festivities for your 'last cigarette' party."

It is clear that at least in some cases tobacco smoke can harm nonsmokers exposed to it. When people are smoking in a room with poor ventilation, for example, the concentration of carbon monoxide can easily reach or exceed the level required to decrease attentiveness and disrupt the thinking processes of nonsmokers. And there is some evidence that passive smoking may result in an increased risk of lung cancer in nonsmokers, but this is still controversial. Any risk to nonsmokers is only a tiny fraction of that faced by smokers themselves.

The best thing nonsmokers can do for friends and family members who smoke is to encourage and support them to take the approaches to smoking control that they, the smokers, think best. Help and encourage them to develop their own plans for smoking control.

Nonsmokers should realize that, given this choice, not all smokers will choose immediate cessation. But nearly all health-concerned smokers will choose to take some steps to reduce their health risks. These steps should be supported and encouraged.

Many will eventually—if not immediately—rid themselves of the habit altogether. And for smokers who are unable to quit, at least for the time being, dose reduction and supplementary pro-health approaches can considerably reduce health risks.

PART VIII THE HOW-TO OF HEALTH CARE

36 **Health Promotion: Your Hospital and You**
Elizabeth Lee, American Hospital Association

37 **A Patient's Rights Primer**
Lori Andrews, J.D.

38 **Medical Tests for Healthy People**
David S. Sobel, M.D.

39 **A Guide to Health Insurance**
Charles B. Inlander, People's Medical Society

40 **Health Risk Appraisals: A Consumer's Guide**
Jonathan Fielding, M.D., and Tracy Rodriguez

36 HEALTH PROMOTION: YOUR HOSPITAL AND YOU

Elizabeth Lee is director of the Center for Health Promotion in Chicago. Established by the American Hospital Association, the Center assists hospitals in developing and implementing patient education, community, and worksite health promotion services.

Consumerism has made a dramatic impact on the health care industry in recent years. Hospitals are now offering new programs designed to help patients avoid hospitalization. We now enjoy HMOs, emergency clinics in shopping centers, wellness programs, and support groups for patients with chronic ailments. How will all this affect us as health care consumers? And what roles will hospitals play in the future? Elizabeth Lee, an advocate of health promotion services, outlines the history of hospital services in the United States and explains how Medicare, economic conditions, and improved health education have forced hospitals to become more resourceful, inventive, and competitive. She also reviews some of the best new programs. ∎

The hospital has always been a place where the sick went to be healed. People in good health usually stayed away, unless they were visiting friends or relatives, seeking care for an emergency, or having babies. It was a place that healthy human beings generally tended to avoid until illness or injury forced them to seek help as patients. Then they would check in, lie back, and wait for physicians, nurses, or other health care professionals to make them well again.

To those who have not been to a hospital in the past several years, their next encounter could come as quite a shock. Not only has the role of the hospital as they knew it changed, but so has the role expected of the patient. In the 1980s, consumerism has made a significant impact on the health care industry, bringing with it the need for a new partnership of care between patients and professionals.

Hospitals are still equipped and staffed to carry out their traditional function as a setting for diagnosis and treatment. Increasingly, however, more of them are offering additional services designed to help people avoid hospitalization in the first place. Responding to recent dramatic changes in the health care environment, hospitals are looking for more efficient ways to both heal the ill and protect the healthy.

In this dual role, hospitals are becoming health care centers in the truest sense of the phrase. Instead of concentrating solely on the treatment of sickness, more hospitals are trying to promote healthier lifestyles, teach patients how to manage their own care more effectively, prepare them and their families to handle more of their recovery time at home, and steer patients with chronic conditions to support groups geared to their needs.

The signs of change are everywhere, even in the settings in which care is provided. No longer is the hospital or the doctor's office the only place where patients can go for treatment. Today, freestanding emergency centers at busy street corners or in shopping centers are treating minor illnesses and injuries 7 days a week. Simple surgical procedures that used to require hospitalization overnight are now being handled in ambulatory centers where patients are admitted

in the morning and released by dinnertime.

For recuperating patients, the disabled, and the frail, the home itself is growing in importance as a setting for health care. According to the U.S. Department of Health and Human Services, almost five million Americans could benefit from the use of some form of health care in the home. Thanks to technological advances and the development of various outpatient services, victims of such conditions as kidney failure no longer need to go into the hospital for the life-sustaining treatment they require.

These changes mean that, whether ill or well, Americans are faced with a broader range of choices and greater responsibilities as health care consumers than they have encountered in the past. As patients, we are going to have to participate more actively in our own care, both within the hospital and afterwards. As consumers, we are going to have to be more aware than ever of the costs and benefits of alternate forms of treatment. And all of use are probably going to have to make some behavioral changes so we can avoid the need for treatment in the first place.

To understand what is happening in hospitals today, it is helpful to examine the way the health care system developed in this country after World War II. During the booming mid-1940s, the federal government launched a number of policies and programs designed to build more hospitals and to upgrade facilities that already existed. A key measure passed in 1946 was the Hill- Burton Act, which made federal funds available for hospital expansion on a massive scale.

As the nation's network of hospitals expanded, so too did the means for more people to take advantage of them. The 1950s brought new tax incentives for employers to provide health insurance for their employees. And they did. Within a single decade, the number of Americans covered by health plans grew from less than 10% to about 70%. When the government enacted the Medicare and Medicaid programs in 1965, virtually all Americans had access to the expanding hospital system.

Growth extended into the 1970s as the federal government continued to fuel the health care boom with funds for professional education and medical research. New medical schools opened and students flocked in, swelling their enrollments in anticipation of physician shortages. Researchers developed increasingly sophisticated—and expensive—medical technology.

As the health care system expanded, so did the nation's investment in health care. In 1950 the nation was spending only about 4% of the gross national product (GNP) on health care—about $12.7 billion. By 1984 that expenditure had grown to more than 10% of the GNP, or some $322 billion. In 1990, that figure is expected to soar to almost $690 billion, keeping health care securely in place as the nation's second-largest industry.

What caused health care costs to skyrocket? Part of the increase came from the double-digit inflation of the 1970s, of course, but the answer is not that simple. One major contributing factor was the fee-for-service arrangement through which private insurance plans and the Medicare and Medicaid programs paid hospitals and physicians for patient care. Under these arrangements, the more time, medicine, and treatment that a patient required, the more that health care providers were paid. This system obviously provided no incentive for providers to be concerned about what was being spent to care for each individual patient. Indeed, the popular and political sentiment that fueled the expansion of the health care system during the postwar years was to provide the best possible care to the greatest numbers of people, without regard to cost.

Another reason was the advent of new technological equipment. The highly sophisticated CAT (computerized axial tomography) scanners used in diagnosis cost up to $1 million apiece, plus another $400,000 a year to operate. Innovative surgical procedures, such as the coronary bypass and kidney transplant, often cost between $18,000 and $25,000 each, and such experimental procedures as liver transplants carried even bigger price tags. Yet these expensive medical marvels became increasingly common.

America's health care system may have been growing bigger and better, but so were the costs of care. By the late 1970s, in a shifting political climate, the health industry's two biggest cus-

tomers—government and business—began looking for ways to slow the rise in costs without damaging the quality of care itself. It was toward that end that the federal government in October 1983 made a dramatic change in the way it paid hospitals to care for the nation's 30 million elderly or disabled Medicare patients.

This new system, known as the prospective pricing system, works this way: the government has categorized patient care into 468 diagnosis-related groups (DRGs) based on the nature of the illness. The price tag on each DRG is an average price based on what it has cost hospitals to treat Medicare patients in the past. Instead of repaying hospitals for the exact costs of treating each individual Medicare patient, the federal government now pays a predetermined amount in relation to the DRG category into which the patient's treatment falls. This means that the treatment for a back injury, for example, carries one standard price, while treatment for diabetes or pneumonia carries another. For any DRG the same amount is paid, whether the patient is in the hospital for 3 days or 30. Hospitals that provide care for less than the established DRG get to keep the difference. Those that do not have to absorb the loss.

The rationale behind this plan is to provide a strong incentive for hospitals to hold down the costs of treating each patient. It is believed that by increasing efficiency, trimming costs per case, and shortening lengths of stay when medically appropriate, the hospital and its medical staff can pare hospital expenses and at the same time help insurers pare theirs. Medicare patients provide hospitals with up to 40% of their revenues. A similar system of payment is currently under consideration for doctors, nursing homes, and other health care providers. It is not unlikely that other insurers will follow the lead of the Medicare and Medicaid programs and redesign the way in which they make payments to hospitals in line with this model.

Other forces have been at work in reaction to rising health care costs. Over the past several years, many businesses have rewritten their employee health policies to encourage the use of alternatives to hospital stays whenever possible. The trend is to emphasize such cost-cutting measures as requiring second opinions before elective surgery and reviewing the need, appropriateness, and efficiency of the medical services, procedures, and facilities being used. A survey of Fortune 500 companies conducted for *Hospitals* magazine in 1985 pinpointed the strategies businesses are considering as cost-cutters. Among the most popular are:

- **Ambulatory Surgery**. More employers are encouraging the use of same-day surgery, where applicable, as an economic alternative to overnight hospitalization. Advances in anesthesia and safer surgical techniques have made it possible for up to 40% of all surgery to take place on an outpatient basis.

- **Outpatient Testing**. Some patients may find it possible to forego hospitalization in favor of a series of outpatient visits during which physicians can study and diagnose their health problems. Even those who are to be hospitalized may find much of what formerly occurred in the hospital now occurring before they are admitted. In a procedure known as preadmission testing, such routine tests as x-rays, blood tests, and urinalyses are often done on an outpatient basis the day before the patient is admitted to the hospital for surgery.

- **Greater Cost-Sharing**. Many people covered by private health plans are being asked to pay greater shares of their doctor and hospital bills. This usually takes the form of a higher co-payment (the percentage of medical bills paid directly out of pocket by the patient) or a higher deductible (the amount a patient must pay before his or her insurance takes effect).

- **Health Maintenance Organizations**. HMOs are medical groups that provide a comprehensive range of health care (anything from office visits to hospitalization) for a prepaid fee. They are currently flourishing and their numbers are expected to surge. Nearly 17 million people belong to an HMO today.

- **Preferred Provider Organizations**. PPOs are groups of physicians and hospitals that contract with insurance companies, unions, or employers to provide health care at nego-

tiated fees. Those enrolled may select an outside provider, but they are given economic incentives such as freedom from co-payments to use "preferred" hospitals and physicians. According to the Fortune 500 survey, the number of companies offering their employees a PPO option rose from 6% in 1983 to 30% in 1985.

As business and government introduced economic incentives such as these into the health care environment, a number of things have begun to happen in hospitals. For starters, the number of hospital admissions has been dropping dramatically. After rising steadily for three decades, admissions began to decline in 1982 and within 2 years had dropped back to what they were in 1978. Moreover, admissions are projected to drop another 10% to 15% by 1995—despite an anticipated increase in the number of elderly patients as the average age of the U.S. population increases.

While the number of admissions has been falling, the length of hospital stays has been shortening. Advanced technology has made it possible to transfer more patient care from hospital beds to other, less expensive settings. Within a year after Congress passed the new prospective payment system, the average length of a Medicare patient's hospital stay had dropped to 9 days—almost a full day less than it was in 1982. By 1985 the average stay had fallen from 7 to 6-1/2 days.

What all of this means to the average hospital patient becomes apparent even before the patient is admitted. To save expensive hospital bed time, patients can expect to have most of their laboratory tests and x-rays done before admission. A surgical patient may not be admitted to the hospital until the morning of surgery, making the patient and family members responsible for presurgery routines, such as adhering to dietary restrictions that formerly were handled by hospital personnel.

Another significant change is often apparent in the days before hospitalization. Because it is likely that a patient will need care after he leaves the hospital, many hospitals are making special efforts to coordinate a plan of care even before the patient is admitted. While this includes preadmission tests, it also is likely to cover the time patients are in the hospital and their needs after they leave. If patients are likely to require special help after they leave, social workers and nurses begin planning this care.

Once in the hospital, the patient's stay is likely to be both shorter and more crowded with activities. Of course, no hospital will discharge a patient without careful medical evaluation and the consent of the patient's physician. In a process known as utilization review, specially trained nurses monitor a patient's hospitalization to help assure that the patient receives the most medically desirable care at the least cost. Still, it is likely that some of the recovery time formerly spent in a hospital bed is likely to occur in another setting, making it doubly important for patients to listen carefully to information provided them and to ask questions so that they can actively participate in their own care after they leave the hospital.

Hospitals have been devising various ways of helping patients deal with these changes. Some hospitals have developed cooperative care units in which patients recovery in more home-like settings and in which friends or relatives can participate in their care. Not only is it less expensive to provide care in these units, but it also provides a learning opportunity for the patient and those who will be assisting the patient at home. While recovering, patients are free to move around and eat in a dining room instead of being restricted to their beds. They also may see their doctors in a central office instead of at the bedside and be responsible for such things as taking their medicines rather than having each dose of medication dispensed to them by a professional. In this way, these units serve as a bridge between the more traditional hospital setting and the home. Pioneered at the New York University Medical Center in 1980, the cooperative care approach has spread to half a dozen cities.

More common are home care programs that provide skilled nursing therapy and health aid services in the patient's residence rather than in the hospital. Less expensive than hospitalization, home care allows patients to recover in a familiar setting among family and friends. Home care

is already the most common alternate service hospitals offer, and the demand for it is expected to increase. There are basically three factors behind this emerging trend:

- **The Availability of New Technology**. Many products and systems have been developed that allow people to get treatment at home that once was available only at a hospital. Such developments as kidney dialysis systems, intravenous nutritional supplements, chemotherapy, and insulin treatments make it possible for patients to be treated at their own residences. To ensure proper care, however, patients or their families require training in the use of the equipment.

- **The Increase of Chronic Diseases**. For the past three decades chronic diseases have been replacing acute illnesses as the principal diagnosis for hospital patients. As Americans live longer, they tend to experience multiple episodes of nonfatal illnesses, which have in the past led to frequent hospitalization. Now, however, adequate care for these illnesses can usually be provided in a less expensive settings, thanks to the technological developments noted above.

- **The Aging of America**.   Americans 65 or older already make up the nation's fastest growing age group, and their number is expected to double to 55 million over the next 50 years. Although this segment of the population presently represents only 11% of the total population, it uses hospital services almost three times as often as any other population group. In addition, illnesses among this age group often are more serious or complicated and therefore take longer to treat and require more nursing services than do those of younger patients.

Patient and family education is the bridge that hospitals use to smooth the transition from hospital bed to other care settings. Within the past several years, such programs have proliferated and increased in sophistication as hospitals have expanded their educational efforts to provide more and better learning opportunities, not only during hospitalization, but before and after as well.

In St. Louis, for example, Barnes Hospital has developed a program that teaches patients with chronic obstructive pulmonary disease (COPD) and their families the skills needed for taking care of that problem at home. Designed to help patients during and after hospitalization, it focuses on the treatment of reversible aspects of the disease and the prevention of complications. Hospital data show a significant drop in length of hospitalization and overall health care costs for 80% of the patients involved in all aspects of the program—classes, home care, and the Barnes Breathing Club, a group of COPD patients who meet regularly for moral support and information sharing.

As part of the trend, many children's hospitals are teaching parents how to care for their youngsters after they go home. For example, parents may stay in their child's room at the University of Chicago Medical Center's Wyler Children's Hospital while their children are hospitalized. This experience is intended to give parents a chance to develop confidence in the use of medical skills they will need at home, such as cardiopulmonary resuscitation or tube feedings, while professional help is still nearby.

Childbirth education programs are also increasingly popular, especially since mothers who used to spend 4 or 5 days in the hospital are now leaving 1 or 2 days after giving birth. To meet this challenge, many hospitals are developing early discharge programs that include follow-up visits by hospital staff members to the mothers at home. Florida Hospital in Orlando has expanded its parenting education program beyond the usual childbirth preparation classes to include information about infant care and interpersonal family relationships. Members of the local La Leche League teach breastfeeding to new mothers, continuing to act as a support group after the mother and child return home. Such efforts are increasing in number.

While the nature of the experience of being a hospital patient is changing dramatically, equally dramatic has been a philosophical shift that is encouraging hospitals to expand their concept of service to include not just the sick, but also the well population of their communities.

All too often in the past, Americans refused to recognize the need to take responsibility for their own well-being. They ate, drank, and smoked too much, exercised too little, then took their diseased bodies to the hospital and expected miracles. Today, recognition of the need for each individual to assume greater responsibility for the state of his or her own health is growing, and hospitals are supporting that recognition by developing a variety of services that go beyond their traditional function of treating disease.

Throughout the country, participants in hospital-sponsored health promotion programs are, among many other things, learning how to read a thermometer, take their own blood pressure, handle depression, lose weight, stop smoking, and overcome the anxieties that led them to indulge too much in the first place. Few and far between as recently as a decade ago, departments specifically designed to provide such health-promoting services to the well population are becoming commonplace in hospitals. St. Vincent Wellness Centers, an affiliate of St. Vincent Hospital and Health Care Center in Indianapolis, typically provides such services to some 10,000 community members a year through an array of programs it offers. The programs are administered through outposts located in three local shopping centers to make them easily accessible to community members. Once unique, this program provides a model that many other hospitals have followed as recognition grows that changes in lifestyle offer the best long-range hope for reducing the incidence of ill health.

In addition to offering such services directly to individuals in their communities, many hospitals are designing health promotion programs that can be offered to groups of employees right at the worksite, where many believe the best opportunity exists for reaching the greatest numbers of people with these health-enhancing activities. Indeed, as the center of health activities in most communities, hospitals are in an excellent position to work closely with local businesses to develop health programs geared to their specific needs. Hospitals have a broad range of resources that few of their competitors can match: health care expertise, personnel, facilities, and services. Generally speaking, programs geared to employers fill the needs for three types of services:

Occupational Health Services. Occupational health programs help businesses meet such tough environmental health standards as the Occupational Safety and Health Act (OSHA) workplace rules. The goal is to help prevent work-related illness or injury and to make it possible for those who do become ill to return to work as soon as possible. Tailored to the needs of the local business community, they can address a broad range of individual problems.

In San Francisco, for example, the Pacific Medical Center has used its many and varied resources to meet all kinds of client needs, both ongoing and those of a one-time nature. City bus drivers have learned how to manage stress on the job and two truck operators—often the first at the scene of a traffic accident—have learned cardiopulmonary resuscitation. When a department store was plagued by a rash of back injuries, the hospital set up a program to teach employees the proper way to lift heavy boxes. To help a local lead battery plant meet OSHA testing standards, a program was set up to ensure that the respirator masks worn by plant employees are regularly checked for defects.

Occupational health services have been around for a long time in the form of annual physical checkups and pre-employment exams, but the demand increased in recent years after the government established OSHA to reduce the estimated 14,000 deaths and millions of disabling injuries that occur annually on the job, costing the nation more than $47 billion a year. Because many employers are too small to afford in-house programs, many hospitals are filling the gap with programs that draw together a variety of resources, making them, in effect, a one-stop shopping center for occupational health services.

Employee Assistance Programs. Frequent absenteeism, reduced effectiveness, deteriorating job performance, and accidents on the job can be symptoms of anything from alcoholism or drug abuse to problems with finances, health, or the family. These programs provide counselors who can teach supervisors how to recognize the problem and guide employees to the appropriate place for confidential care.

The motivation for such programs is strong enough. Statistics show that 10% of all U.S. employees have personal problems serious enough to affect their performance on the job. The resulting absenteeism alone costs American industry an estimated $20 billion a year, not to mention the losses in productivity and quality of work that usually accompany such problems.

Lifestyle Programs. Hospital-based worksite health promotion programs are typically designed to help employees assume responsibility for their own well-being and to provide them with the tools they need to change bad health habits. Participants typically can find assistance and encouragement through these programs to exercise more, maintain appropriate weight, stop smoking, and manage stress better. Such changes, experts say, could help to reduce seven of the ten leading causes of death among Americans today.

They could also go along way toward improving the *quality* of a person's life. Not only do they promise to help reduce the cost of health care and add years to life, but they can also add a lot of enjoyment. In Newport News, VA, for example, the Riverside Hospital has developed the Peninsula Wellness and Fitness Center. The center is backed by the professional expertise of an exercise physiologist, a nutritionist, a registered nurse, two clinical psychologists, and four physicians. The center itself, located four miles from the hospital, provides some 70,000 square feet of space where 3400 members share the use of nine indoor and outdoor tennis courts, eight racquetball courts, an indoor swimming pool, basketball and volleyball courts, running tracks, a general exercise area, 28 Nautilus strength-training machines, stationary bicycles, rowing machines, treadmills, saunas, and whirlpool tubs. Membership is open to both corporations and individuals. As attractive as the most plush and expensive health club, the hospital-affiliated fitness center offers the bonus to its clients of scientifically sound programming planned and supervised by professionals who meet the hospital's high medical standards.

The Peninsula Wellness and Fitness Center is just one of more than 250 such hospital-affiliated fitness facilities in the U.S., and their numbers are growing. But that figure does not begin to indicate the magnitude of the trend toward the development of health promotion programs in hospitals. A 1984 American Hospital Association Center for Health Promotion survey indicated that among 3578 hospitals that responded to the survey, almost 85% were providing health promotion services in an organized form to patients and community members. Of these, almost 2400 indicated that they provided such services directly to community members, and 1200 offered them through businesses. In addition, 2500 had organized programs for another important segment of the well population—their own employees.

Smaller hospitals are also getting into the act. In northern Wisconsin, for example, the Eagle River Memorial Hospital, which has only 41 beds, serves a three-county rural community with a variety of programs ranging from health improvement to cardiac rehabilitation. Operating out of borrowed gymnasiums, classrooms, and community halls, the hospital sponsors workshops in healthy living, exercise classes, stop-smoking clinics, and courses in nutrition and stress management.

Some hospitals are going even further to address the root causes of ill health. One, Brooklyn's Lutheran Medical Center, has directed its health-promotion efforts at the illnesses of poverty and blight in its inner city neighborhood. Forging coalitions with community groups, the hospital operates on the principle that the health of the individual often reflects the health of the community. To care for both, the medical center works with its neighbors to do such things as upgrade housing, improve garbage collection, and increase police protection.

The hospital of today has become much more than a refuge for the sick. Whether it is serving the community, protecting employees' health at the worksite, or helping patients bridge the gap between the hospital bed and recovery or continued care at home, the hospital has become an important partner in the health of the nation. The other partner is you. By taking responsibility for our own health, by both understanding what causes medical problems and being willing to change the behavior that causes them, each of us can help lower the cost of health care and increase the richness of life.

37

A PATIENT'S RIGHTS PRIMER

Lori Andrews, J.D., a Yale Law School graduate, is a project director in medical law at the American Bar Foundation. She has testified in Congress on medical legal issues, and she has advised state legislators, the Department of Health and Human Services, the Office of Technology Assessment of the U.S. Congress, the Centers for Disease Control, the World Health Organization, and the Institute of Medicine of the National Academy of Sciences. She is the author of *New Conceptions: A Consumer's Guide to the Newest Infertility Treatments* (Ballantine, 1985).

As people have become more involved with their own health care, they have grown increasingly aware of their legal rights as patients. The informed health care consumer is better able to choose a physician, hospital, or procedure. And although hospitals and physicians have frequently required patients to sign waiver agreements agreeing not to sue as a result of treatment, this has rarely been upheld as valid in the court system. As attorney Lori Andrews points out, patients have many legal rights, but it is each individual's responsibility to ensure that they are enforced. Unfortunately, when a person is ill, it is difficult to discuss legalities. It is critical, therefore, that the healthy work to ensure the rights of every patient.■

People have begun to take more control over their health, paying attention to nutrition and fitness, recognizing the influence of lifestyle and the environment on health, and actively seeking the most appropriate practitioner and procedure for what ails them. Individuals exercise their bodies to keep them fit, but they seldom realize the effect of exercising their legal rights on protecting their health as well.

Consequently, the legal rights of health care consumers are getting flabby. Existing rights, such as the all-important right to informed consent, are so seldomly exercised that they are now flagrantly disregarded. Lack of exercise has also impeded the expansion of health care rights to parallel the expansion of consumer control of and interest in health.

The law can be used to gain access to information necessary for health promotion, to make choices among practitioners, institutions, or procedures, or to seek recompense for health care errors. Exercising these rights can help improve the quality of information and care received. For those reasons, it is important to explore what health care rights exist and how they might be enhanced to meet today's health needs.

THE CHOICE OF PRACTITIONER

There are at least 125 different types of health care practitioners as well as a panoply of other types of individuals—from aerobics instructors and vitamin dealers to mutual aid group members—who contribute to health promotion and disease care. In recent years, health care consumers by case law and statute have gained rights to consult an increasing variety of health care purveyors.

A 3-year study by the California Board of Medical Quality Assurance found that "consumers are becoming wiser about health care, and more critical in their choices of practitioners." The study attributed the increased popularity of alternative practitioners to people's dissatisfaction with doctors' invasive and sometimes hazardous techniques, peoples' preference for health care methods emphasizing the body's innate healing abilities, and their desire for a relationship with a health care provider in which they could take a more active role.

Consequently, statutes that give physicians a monopoly on the provision of health care services are coming under fire. All states have medical practice acts that allow only licensed physicians to provide health care in any form—from offering health care advice to diagnosing or treating a person's mental or physical condition. Yet it is questionable whether physicians should have a monopoly in fields such as health promotion, since they are not adequately trained to advise people about nutrition or lifestyle threats to health. Even in areas of traditional medical care, empirical research has demonstrated that between 75% and 80% of adult primary care and 90% of pediatric primary care services could safely be delegated to alternative health professionals. Not only have nonphysician health care providers (such as nurse practitioners) fared well on such assessments of quality, they offer savings as well. One study estimated that if alternative practitioners provided the readily delegable portions of adult and pediatric primary care, the cost savings would range from one half billion to one billion dollars, slashing 19% to 49% of the total primary care provider costs.

In one Texas court case, people wanted access to acupuncturists. But the medical practice act gave licensed doctors a monopoly on the provision of treatment so only doctors could perform acupuncture. This meant that people trained and experienced in acupuncture could not offer it because they had no medical license. Licensed medical doctors could perform acupuncture under the law, but they had no training in it and very few offered the procedure. The court held that the medical licensing requirement was an unconstitutional infringement on the consumer's right to make health care decisions, and it granted people the right to consult acupuncturists.

Another challenge to the physician monopoly occurred in a suit against Blue Shield of Virginia, in which the insurance company refused to pay psychotherapist's fees unless the services were billed through a physician. Blue Shield argued that the rule was necessary to prevent needless psychotherapy when the health problems had a physical basis. The court, however, ruled against the restriction, finding it did not in fact fulfill that goal, since the Blue Shield policy allowed the service to be billed through any physician, not just those who regularly treat mental and nervous disorders. The U.S. Supreme Court in June 1982, considering another case based on the same insurance provisions, said that consumers have a right to bring suit against the insurer when they are forced by the insurance plan to consult a physician before getting access to a psychotherapist. Such cases may help lead to insurance reimbursement for a wider variety of nonphysician practitioners.

A case for access to nonphysician practitioners has been made in state legislatures as well. Some states have established Holistic Health Boards to license holistic practitioners as alternatives to traditional doctors. Over the past decade, at least 45 of the 50 states amended their nursing practice acts to expand the role nurses could play in diagnosis and treatment. Fifteen states enacted some form of direct reimbursement for nurses. Similarly, physician assistant laws have been passed in at least 43 states.

The predicted oversupply of physicians, however, is leading organized medicine to lobby against legal recognition of nonphysician practitioners. So, unless people continue to press for the right to consult nonphysician practitioners, that right might be curtailed.

THE CHOICE OF A PROCEDURE

The most important legal protection of patients is the doctrine of informed consent. A physician must provide sufficient information to a patient so that he or she can make a knowledgeable decision whether or not to proceed with a proposed procedure. The idea that competent adult patients should have a right to decide what is to be done to their bodies is firmly grounded in the case law. These judicial and legislative precedents generally establish that the physician must tell the patient the nature of the condition, the risks and benefits of proposed diagnostic procedures or treatments, and the availability, risks, and benefits of alternatives. In addition, the court in at least one case has found that physicians should inform patients of the risk of not undertaking a medical procedure. The Supreme Court of California held that a physician could be found liable for not informing a woman that failure to undergo a Pap smear might prevent cancer detection.

Furthermore, patients have the right to know how they are progressing. In one case, a physician failed to inform the patient that the prescribed treatment was not working. The court held that the physician had a duty to monitor the treatment, to inform the patient at the earliest possible time that a given treatment method was not working, and to advise the patient as to other treatment possibilities.

Informed consent not only protects an individual's freedom to make health care decisions; according to empirical studies, the provision of information can provide a physical and psychological benefit to the patient. Patients who receive information about the nature of a proposed diagnostic or treatment procedure more readily adjust to the stress of the procedure, need fewer pain killers afterward, and have a quicker recovery period. This has lead psychologist Irving Janis to describe disclosure in terms of an "emotional inoculation" that prevents the patient from being overwhelmed by the threatening events and sensations accompanying a medical procedure.

Despite its potential benefits, true informed consent is rarely encountered in practice. People are less satisfied with the information given to them by physicians than with any other aspect of health care. An observational study carried out for the President's Commission for the Study of Ethical Problems in Medicine and Biomedical and Behavioral Research found "that it was common in the hospitals studied for physicians to fail to inform patients about the nature, purpose, and risks of planned procedures in a way that would enable them to make meaningful decisions."

Informed consent is a right that has been weakened because patients don't exercise it. Whenever a patient's physician advocates a procedure, he or she should ask the following questions to protect that right: What does the procedure entail? What is my prognosis with or without it? What alternatives are available?

Answers to these questions can help combat the medical tendency to intercede even when a disease may run its course without the intervention. It can also help the patient to reject a procedure that is being advocated more for the benefit of the practitioner than the patient. By being required to provide information about alternatives, the physician will be forced to keep up with the literature and will be less able to foist upon the patient a particular specialty bias (e.g., the tendency for surgeons to recommend surgery for a particular disorder, while internists recommend medication for the same condition).

Particular abuses in the informed consent area have led to specialized legislation. For example, many women with breast cancer were advised by their physicians to undergo a radical mastectomy without being told of the availability of an equally effective alternative, the partial mastectomy. In other instances, the woman would consent to a breast biopsy only to wake up with her entire breast removed. Situations such as these led to state legislation such as a law in California that requires doctors to inform breast cancer patients in writing of the alternative treatment techniques. (Note that the patient's general informed consent right *already* requires physicians to inform patients about treatment alternatives. But apparently so few physicians do so—and so few patients ask for that information—that special legislation was necessary.) In New Jersey, a law was enacted requiring a doctor to obtain written consent from a woman on a form that allows her to choose whether she consents solely for a biopsy or for a biopsy and, if it seems necessary in the eyes of the physician, surgery as well.

THE CHOICE OF A HOSPITAL

Your choice of a practitioner or a preventive, diagnostic, or treatment procedure is limited by a lack of information and the law's tendency to grant a monopoly to standard medical practitioners and procedures. But your choice of a hospital is even more limited. Generally consumers cannot contract directly with hospitals but rather must go where their physician has admitting privileges.

Even if your physician has admitting privileges at several hospitals, you may not know how to choose among these institutions. The most vital information is shielded from view. It is difficult to learn the infection rate at a given hospital, the Caesarean section or hysterectomy rate, or the cost of particular procedures in comparison to other hospitals. Although hospital pathology departments assess whether supposedly diseased tissues and organs removed during surgery are actually diseased (thus giving an idea whether a particular doctor is fraudulently or incompetently undertaking unnecessary surgery), those reports are not available to people wishing to make a choice regarding hospitals or doctors.

There are two tactics for getting such vital information. The first is to lobby for passage of a law requiring hospitals to publish this data. Compliance with such a law will not require much additional effort on the part of the institution since such information is already collected for internal review purposes or for filing with the state.

Alternatively, consumer groups could demand such information from hospitals. With declining admission rates, hospitals are now competing for patients. They are beginning to advertise no-wait emergency rooms, limo service, or birthing rooms as a way to lure patients. If it were clear that patients wanted information about infection rates, surgery rates, prices, and so forth, hospitals with good track records in these areas might begin to advertise them, forcing other hospitals to follow suit. As a first step for consumers to demonstrate their desire for such information, HMOs should require such disclosures from participating hospitals. Medicare and Medicaid contracts should not be awarded without such disclosures.

EMERGENCY CARE

Sometimes a patient is in no condition to choose a hospital. When an emergency exists, he or she may be taken to the nearest facility. In fact, twice as many patients are handled in emergency rooms as are admitted to hospitals each year. A hospital with an emergency room must see all emergency patients and must do so within a reasonable amount of time. Before an emergency patient can be transferred to another institution, he or she must receive adequate treatment and the condition must be stabilized. An emergency patient must be given care even if he or she cannot produce evidence of the ability to pay. In one New York court case, for example, an emergency room nurse turned away a heart attack victim because he couldn't demonstrate that he had the proper health insurance. The hospital was held liable.

IN-PATIENT CARE

Many hospital patients feel that their dignity, privacy, and sense of control are stripped away along with their street clothes when they enter a hospital. This need not be the case, however, since patients possess an arsenal of legal rights while in the hospital.

A hospital patient has the legal right to refuse to be examined or treated by any doctor or student. In one case affirming that right, a pregnant woman about to give birth refused to be examined by a medical student. Nevertheless, after a doctor performed a rectal and vaginal examination on her, 10 or 12 men who were apparently students each performed the same examination two or three times on her. "Whenever I screamed and protested they just laughed, told me to shut up," she testified. The court held the hospital liable.

In a teaching hospital, a barrage of physicians, residents, interns, medical students, and consultants are paraded through patient's rooms. New York lawyer Morris Abram, chairman of the President's Commission for the Study of Ethical Problems in Medicine and Biomedical and Behavioral Research, was hospitalized with cancer. The endless stream of doctors—often asking repetitious questions—wore him out. He finally designated one doctor as the only one he would talk to and he had her coordinate all his care.

A patient also has the right of informed consent to know his or her condition and to know what types of tests and procedures are scheduled. The patient may refuse any test or procedure. It makes sense to ask for the informed consent form before entering the hospital in order to have time to read it closely at home. When patients scheduled

for radiation treatment at a cancer center were allowed to take their consent forms home before surgery, they demonstrated a greater understanding of the nature and risk of the proposed procedure.

In one case, a neurosurgeon suggested that one of his female patients have a nerve operation. Rather than getting her consent while she was at his office, he admitted her to the hospital where a foreign-born resident explained the procedure and obtained her signature on the consent form. The surgery proceeded badly, necessitating a second attempt. The woman sued, claiming that she hadn't comprehended what she was agreeing to because she didn't understand the resident's accent and the hospital was no place to reflect on the information that was presented. The jury voted her a $15,000 award.

Information is not generally accorded the patient in the hospital, even though it is within his or her clear legal rights. For that reason, the patient will have to ask for information. Some patients wonder whether the blanket consent form they sign when they enter the hospital deprives them of the right to question and veto a procedure later on. Although hospital personnel try to convince patients that this form has great weight, courts have held it to be merely a consent to routine procedures (such as blood tests). Each time an additional diagnostic or treatment procedure is undertaken, informed consent is required. The patient should be told the benefits and risks of the proposed procedure and its alternatives, and should be asked to sign a specific consent form about that procedure. Even if he or she has signed either a broad or specific consent form, the patient can revoke the consent at any time before the procedure is performed.

The patient's right to refuse treatment allows the patient to turn down even life-saving treatment. The hospital cannot abandon a patient just because he or she refuses a particular surgery, for example, but rather, according to Boston University health law professor George Annas, the hospital is "legally obligated to continue to render the best medical care possible within the limitations imposed by the patient's refusal."

The terminally ill patient has a right to a death with dignity. At least 13 states and the District of Columbia have natural death acts or living will statutes which allow people to record in advance that they do not wish to have their dying extended by technological means. Of course, patients can change their minds and request extraordinary treatment later on if they so desire.

In order to discharge a patient, a hospital must have a written order of a physician who is familiar with the patient's case. On the other hand, patients have a right to leave the hospital at any time, even against doctors' orders and even without paying the bill. Hospital staff members are liable for false imprisonment if they use threats of harm to keep a patient against his or her will. In one case, a court held that a woman who was kept in the hospital 11 hours for not paying her bill could sue for false imprisonment.

MEDICAL RECORDS

An important check on the quality of your health care is to look at your medical record. In a majority of states, patients have a right to see their medical records. Patients should ask to see the ongoing hospital record to keep abreast of what tests are ordered and to see that their symptoms are correctly recorded in the charts. When a patient undergoes surgery and is discharged from the hospital, he or she should request the subsequent pathology report. If enough patients do this, unnecessary surgery rates will fall since doctors will be aware of the consumer check on their recommendations.

Information about a patient that health care personnel receive in the course of caring for that patient is confidential. Except in rare instances where disclosure is required by the state (such as in the case of venereal disease reporting), the patient can sue the practitioner if private information is disclosed to a third party, such as the patient's employer, relatives, or spouse.

ABANDONMENT

Once a doctor-patient relationship is established, the doctor cannot abandon the patient unless the patient consents to termination of the relationship

or the doctor withdraws after assuring that the patient has a reasonable opportunity to receive care elsewhere. Similarly, hospitals are liable for wrongful discharge of a patient if he or she is sent home prematurely.

Unless specifically terminated, the doctor-patient relationship can be viewed as extending indefinitely. Recent cases have held that a doctor's duty to his or her patient continues even if years pass without the patient consulting the doctor. For example, a physician who inserted an IUD in a woman has been held to have a responsibility to recontact that woman years later to warn her of the dangers of the IUD.

REDRESSING GRIEVANCES

If your legal rights are being ignored, you are unsatisfied with your care, or you are the victim of malpractice, there are several options. If you are in the hospital and your physician is not answering your questions, contact the chief of service (the head physician for that particular specialty area of the hospital), the chief of staff (the head physician for the entire hospital), or the hospital administrator (the chief executive of the hospital).

Another alternative is to register your complaint with the state disciplinary board. Every state has laws forbidding physicians to engage in unprofessional conduct. If the physician does not meet those standards, he or she can be subjected to disciplinary board action, such as the suspension or revocation of his or her medical license, payment of a fine, or a requirement that he or she take extra courses or practice under the supervision of another physician.

Laws vary from state to state in what is considered to be unprofessional conduct. In 37 states, incapacity, incompetence, or failure to conform to a minimum standard of care is prohibited. In 19 states, betrayal of confidential patient information is prohibited. In 13 states, failure to maintain records is a grounds for discipline. In 11 states, abandonment is prohibited. In 33 states, it is considered unprofessional conduct for a physician to make untrue, improbable, or fraudulent statements.

A patient who receives negligent treatment

from a health care practitioner also has the option of bringing a malpractice suit. To prevail in such litigation, the patient must prove that the practitioner did not live up the prevailing standard of care and that the negligence caused the patient harm.

Hospitals and physicians, cognizant of the possibility of lawsuits, have often required patients to agree not to sue as a condition of treatment. In some cases, such release clauses have even purported to make the hospital and physicians immune from suit for falling below the standard of care all physicians must adhere to—that is, for their own negligence. Courts have either held such releases to be invalid or have construed them strictly.

In one leading case, the California Supreme Court held that when the hospital or physician provides needed services, exercises a decisive bargaining advantage over the patient, and provides no choice for the purchaser to obtain protection against negligence, such release clauses are invalid. Though that case involved a clause protecting a charitable hospital from suits for its own negligence, its logic has been applied in cases covering a wide variety of exculpatory clauses.

During the 1970s, lobbyists for the medical profession were successful in getting statutes passed to limit patients' rights to bring suits and collect damages for negligence. These laws included shortened statutes of limitations (giving patients less time to bring suits charging medical malpractice), requirements for pretrial screening panels to assess the validity of patients' claims, provisions for binding arbitration, limits on attorneys' fees, limits on damage awards, and provisions permitting the periodic payment of damage awards rather than the traditional lump sum award.

Although the restraints on patients' rights in the medical malpractice area have been declared unconstitutional in some states, they have been upheld in other states. The medical profession is again claiming that there is a medical malpractice crisis and alleging that laws should be enacted to further limit patients' rights to sue. To assure that consumers continue to have rights to litigate malpractice claims and to be compensated for negligence, it may be necessary to confront legislators with the consumer viewpoint.

Patients have a variety of legal rights. However, these rights are not self-enforcing; they require initiative on the patient's part. Because patients may be alone, unsure, vulnerable, unaware of their rights, or overwhelmed by the expertise or authority of physicians or hospitals, these rights are often not enforced. Furthermore, the medical profession's lobbyists have done much in recent years to persuade legislatures to limit these rights. Unless individuals both healthy and ill continue to work toward keeping those rights, health care rights may themselves be on the critical list.

38 MEDICAL TESTS FOR HEALTHY PEOPLE

David S. Sobel, M.D., M.P.H., is director of patient education and health promotion for Kaiser Permanente Medical Care Program in Northern California and chief of preventive medicine at the Kaiser Permanente Medical Offices in San Jose. He is a contributing editor to *Medical Self-Care* and a recipient of awards from the American Heart Association and the American Film Festival. He is co–author (with Tom Ferguson, M.D.) of *The People's Book of Medical Tests* and of *The Healing Brain*.

When we're sick, we usually agree to any medical tests that our physician recommends. We will agree to any procedure that will help us to recover. But when we're healthy, a different approach seems warranted. Most of us know very little about the tests prescribed for us, including their purpose, their level of accuracy, and possible side effects. Yet most of us are subjected to medical tests throughout our lives, and tests are usually costly. Dr. David Sobel describes basic medical tests that are administered to healthy people, answers some important questions, and lists criteria by which we can decide whether or not to undergo such testing. ▪

Adapted from The People's Book of Medical Tests by David S. Sobel and Tom Ferguson, New York: Summit Books, 1985.

Each year patients faithfully flock to their doctors for their annual physical exam and testing. They are questioned, tapped, probed, bled, and x-rayed, all in the name of health. But is all this testing really necessary? If you are generally healthy and without symptoms, should you undergo medical testing, and, if so, which tests should you have? In order to answer such questions, you need to understand the uses and limits of medical tests.

Medical tests are performed for several reasons. If you have symptoms, tests can help evaluate these symptoms and diagnose disease. If you have a known disease, tests can be used to follow the progress of treatment and management. And finally, even if you don't have symptoms or a known disease, medical tests can be used to screen for hidden disease.

At first glance, it may seem like a great idea to undergo batteries of screening tests on a periodic basis. Then diseases can be detected even before the symptoms develop and you can be treated at an earlier, more curable stage in the disease. On this basis doctors and patients alike tend to assume that if a few tests are good, more must be better. Unfortunately, very few screening tests have been shown to be of benefit. In fact, screening tests can actually do harm.

FALSE POSITIVES: WHEN "ABNORMAL" DOES NOT MEAN "DISEASE"

There is a significant problem with false positive test results, that is, "abnormal" results in a healthy person. When confronted with an abnormal test result, the natural tendency is to assume that you are sick. However, this is often not the case.

First of all, the abnormality may be a statistical fluke. Due to the way normal values for tests are determined, a certain percentage of healthy people will automatically have abnormal results. For example, the "normal" or reference values for many blood and urine tests are established by testing healthy volunteers, often young laboratory workers, medical students, or blood donors. The "normal" range of values is then constructed to include 95% of those "healthy" people. However, this means that 5% (one in 20) of all healthy peo-

ple will have abnormal values on any given lab test. So, if you perform 12 separate tests, you stand about a 50% chance of having an "abnormal" result—even though you are perfectly healthy.

Furthermore, the range of normal values used may not be appropriate for you. Since these reference values are usually set up by testing young, white, healthy volunteers, the results may not apply if you are older, of a different race, obese, or different in some other significant way from the reference population. Your "abnormal" results may, therefore, mean that you are different from the norms but not necessarily diseased.

False positive results may also be due to other factors that can influence lab test results, such as the use of certain drugs or medications, exercise, stress, meals, time of day, or improper handling of the lab specimen. Even in the best-managed laboratories, 2% to 5% of results may be in error due to variation in the test reagents or clerical errors such as mislabeling the test specimens.

False positive test results can be harmful. They can cause unnecessary anxiety and concern. They can result in mislabeling someone as being diseased when in fact he is healthy. Sometimes repeat or further testing is necessary to sort a true positive from a false positive, and this can be costly, inconvenient, and at times involve riskier tests.

FALSE NEGATIVES: WHEN "NORMAL" DOES NOT MEAN "HEALTHY"

Screening tests can also cause problems when they fail to detect abnormalities that are in fact present. The test may read normal, but the patient is sick. Sometimes the test is just not sensitive enough to detect the abnormality.

Many tests require subjective interpretation and are therefore more likely to miss important abnormalities. For example, in a study of the reading of chest x-rays, over 70% of reports contained disagreements among experienced radiologists. In 25% of the reports, important findings were missed. Other researchers have found that radiologists failed to spot 20% to 50% of lung cancers visible on chest x-rays.

False negative results can be harmful when

important diseases are missed. But they can also be harmful when "normal" results falsely reassure a patient. For example, a chest x-ray is not a very sensitive test for detecting early lung cancers or lung damage due to cigarette smoking. Therefore a great disservice is being committed when a smoker is reassured by a "normal" chest x-ray and continues to smoke.

Finally, normal usually means average—that is, you will be compared with average values characteristic of the population. However, normal in this sense does not necessarily mean optimal, healthy, or desirable. For example, you might have a normal (average) blood pressure or cholesterol level, but lower levels may actually be healthier. As one observer commented, "It is 'normal' to die of heart disease in the United States."

For these and other reasons, it is important to carefully select only those screening tests that might be useful for you. To help you know better which tests to have, consider the following questions:

1. **Is the disease or condition being tested for an important health problem?** It doesn't make much sense to screen for a trivial health problem. You should be more interested in tests that detect conditions significantly influencing the quality and quantity of your life. So a screening test for discerning pitch is unlikely to be of much benefit (unless you are a musician), while one for cancer or heart disease is more promising.

2. **Are you at significant risk for the disease or condition being tested for?** Many diseases occur primarily either in men or in women, in certain ethnic groups, or at certain ages. If you are not at increased risk due to your age, sex, or medical history, then the proposed test is unlikely to benefit you. For example, colon cancer tends to occur in people over the age of 45 or 50, so in younger people there is little reason to screen for the disease unless special risk factors (such as family history of polyps or colon cancer) make the disease more likely.

3. **Can the proposed screening test detect the disease or condition before symptoms alert you that something is wrong?** Most diseases announce their presence with characteristic symptoms which, when evaluated, can lead to a diagnosis. For some diseases, however, waiting for symptoms to develop can mean that the disease will spread and perhaps become incurable. For example, early diagnosis of cervical cancer is very desirable, since a Pap smear can detect the cancer when it is most easily cured, before symptoms appear. On the other hand, you don't really need a screening test for appendicitis, since the condition is usually announced promptly by the symptom of abdominal pain.

4. **Do early diagnosis and treatment favorably alter the progress of the disease?** It makes little sense to screen for a disease for which there is no effective treatment. However, even if an effective treatment is available and acceptable, it must be shown to be more effective when applied in the stage before symptoms develop. For example, if an incurable lung cancer is discovered 6 months before symptoms would have announced its presence, the person doesn't actually survive any longer as a result of early diagnosis and treatment. The test merely informs the person of the cancer 6 months earlier. The result is that the person lives 6 months longer knowing that he or she has an *incurable* disease, but actual survival is not enhanced by the screening effort. Similarly, the laboratory diagnosis of arthritis before symptoms develop is not useful, since available treatments are not any more effective when started in the early stages of the disease. Fortunately, there are a few diseases, such as high blood pressure, breast cancer, and colon cancer, for which early diagnosis and treatment do make a difference.

5. **Is the proposed screening test reasonably accurate, acceptable, and inexpensive?** One

of the greatest stumbling blocks to effective screening programs is the lack of accuracy of the tests. If a test is not sensitive enough to identify the people with the disease in question, then many diseased people will be missed (false negatives). On the other hand, if the test is positive in many healthy people (false positives), mistaken diagnoses may occur and further testing is usually required to sort this out. Unfortunately, no test is 100% accurate, so we must choose the best available.

The proposed test must also be acceptably comfortable and safe. While examination of the colon with a long, flexible viewing instrument (colonoscope) may be the most effective way to detect early colon cancer, it is unlikely that this would be acceptable as a routine screening test for healthy people because of the discomfort, risk, and expense.

The expense of even low-cost tests can mount rapidly. The cost of a screening program also includes the cost of follow-up investigations of those who demonstrate positive results on screening. Since medical resources are not unlimited, it is generally agreed that screening tests should be shown to offer significant savings in terms of prolonged life or decreased suffering to justify the effort. Otherwise, health resources would be better spent elsewhere.

In summary, for a screening test to be worthwhile, it must reliably detect a significant disease before symptoms develop; the treatment must be more effective when begun before symptoms arise; and the detection and treatment must be accomplished at an acceptable risk and cost. Very few tests currently meet these requirements.

So back to the original question: which tests should generally healthy people have and how often should they have them? Nearly everything you read and every doctor you ask will give you a different opinion. Some say you should have regular electrocardiograms (EKGs), others disagree. Some argue for many blood tests, others shun them. While many experts may agree on the value of a certain test, they may disagree on who should

have it or how often. In truth, we often lack the kind of controlled scientific data that would allow us to know with much certainty which tests should be performed.

Despite these limitations, I can offer some rough guidelines in the chart that follows to help you select which medical test to have and approximately how often they should be performed. These recommendations are intended for generally healthy adults. They are based for the most part on several large studies and reviews by panels of medical experts. You will notice that instead of recommending the same tests for everyone, there is an attempt to individualize the tests to some degree, depending upon age and sex. Some of the recommended tests have not been shown definitively to meet the most stringent requirements for effective screening tests, and yet they are included because it seems likely that their benefits outweigh their risks. (See table 38-1.)

These guidelines represent the minimum tests recommended for people *without symptoms*. If you have symptoms or are at increased risk for certain conditions due to your medical or family history, additional tests may be advisable. Use these guidelines as a starting point, and discuss your particular needs with your doctor.

Remember:

- Don't have tests you don't need.
- If you have an abnormal result, don't panic. Many times retesting, reinterpretation, further testing, or a second opinion will "cure" the "disease" and prove that you are healthy. No test is 100% accurate. In interpreting any test result it is important to remember that medical tests are only one part of the picture and often not the most important part. Your tests must always be viewed in the context of other information available about you: your past medical history, family history, age, sex, habits, use of medications, symptoms and previous test results, and the results of physical examinations.
- If you have a normal test result, still remain on the alert for signs or symptoms that may suggest disease. Although carefully selected

TABLE 38-1.
MEDICAL TESTS FOR HEALTHY PEOPLE

Test and Conditions	Age 18–39	Age 40–49	Age 50–59	Age 60–69	Age 70 +
HISTORY AND PHYSICAL EXAMS For various disorders and risks	Every 5–10 years	Every 3–5 years	Every 2–3 years	Every 2–3 years	Every 2–3 years
BLOOD PRESSURE MEASUREMENT For hypertension	Every 2–3 years	Every 2–3 years	Every 2–3 years	Every 2–3 years	Every 2–3 years
VISION TEST For vision problems	Every 5 years Every 2–3 years if correction lenses worn	Every 5 years Every 2–3 years if corrective lenses worn	Every 5 years Every 2–3 years if corrective lenses worn	Every 5 years Every 2–3 years if corrective lenses worn	Every 5 years Every 2–3 years if corrective lenses worn
TUBERCULIN SKIN TEST (PPD) For tuberculosis	Every 5 years until age 35 or every 1–2 years if high risk				
URINALYSIS For kidney and urinary tract disease, liver disease, diabetes, metabolic disorders	Every 10 years	Every 5–10 years	Every 5–10 years	Every 5–10 years	Every 5 years
HEMATOCRIT For anemia	Every 3–5 years (women) Every 10 years (men)	Every 3–5 years (women) Every 5–10 years (men)	Every 5–10 years Every 5–10 years	Every 5–10 years	Every 5 years
BLOOD GLUCOSE For diabetes	Every 10 years	Every 5–10 years	Every 5–10 years	Every 5–10 years	Every 5 years
CHOLESTEROL For heart disease risk	Every 5–10 years	Every 5–10 years	Every 5–10 years	Every 5–10 years	
GLAUCOMA TEST (TONOMETRY) For glaucoma		Every 3 years	Every 3 years	Every 3 years	Every 3 years

(Table 38-1. Cont'd)

Test and Conditions	Age 18–39	Age 40–49	Age 50–59	Age 60–69	Age 70+
HEARING TEST For hearing impairment			Every 3–5 years	Every 3–5 years	Every 3–5 years
TEST FOR HIDDEN BLOOD IN THE STOOL For bowel cancer			Every year	Every year	Every year
SIGMOIDOSCOPY For bowel cancer			Every 5 years	Every 5 years	Every 5 years
For men add: **TESTICULAR SELF-EXAM** For testicular cancer	Monthly				
For women add: **PAP SMEAR** For cervical cancer	Every 3 years after 2 normal yearly exams	Every 3 years after 2 normal yearly exams	Every 3 years	Every 3 years	Every 3 years
BREAST SELF-EXAM For breast cancer	Monthly	Monthly	Monthly	Monthly	Monthly
BREAST EXAM BY DOCTOR For breast cancer	Every 2–3 years	Every 1–2 years	Every 1–2 years	Every 1–2 years	Every 1–2 years
MAMMOGRAPHY For breast cancer	Once between the ages of 35–39	Every 1–2 years	Every 1–2 years	Every 1–2 years	Every 1–2 years
RUBELLA ANTIBODY TITER For immunity to German measles	Once				

screening tests can help you protect your health, remember that the most important factors that determine your health do not show up on medical tests at all. In truth, choosing not to smoke, drinking alcohol moderately or not at all, wearing seat belts, exercising regularly, eating wisely, and managing stress effectively will do more to protect and promote your health than all the tests in the world.

39 A GUIDE TO HEALTH INSURANCE

Charles B. Inlander is the president of The People's Medical Society, the largest consumer health organization in the United States. He also is a lecturer at the Yale School of Medicine and a contributing editor to *Medical Self-Care*. Mr. Inlander is co-author (with Ed Weiner) of *Take This Book to the Hospital with You* (Rodale Press, 1985), and *Medical Mistakes: How Not To Be One* (Rodale Press, 1987). He frequently appears on television talk shows.

For a long time, critics of medical care, whether constructive or not, were either radical physicians, social analysts, or lonely victims of medical malfeasance. The formation of The People's Medical Society a few years ago changed all that. Now the lonely voices have an advocate. Charles Inlander describes the pioneering work done by the Society in a wide range of health policy issues, then focuses on the confusing area of health insurance. He explains for the average consumer the purpose of health insurance, its values, and its limitations. This article offers a wealth of cogent information from an organization independent of the health insurance industry.∎

Recently, the U.S. Department of Health and Human Services released a study indicating that one out of four Americans under the age of 65 has no health insurance coverage at least part of the year or has a private health insurance policy that fails to cover major health costs.

While the study concentrates on those under 65 years of age, the problem of inadequate health insurance coverage has had a dramatic impact on America's over-65 population as well. The fact that Medicare is paying less than 50% of the average senior citizen's annual medical bill means that Medicare recipients must carry a supplemental insurance policy to be fully protected from potential financial ruin. Often, though, the cost of supplemental insurance is out of reach for a senior citizen living on a fixed or small income. (See table 39-1.)

Compounding this problem is the difficulty most Americans have trying to understand health insurance. The terms are hard to understand; the provisions are not explained in comprehensible language. The policies themselves seem to be cluttered with jargon that appears meaningless when first read but becomes vitally important when making a claim against the policy.

Medical care is very expensive. You can expect to pay at least $250 a day for just for the hospital room and up to $700 a day if you require intensive care. Even during a short stay in the hospital, you could accumulate a bill of $20,000 or more. If your family were faced with these enormous expenses, the resulting economic loss could be catastrophic. Perhaps your insurance will cover the majority of your expenses and you will need to pay only a few dollars out-of-pocket. But with the wrong type of coverage you could be facing serious financial loss. Health insurance is supposed to protect against such loss. It is imperative that you have the proper health insurance coverage; this means having the right policy or policies.

Too often people have gone into the hospital confident their health insurance would cover their expenses, only to discover this was not the case. Thus, having the maximum amount of information concerning health insurance will increase your chances of selecting the proper coverage.

The basic types of health insurance policies cover services that are provided by hospitals and by doctors. You will often see these policies listed as Hospital insurance, Medical insurance and Surgical insurance. You may sometimes see Medical and Surgical insurance combined as Medical-Surgical.

Another type of insurance that is very important is Major Medical, also called "catastrophic" insurance. Major Medical covers the costs of medical care that you would require should you become very ill or have a serious accident. It pays the bills that basic health insurance does not cover. If you cannot afford both basic and Major Medical, you should consider purchasing at least a Major Medical policy.

THE VOCABULARY OF HEALTH INSURANCE

There are certain very important terms you should understand before beginning to read through different insurance policies. By understanding how these terms are used and what they mean, you will be in a much better position to select health insurance that meets your needs.

Definitions

Assignment: When you instruct your insurance company to pay the hospital or doctor directly for services you received. Your policy may normally pay you, but in this instance you would have the payment sent to the hospital or doctor.

Benefit: The amount of money or services an insurance company will pay you under the provisions of the policy. These benefits may be payable either directly to you or to the provider (hospital, doctor, medical supplier).

Claim: When you, your doctor, or your hospital notifies your insurance company that you have received a medical service and are requesting payment of benefits. The claim must normally be filed on a form supplied by your insurance company.

Co-Insurance/Co-Payment: A provision found in some health insurance policies that specifies how you and your insurance company will share the payment of covered services. For example, you are responsible for the first 20% of a covered expense, while the insurer pays the

TABLE 39-1.

THE MEDICARE PROGRAM—WHAT IT PAYS . . . WHAT YOU PAY

Medicare Services	Benefit Period	Medicare Pays	You Pay
PART A: HOSPITAL INSURANCE		All but	Deductible
Semi-private room rate	First 60 Days	deductible	$400
Miscellaneous hospital services & supplies			
Dietary & meal services		All but	
Special care units	61st to 90th Day	$100 per day	$100 per day
Diagnostic procedures, x-rays, etc.			
Laboratory services		All but	
Operating & recovery rooms	90th to 150th Day	$200 per day	$200 per day
Anesthesia			
Rehabilitation services	Beyond 150 Days	NOTHING	ALL COSTS
SKILLED NURSING CARE	First 20 Days	All Costs	Nothing
In approved facility after 3-day hospital	21st to 100th Day	All but $50/day	$50 per day
stay and enter the facility within	Beyond 100 Days	NOTHING	ALL COSTS
30 days of discharge			
Home Health Care	Unlimited as medically necessary	ALL COSTS	NOTHING
Hospice	Two 90 day periods and one 30 day period	All costs but outpatient drugs and respite care	Limited drug costs and respite care
Blood	As needed	All but first 3 pints	First 3 pints
PART B: PHYSICIAN INSURANCE			
Physician & surgeon fees	As medically	80 % of approved	$75 deductible &
Physical/speech therapists	necessary	amount after	20% of balance
Diagnostic tests		$75 deductible	(you also pay any
Medical supplies			charge above
Inpatient & Outpatient services			approved amount)
Ambulance service			
Home Health Care	Unlimited as medically necessary	ALL COSTS	NOTHING
Outpaitent Hospital Treatment	Unlimited as medically necessary	80% of approved amount after $75 deductible	After deductible 20% of balance
Blood	As needed	80% of approved amount after 3 pints	First 3 pints and 20% of balance

Figures quoted are effective January 1, 1985. Deductibles and Medicare allowances are subject to change on a yearly basis. For the most recent information consult a current copy of *Your Medicare Handbook*.

remaining 80%. This should not be confused with deductible, which is what you pay before your insurance begins to pay benefits. Some policies, such as Major Medical, also have a ceiling on your total out-of-pocket expenses. This ceiling is called the stop-loss and is listed in the policy.

Conversion Clause: The privilege granted by a group policy to convert to an individual policy upon termination of group coverage.

Coordination of Benefits: The specific term used to designate the process used by health insurance companies to avoid paying duplicate benefits to an individual covered by more than one group policy. The companies determine how much of a claim each one will pay. This prevents a policyholder from making a profit as the result of an accident or illness.

Deductible: The amount of money you must pay before your insurance benefits begin. The insurance company will pay benefits only on costs above the amount of your deductible.

Effective Date: The date on which coverage provided by an insurance policy begins. This is the first date on which you as a policyholder could file a claim and have it paid.

Exclusions: Specific conditions or circumstances under which a policy will not provide benefits. The specific services excluded from a policy may be found in the schedule of benefits. (See Schedule of Benefits.)

Indemnity Benefits: The payment of a specific dollar amount for each day of hospitalization. Payment is made directly to you and not to the hospital or doctor unless you specifically instruct your company to do so. For example, you may have a policy which pays you $100 a day for room and board, nursing care, and other services. Should the cost of your care be more than your policy pays, you are responsible for the difference. Amount and days of coverage may vary depending on your policy. We offer some suggestions later on how you can determine if indemnity benefits will cover hospital costs in your community.

Pre-Existing Condition: A physical and or mental condition which you have or had prior to purchasing health insurance. Usually, benefits will not be paid for services related to pre-existing conditions. Each company determines which con-

ditions are considered pre-existing and specifies if the condition will ever be covered by the policy. Many companies offer coverage of these conditions after a certain time period, for example, 2 years.

Premium: The amount you pay to purchase the insurance and keep it in force. You may pay premiums monthly, quarterly, semiannually or anually.

Renewal Clause: A clause which indicates the provisions under which the policy may or may not be renewed. Since many individual health insurance policies are written for a limited time, usually one year, they must be renewed at the end of each term. The provisions you are most likely to encounter are:

Guaranteed Renewable: The company guarantees your right to renew your policy to a specific age. For most health insurance policies, it is 65. (Obviously Medicare Supplemental Insurance is usually not purchased until age 65 and some policies may be renewed for life.) A guaranteed renewable policy may also have a guaranteed premium which will not be raised during the term of the insurance.

Conditionally Renewable: You may renew your policy until you reach a certain age, usually 65, provided you have complied with the other conditions of your insurance policy.

Optionally Renewable: The company may decline to renew your policy on the anniversary date. For instance, you may be hospitalized at the time your policy is to be renewed and the company may not renew your policy.

Schedule of benefits: The list of medical services that a particular insurance policy will cover. Every health insurance policy has a schedule of benefits.

Waiting Period: The length of time a policyholder is required to wait from the effective date of the policy until benefits for certain conditions are provided. This time is usually indicated in the contract agreement. Some policies have a waiting period of 15 to 30 days before any illness will be covered. This may also be referred to as the probationary period.

The following terms describe how insurance may be purchased.

Individual Insurance

Individual insurance is coverage for you or your dependents, purchased independently of any group. You may want to consider purchasing an individual insurance policy if you have no group coverage, if your group coverage is not complete or comprehensive, or if through a group policy you cannot cover your dependents. However, you should know that you may pay a rather steep premium for this coverage, and the deductible and co-insurance/co-payment may mean a large out-of-pocket expense.

Another major disadvantage, and something a purchaser should be alert to, may be the temporary nature of some individual health insurance policies. You may not be able to buy coverage for more than 90 to 180 days for basic Hospital and Medical-Surgical insurance. (However, Major Medical policies may be purchased on a year-to-year basis.)

Group Insurance

Group insurance is coverage bought at lower cost through an employer or organization. Since a large number of people are being covered by one overall policy, insurers reduce the premiums.

If you are eligible to join a group and purchase group insurance, by all means do so. Group insurance that is provided by an employer is by far the best way to obtain health insurance coverage. However, there may be ways of joining groups other than through an employer. For instance, many associations make group insurance available to their members, and you may be eligible for membership.

If group insurance is provided by your employer, you can usually extend coverage to a spouse or dependents. However, your employer might not be willing to pay the addition premium to cover them—in which case you must pay the extra premium yourself. Though an additional expense, the inclusion of a spouse and dependents to a group plan is still lower than purchasing individual policies.

Also note the effective date of coverage. Some policies cover you immediately upon employ-ment, while others require a waiting period. It is not uncommon to find group policies which require a 30-day waiting period before you become eligible to file a claim.

Should you find yourself about to become unemployed, you may still be able to retain some health insurance coverage. Group policies usually contain a conversion clause which permits you to convert to individual coverage when you are no longer part of the group. You will be responsible for paying the premium, but at least you will have health insurance. However, coverage may not be as extensive as it was under the group policy. Furthermore, you may pay a larger deductible and increased co-insurance/co-payment. Be sure to inquire into the amount of coverage you would have if you convert your group coverage to individual coverage.

Franchise Insurance

Another way to purchase insurance is through a group or association which offers franchise insurance. Individual policies are issued to the members of the group and coverage may include your spouse and dependents. With a franchise policy, the group or association agrees to collect the premiums for the insurance company.

Some employers who do not pay for their employees' health benefits may offer franchise insurance as an alternative. The franchise policy may have rates that are lower and benefits that are better than those found in a similar individual policy.

There are several types of policies available.

Hospital Insurance, Medical-Surgical Insurance and Major Medical Insurance

Hospital Insurance: Provides coverage for in-patient and outpatient hospital services. For in-patient services, these policies usually provide coverage for a specific number of days of hospitalization and also specify dollar limits on total benefits payable. These policies also cover procedures that you receive at the hospital even though you are not admitted and do not occupy a bed.

Medical-Surgical Insurance: The medical portion of this type of insurance pays for doctor visits to the hospital and may pay for office visits. Other medical services covered include drugs, x-rays, anesthesia, and laboratory tests performed outside of the hospital. The surgical portion covers the cost of surgical procedures, whether performed in the hospital, a doctor's office, or an ambulatory surgical center. The surgeon is paid according to a schedule of surgery determined by the insurance company and the doctor. The schedule of surgery indicates the maximum allowable payments for specific procedures.

Major Medical Insurance: This insurance is often referred to as catastrophic insurance because it protects you from the high cost of medical care associated with a serious illness or accident. Major Medical provides much broader coverage than basic Hospital and Medical-Surgical insurance policies. In addition, you collect more benefits for a longer period of time. These policies usually require a yearly deductible that must be paid before coverage begins. Deductibles will vary from one policy to another.

After the deductible is paid, Major Medical insurance pays up to a certain percentage of covered expenses. For example, many policies pay 80% of covered expenses with the remaining 20% paid by the policyholder. This is co-insurance/co-payment.

Once your out-of-pocket expenses, including the deductible and co-insurance/co-payment, reach a certain amount, many Major Medical policies protect you from further out-of-pocket expenses. This is known as the stop-loss provision, and it means that once you have paid out, for example $2500, that is all you will pay. Your policy pays the remaining covered expenses up to the maximum limits. You may want to consider purchasing a Major Medical policy if you can only afford one type of health insurance.

It is important to remember that Major Medical insurance is usually cheaper than Hospital or Medical-Surgical insurance. This is because of the large deductible these policies carry. They may require you to pay $500 before they take effect. But once the policy requirements are met, Major Medical can cover the majority of costs.

Other Types of Policies

The following policies provide coverage for very limited services or conditions; therefore, they are not generally recommended as a substitute for basic Hospital, Medical-Surgical, or Major Medical insurance.

Accident: This type of health insurance is very limited in its coverage and may not be the proper type of insurance for you. It excludes illness, but it will cover medical expenses that result from an accident. Because this type of policy provides limited coverage, we do not recommend it.

Dental: Routine dental care is usually covered under dental policies in addition to crowns, bridges and root canals. Some dental policies also cover orthodontic services, but only if the service is not cosmetic. Because the premium for dental insurance is very high, it is more commonly available on a group basis. Therefore, your best opportunity to acquire dental insurance is usually through an employer-provided group plan.

Disability Income Insurance: While technically not health insurance, disability income insurance is often included in some health insurance benefits packages. This insurance provides you with income when you are unable to work because of illness or accident. If your disability was the result of a job-related accident, you are probably covered by your state's Worker's Compensation Insurance.

Depending on the provisions of the policy, the degree of your disability could have a significant impact on whether or not you receive benefits. The insurance company makes the decision as to whether or not your disability would be covered. The more common types of disabilities are:

Occupational. The company defines your disability with regard to your inability to perform the duties of your occupation.

General disability. The company defines disability with regard to your ability to perform the duties of any occupation for which you may be suited as a result of education, training, or experience.

Combination Disability. The company defines your disability in terms of a specified time during which you are unable to perform the duties of your occupation. This may range from 10 days to 6 months. You may purchase disability income insurance policies on a long or short-term basis. You should know, however, that these policies usually have a waiting period (for example 7 to 14 days or longer) before any benefits are paid. The longer you wait for benefits, the lower the premium cost.

Disease-Specific: You may have seen this type of insurance advertised on television or in a newspaper supplement. This insurance usually covers one disease (for example, cancer or heart disease). We do not recommend disease-specific insurance. These policies pay limited benefits and may duplicate what you already have or may be ready to purchase. Your dollars would be better spent on more comprehensive types of policies.

Long-Term Care: This insurance may also be known as nursing home insurance since it covers the services provided by a skilled nursing facility. The most important thing to remember is that this insurance will pay benefits only if you receive skilled nursing care. In addition, your need for skilled nursing care must be certified by a physician as being medically necessary. If you should no longer require care at the skilled level, your benefits may cease. Most policies do not cover services provided by intermediate or custodial care facilities. Most patients in nursing homes are receiving custodial care rather than skilled nursing care.

We do not recommend that you purchase this type of insurance.

Travel Insurance: Again, this is not specifically health insurance. You have probably seen this type of insurance offered at airports or through automobile clubs and some credit card companies. These policies offer to pay a certain amount of benefits if you are injured or killed as the result of a travel accident. The benefits are for a limited time only and probably duplicate coverage that you already have or may purchase. These policies are more specifically a form of life insurance, and the money they pay is not necessarily intended to pay for the cost of medical services.

How Benefits Are Paid

Before you begin to review different health insurance policies, you should be aware of how benefits are paid to policyholders. There are generally two types of benefits, the indemnity benefit and the service benefit.

Indemnity Benefits: This type pays a specific amount for each day of hospitalization. The payment is made directly to you and not to the hospital or doctor unless you specifically instruct your company to do so. For example, a policy may pay you $100 a day which you would then use to pay the hospital room and board, nursing care, and other services. However, you are not obligated to use the money for expenses related to your hospitalization. The benefits would be payable for a set period of time which is clearly indicated in the policy.

If the cost of your care is more than your policy pays, you are responsible for the difference. Furthermore, the amount it pays per day of hospitalization is usually much less than your actual cost per day.

Know when the benefits become payable under an indemnity plan, because these policies may not pay benefits for your first day in the hospital. It is a good idea to find out the current hospital room rate in your area before considering any insurance policy that pays indemnity benefits.

Service Benefits: The service benefits pay the hospital or doctor directly for the services you receive. The insurance company negotiates with the hospitals and doctors to determine the reimbursement rate for services. Once these rates are determined, the hospitals and doctors agree to accept the reimbursement and will not bill you for any additional fee. The hospitals and doctors who agree to accept the insurance company's terms are referred to as participating, or member, providers. Should you obtain medical services from a doctor or hospital who is not a participating member, you may incur an out-of-pocket expense. For example, if you are a Blue Cross member and obtain medical care at a nonmember hospital, Blue Cross may require you to cover a portion of your expenses. Check your particular plan for specifics on receiving care at nonmember hospitals. When you purchase an insurance policy that pays service benefits, the company will give you the names of the participating providers.

Blue Cross/Blue Shield are examples of service benefits plans because they sign contracts with hospitals and doctors to pay the "usual, customary, and reasonable" (UCR) fees of the providers in your area. If you are covered by one of these plans, you may have noticed the letters "UCR" on your identification card. Commercial companies also provide service benefits plans. Service benefits are more comprehensive than indemnity benefits, and for this reason we recommend that you purchase a health insurance policy that pays service benefits. However, you may encounter a service benefit plan that requires a deductible or has a co-insurance/co-payment provision.

"Which insurance policy is the best for me?" Probably the best advice in answering this question is to shop around. The following questions will help you evaluate the coverage provided by the policies you are considering.

Hospital Insurance

- Does the policy pay indemnity benefits or service benefits? (Service benefits tend to be more complete and are preferable.)
- Does the policy cover the daily room and board rate of the hospitals in your area? (Contact the hospitals in your area to determine their daily room rates, or call your state's Hospital Association.)
- How many days of hospitalization does the policy cover? (If under 30 days, you may not want to consider the policy.)
- Does the policy have a waiting period or elimination period before hospital benefits are provided? (We do not recommend hospital policies with long waiting periods, for example, 7 to 10 days.)
- Does the policy cover pre-existing conditions? (Remember, some conditions may be excluded for a period of time and covered

later. Avoid policies that may never cover these conditions.)
- Does the policy pay for medicines and other services such as x-rays, laboratory services, treatments, etc.?
- Does the policy cover the costs associated with an operation such as the operating room fee, recovery room, or other specialty rooms? (Look for a policy in which these services are included.)
- Does the policy cover specialty care such as intensive care, coronary care, or burn care? (With specialty care costs running at almost $700 per day, any policy that does not pay at least a portion of them should be avoided.)
- Does the policy cover inpatient and outpatient psychiatric care?
- Does the policy cover outpatient services that you receive at the hospital or at a free standing ambulatory care center? (With more services becoming available on an outpatient basis, this should be covered.)
- Does the policy cover the expenses associated with an emergency room visit?
- Does the policy require you to use one particular hospital, or may you choose your own hospital? (If you want the option of choosing a hospital, avoid policies that limit your choice.)
- Does the policy pay anything toward the services you may receive in a hospital that does not have an agreement with your insurance company? (Sometimes insurance companies may pay a portion of your expenses in what are called noncontracting facilities.)
- Does the policy require you to pay a deductible or make co-payments towards expenses? (The fewer out-of-pocket expenses you pay, the better. Avoid hospital policies that require deductibles and co-payments.)
- Can the policy be renewed? (We recommend a policy that is guaranteed renewable and also guarantees the premium not to change during the life of the contract. Review renewal clauses for more information.)
- Can the benefits provided by the policy be changed at the option of the company? (A

policy in which benefits can be changed should be avoided.)

Medical-Surgical Insurance

You may also see this listed as Medical Insurance and Surgical Insurance. However, the following questions apply to both.

- Does the policy require you to share in the cost of your care through a deductible and co-payment? (We recommend policies that do not require out-of-pocket expenses for basic services.)
- How much does the policy pay toward doctor visits when you are in the hospital? (Check with your doctor to find out if this amount covers his usual fee.)
- How many visits does the policy cover when you are in the hospital? (If you have an extended illness, your benefits could be used up quickly.)
- Does the policy cover office visits or home visits by your doctors? If so, how many of each type?
- Does the policy cover diagnostic tests performed in the doctor's office?
- Does the policy cover lab services in conjunction with tests ordered by your doctor?
- Does the policy cover second opinion surgical consultations? (Many policies now require a second opinion before a surgical procedure will be covered.)
- Does the policy have a surgical schedule that pays one lump sum regardless of the surgeon's fee, or does it pay the "usual, customary, and reasonable fee" of the surgeons in your area? (Policies that pay benefits in line with surgeons' fees in your area are preferred.)
- Does the policy pay for your surgeon to bring in a consultant on your case?
- Does the policy cover the cost of an assistant surgeon? (You should pay close attention to this, since some policies only pay for the primary surgeon and you must pay for the assistant surgeon.)
- Does the policy cover surgical procedures performed at an ambulatory surgical center or one-day surgery in the hospital? (Many insurance companies now recognize the cost effectiveness of one-day surgery and will cover it. You should look for a policy that has this benefit.)
- Can you pay the premium on an annual basis?
- Can the policy be renewed; if so, under what conditions? (A guaranteed renewable policy is best. See page 333 for renewal conditions.)

Major Medical Insurance

- What is the maximum dollar amount of coverage provided by the policy you are considering? (You should try to purchase a Major Medical policy with a maximum limit as high as possible, if you can afford the premium.)
- Does the policy have a deductible that you can afford? (Major Medical policies usually have a deductible that is much higher than basic Hospital and Medical-Surgical insurance.)
- Does the deductible apply to a benefit period such as one year, or does it apply each time you file a claim? (To avoid excessive out-of-pocket expenses, choose a policy that has a yearly deductible, as opposed to one that has a per-incident deductible.)
- Are the co-insurance/co-payment provisions of the policy at least 80:20 or better? (The more the company will pay, the less you will need to pay. A co-insurance/co-payment of 80% by the company is very common among Major Medical policies.)
- Does the policy restore any portion of the maximum benefits once you are well and can submit medical evidence to establish your improved health? (Some policies restore a portion of your maximum benefits provided you have not made claims for a certain period of time. This is a good provision to have in any Major Medical policy.)
- What is the stop-loss amount at which point you stop paying anything towards your medical expenses? (It is very important that you know the stop-loss provision of any Major

Medical policy since this determines your maximum out-of-pocket expense.)

- Does the policy cover all hospital and doctor expenses associated with your care, or are there services which are excluded? (The more complete the coverage, the less you need to worry about paying these costs yourself.)
- Can the policy be renewed, if so, under what conditions? (The guaranteed renewable policy is preferred.)

By now you should have a very good idea of which policies meet your specific needs and which ones you can afford. Before making any final decision, you may want to consider the following warnings and then review the policies one more time.

Warnings

Mandated Benefits. Some states require that all health insurance policies sold within their boundaries provide certain benefits. These regulations may apply to both group and individual policies. Check with your state insurance department to determine if there are certain minimum benefits that must be provided by all health insurance policies. (A complete list of state insurance departments may be found at the end of this chapter.)

Exclusions. Knowing which services are excluded from a policy might be more important than knowing what is covered. In fact, the first thing you might want to read is the exclusion clause found in the schedule of benefits. You may discover that a policy you had been considering has so many exclusions that it does not provide the coverage you desire. If there is any doubt as to whether or not a service is covered, check with the agent or the insurance company.

Another aspect of the exclusion clause is that injuries or illnesses that would ordinarily be covered may be excluded if they occur under the following circumstances:

- Attempted suicide or self-inflicted injuries.
- Injury or illness covered under Workers' Compensation.
- Injury or illness resulting from war or military service.

- Treatment received in government hospitals (VA, military or federal institutions.

Coordination of Benefits. If you are covered under more than one group plan, you cannot collect duplicate benefits. Under the provision known as coordination of benefits, insurance companies determine the percentage of your claim each company will pay. In no case will total payment of benefits exceed the actual expenses of your medical care.

Changing Policies. Do not under any circumstances cancel an existing policy before you have purchased a replacement policy. The last thing you want is to be left without any health insurance coverage. If you have questions regarding your present policy, it is best to contact your agent and ask if you can upgrade the coverage you have.

Completing the Application. Give a complete, accurate medical history. If you omit something, it may delay the start of your coverage. If you deliberately omit something, it could be grounds for cancelling your policy or denying you benefits should you file a claim.

A condition that you have or had may not be eligible for coverage under health insurance. This is called a pre-existing condition. The insurance company will usually determine (based upon your medical history) if it will provide coverage for this condition.

Some policies consider a condition pre-existing even if you did not know that you had the condition before you bought the policy. Also, you need to know how many years the company will go back in looking for pre-existing conditions. Some companies may go back as far as birth; others go back 2 years.

Policies vary as to how long they exclude benefits for pre-existing conditions. Usually, policies will not pay for pre-existing conditions for 1 or 2 years after the effective date of the policy, but some policies may have longer or shorter periods.

Never allow the insurance agent to process the application for you without thoroughly reviewing it. Remember, an insurance agent cannot alter any provisions of a policy; only the company can do that through a rider to the policy.

Free Look Provision. After you have signed the application and paid the premium, your state may permit you to review the policy for a certain number of days before you decide to keep it. If you have questions, contact your agent at once. Should you decide not to keep the policy, simply return it to the company within the time allotted and request a full refund of any premium. In the event you have a problem returning the policy within the specified time, contact your state insurance department for assistance.

Consumer Protection. Should you have any problems with an insurance company, you may want to contact your State Insurance Department for assistance.

We have prepared a list of insurance departments and a guide to filing a complaint at the end of this chapter. Insurance companies are regulated by the states, and it is the responsibility of the insurance department to investigate consumer complaints.

Shopping Tips

Do

- Purchase insurance from a reputable company. (To find out if any complaints have been filed against a particular company, check with your state insurance department. Also check the rating given the company and its policies by A.M. Best Company. You can find the Best directory at your local library.)
- Be careful when purchasing mail order insurance. (Check with your state insurance department to make sure the company is licensed to sell policies in your state.)
- Avoid "disease-specific" policies (for example, cancer insurance). (Disease-specific policies may duplicate the coverage you have and may pay limited benefits.)
- Make sure the salesperson clearly explains your premium costs. (You may save money if you can afford to pay annually.)
- Make sure the salesperson gives you a complete schedule of benefits for the policy. (Do not purchase any policy until you know

which services are provided and which services are excluded.)
- Be aware of any exclusions, pre-existing conditions, and waiting periods. (These items generally limit your coverage, so avoid policies that exclude too many services and conditions, as well as those that make you wait too long before you can begin to file claims.)
- Double-check all your entries on the application before you sign. An accidental omission might delay the start of coverage or could lead to a claim being denied.
- Pay your premium by check and make it payable to the insurance company—not to the agent.
- Take advantage of any "free look" as mandated by your state insurance department. (If you do not know if your state has any "free look" provision, contact the insurance department.)

Don't

- Don't be alarmed by claims of "last chance," "limited enrollment period," or other scare tactics. (Reputable insurance companies and salespersons will not use these pressure tactics.)
- Don't be fooled by the "government" look—the federal government does not sell health insurance.
- Don't be misled by celebrity endorsements. You should examine these policies as carefully as others. (Remember, the person making the endorsement is being paid to say nice things about the company.)
- Don't pay cash to the salesperson. If you pay cash, you have no record to prove that you paid the premium.
- Don't purchase more policies than you need. Duplicate policies only mean added expense for you.
- When you purchase a new policy, don't cancel your existing policy until the effective date of the new policy. (Make sure you clearly understand when your new policy becomes effective.)

MEDICARE

Some of the worst cases of under-insurance or over-insurance have occurred among senior citizens. Furthermore, out-of-pocket expenses for those on Medicare have been growing each year. To avoid large out-of-pocket expense, it is more important than ever to select the right supplemental insurance policy from the many different types on the market.

The federal Medicare program was intended to make health care accessible and affordable to senior citizens, not to provide 100% coverage.

Medicare is divided into Part A: Hospital Insurance and Part B: Medical Insurance. Part A provides coverage for hospital services, post-hospital skilled nursing care, home health care, and hospice services. When you turn 65 and are eligible for Medicare, you are automatically covered under Part A. You do not pay a premium for this coverage.

Part B: Medical Insurance is optional and provides coverage for physician's services, inpatient and outpatient medical services and supplies, home health care, outpatient hospital treatment, and the services of various therapists. (See Table 39-1 for specific benefits provided.) *Your Medicare Handbook*, available at any Social Security Administration office, contains complete information.

A major deficiency in the program is that many physicians and medical suppliers do not accept the approved medicare reimbursement rate as full payment. In those cases you have to pay the difference between the rate the physicians or suppliers charge and that which Medicare pays. You can avoid this extra out-of-pocket expense if your physician or supplier accepts Medicare Assignment. This means accepting Medicare's approved amount as full payment for services rendered. To find out which physicians in your area accept Medicare Assignment, contact your local Social Security Administration office. Also, be sure to ask any doctor you use or are considering using if he/she accepts assignment.

Even if the physician or supplier accepts Medicare Assignment, you pay a portion of your expenses through a deductible and co-insurance/co-payment. These are the gaps in Medicare coverage that you are responsible for paying.

Medicare Supplemental Insurance, sometimes referred to as "Medi-gap" insurance, can help you close some of these gaps. However, few policies cover all of your expenses.

To evaluate supplemental insurance policies, first gather the schedule of benefits for several policies. Many commercial insurance companies and Blue Cross/Blue Shield Association sell supplemental insurance. Some of the companies that sell health insurance may be very familiar to you because of their advertising. You have probably seen ads for them in magazines, newspapers or on TV, or received direct mail advertisement. Even some unions sponsor supplemental insurance. To find several different policies, we suggest that you contact insurance agencies or agents in your area. They should be able to provide you with complete information on the types of supplemental policies they sell.

When shopping for Medicare Supplemental Insurance you want to look for a policy that covers at least the deductibles and co-payments that are required from the 61st through the 150th day of hospitalization. You also want the policy to cover the co-payment associated with skilled nursing care from the 21st through the 100th day. Under Part B, the supplemental policy should cover the deductible and the 20% co-payment.

Some supplemental policies may provide more coverage such as prescription drugs, additional physician visits, private duty nursing, and some nursing home care. The extra services may be nice to have, but the premium may be prohibitive.

Always purchase a policy that gives you the right to renew. Renewal conditions vary from policy to policy.

Other Options

A new approach to providing additional coverage for Medicare recipients is the Medicare Health Maintenance Organization (HMO). HMOs for Medicare recipients have recently been approved by the Health Care Financing Administration (HCFA), the agency that administers the Medicare program.

Medicare recipients living in selected areas have the option of joining an HMO that has a contract with HCFA to provide services to Medicare enrollees. (There may be other HMOs that will enroll Medicare recipients even though they may not have an HCFA contract. Contact those in your area to determine if they do enroll Medicare recipients.) The monthly enrollment fee would be paid by Medicare; however, recipients would be required to maintain their Medicare Part B insurance and to pay the monthly premium. In addition, some of these Medicare HMOs may require recipients to pay a monthly fee for services over and above those covered under regular Medicare.

One advantage of the Medicare HMO is that claims no longer need to be filed and the deductibles and co-payments may be waived. However, check the exact requirements with the Medicare HMO in your area. Some Medicare recipients have been able to cancel their supplemental insurance as a result of joining the HMO.

Remember, if you join the HMO you will be required to receive all your medical services from the doctors on the staff of the HMO. Some people do not like the idea of not being able to retain their own doctor, and for these people the HMO may not be the best option.

Do not enroll in a Medicare HMO unless you clearly understand how it operates. Ask plenty of questions, especially about your right to return to the regular Medicare program if you do not like the HMO. There may be penalties and waiting periods involved should you decide to make the change. A Medicare HMO might be the right choice for some people, but do not make a hasty decision. Should you have any questions concerning any aspect of a Medicare HMO, contact your Social Security Administration office or your State Insurance Department.

NEW APPROACHES TO PROVIDING HEALTH CARE BENEFITS

As business and individuals search for new methods to control the cost of health care, HMOS, Preferred Provider Organizations (PPOs), and Self-Insurance are becoming popular options.

Health Maintenance Organization

A Health Maintenance Organization is a prepaid group health plan that provides direct medical services. It emphasizes wellness and health promotion to its members. HMOs usually offer their services to groups; however, individuals may have the opportunity to join an HMO during an open enrollment period.

Your employer may pay the required monthly charge or may require you to share a portion of the cost. In addition, you may be expected to pay a portion of the monthly fee to extend coverage to a spouse and dependents.

Depending upon the organizational structure of an HMO, you may need to give up your private physician if you join. These HMOs have their own facility and provide services under one roof. If you join this type of HMO, you would be required to receive all your medical care from the practitioners who are employed by the HMO.

A variation of the HMO is the Individual Practice Association (IPA), which permits physicians in private practice to offer prepaid health care plans. You would continue to use your physician for all your medical care and would not be billed at the time services are rendered. The physician would bill the HMO for the care provided.

Preferred Provider Organization

This is a group of doctors or hospitals who agree to provide medical services to employees of one or more companies. The PPO operates on the concept that employees will use only those providers who are members of the PPO for all their medical care. The providers in the PPO reduce their fees for a guarantee of patient volume. When an employee uses a doctor or hospital outside of the PPO, he must pay the difference between what the PPO would allow for the service and the charge by the nonmember provider. In addition, employees may be required to pay a deductible if they use nonmember providers.

Self-Insurance

When an employer decides to offer a Self-Insurance plan to employees, it means the employer will pay for employees' medical care up to a certain dollar limit. Employees may still be responsible for any deductible and co-payment that is part of the Self-Insurance plan. Instead of issuing Hospital and Medical-Surgical policies, the employees may contract with an insurance company to process employee claims.

Insurance companies who help businesses administer Self-Insurance plans usually have an Administrative Services Only contract to handle employees claims. Many companies that self-insure also offer their employees a Major Medical policy so they are not without catastrophic coverage.

Self-Insurance permits businesses to gain some control over the cost of providing health care benefits to employees.

STATE INSURANCE DEPARTMENTS

Insurance departments in every state play an important role in regulating insurance companies. The department is headed by a commissioner who is the chief administrative officer. The commissioner is responsible for directing the activities of the department and enforcing the laws governing the insurance industry.

The department is responsible for writing the regulations that accompany the insurance laws. It also licenses companies and agents to sell insurance, approves the policies that are sold, and mandates certain minimum benefits for each type of policy.

The department has the power to conduct investigations, take testimony, hold hearings, render verdicts, and impose punishment consistent with its responsibilities. The punishment is usually in the form of fines, suspensions, and revocations of licenses. In some extreme cases, a company could be banned from selling its policies in your state.

Your state insurance department may also be able to help you if you have a problem with your insurance company or an agent. If you file a formal complaint with the department, it will be investigated and an attempt made to resolve the problem. The department cannot act as your legal counsel, but it can advise you of your rights under the insurance laws.

How to File a Complaint

Should you have a problem with your insurance company, you can file a complaint with your state insurance department. Your complaint should be in writing and contain the following information.

1. Your name, address, and telephone number.
2. The name, address, and telephone number of your insurance company.
3. The identification number of your policy.
4. The type of policy.
5. The nature of your complaint. Are you complaining about the premium, coverage, a claim, or the actions of your agent?

Make sure that you keep copies of everything you send to the insurance department. The department will investigate your complaint to determine if there is anything it can do to resolve the problem. You must be willing to follow through on your complaint and appear at any hearings if so directed. If the law and the facts are on your side, then the Insurance Department can usually help you resolve the problem.

Alabama
DEPARTMENT OF INSURANCE
135 South Union St.
Montgomery, AL 36310
(205) 269-3550

Alaska
DIVISION OF INSURANCE
3601 C St.
Suite 722
Anchorage, AK 99503
(907) 562-3626

Arizona
INSURANCE DEPARTMENT
Commerce Building
1601 W. Jefferson St.
Phoenix, AZ 85007
(602) 255-4862

Arkansas
INSURANCE DEPARTMENT
Department of Commerce
12th & University Ave.
Little Rock, AR 72204
(501) 371-1325

California
DEPARTMENT OF INSURANCE
600 South Commonwealth Ave.
Los Angeles, CA 90005
(818) 736-2551

Colorado
DIVISION OF INSURANCE
Department of Regulatory Agencies
First Western Plaza
303 West Colfax, 5th Flr.
Denver, CO 80204
(303) 866-3201

Connecticut
INSURANCE DEPARTMENT
165 Capitol Ave.
Hartford, CT 06106
(203) 566-5275

Delaware
DELAWARE INSURANCE
   DEPARTMENT
Robert Short Memorial Bldg.
21 The Green
Dover, DE 19901
(302) 736-4251

District of Columbia
DEPARTMENT OF INSURANCE
512 North Potomac Bldg.
614 H St., N. W.
Washington, DC 20001
(202) 727-1273

Florida
DEPARTMENT OF INSURANCE
The Capitol
Tallahassee, FL 32301
(904) 488-3440

Georgia
DEPARTMENT OF INSURANCE
238 State Capitol
Atlanta, GA 30334
(404) 656-2056

Hawaii
INSURANCE DIVISION
Department of Commerce
1010 Richards St.
Honolulu, HI 96811
(808) 548-6522

Idaho
DEPARTMENT OF INSURANCE
State Office Bldg.
700 West State St.
Boise, ID 83720
(208) 334-2250

Illinois
DEPARTMENT OF INSURANCE
Bicentennial Bldg.
320 W. Washington St.
Springfield, IL 62767
(217) 782-4515

Indiana
DEPARTMENT OF INSURANCE
509 State Office Bldg.
100 N. Senate Ave.
Indianapolis, IN 46204
(317) 232-2386

Iowa
INSURANCE DEPARTMENT
Lucas State Office Bldg.
E. 12th and Walnut Sts.
Des Moines, IA 50319
(515) 281-5705

Kansas
INSURANCE DEPARTMENT
State Office Bldg.
Topeka, KS 66612
(913) 296-3071

Kentucky
DEPARTMENT OF INSURANCE
151 Elkhorn Ct.
Frankfort, KY 40602
(502) 564-3630

Louisiana
DEPARTMENT OF INSURANCE
Insurance Bldg.
950 N. 5th St.
Baton Rouge, LA 70804
(504) 342-5328

Maine
BUREAU OF INSURANCE
Department of Business
   Regulation
State House, Station 34
Augusta, ME 04333
(207) 289-3101

Maryland
INSURANCE DIVISION
Department of Licensing &
   Regulation
Stanbalt Bldg.
501 St. Paul Pl.
Baltimore, MD 21202
(301) 659-6300

Massachusetts
DIVISION OF INSURANCE
Department of Banking &
   Insurance
Leverett Saltonstall State Office
   Bldg.
100 Cambridge St.
Boston, MA 02202
(617) 727-3333

Michigan
INSURANCE BUREAU
Department of Licensing &
   Regulation
1048 Pierpoint St.
Lansing, MI 48909
(517) 373-0220

Minnesota
INSURANCE DIVISION
Department of Commerce
500 Metro Square Bldg.
St. Paul, MN 55101
(612) 296-6907

Mississippi
INSURANCE DEPARTMENT
1804 Walter Sillers Bldg.
550 High St.
Jackson, MS 39205
(601) 354-7711

Missouri
DIVISION OF INSURANCE
Dept. of Consumer Affairs,
   Regulation & Licensing

515 E. High Street
Jefferson City, MO 65102
(314) 751-4126

Montana
DEPARTMENT OF INSURANCE
205 Roberts St.
Helena, MT 59620
(406) 449-2040

Nebraska
DEPARTMENT OF INSURANCE
301 Centennial Mall S.
Lincoln, NE 68509
(404) 471-2201

Nevada
INSURANCE DIVISION
Department of Commerce
201 S. Fall St.
Carson City, NV 89710
(702) 885-4270

New Hampshire
INSURANCE DEPARTMENT
169 Manchester St.
Concord, NH 03301
(603) 271-2261

New Jersey
DEPARTMENT OF INSURANCE
201 E. State St.
C.N. 325
Trenton, NJ 08625
(609) 292-5363

New Mexico
DEPARTMENT OF INSURANCE
Corporation Commission
428 PERA Bldg.
Santa Fe, NM 87501
(505) 827-2451

New York
INSURANCE DEPARTMENT
Two World Trade Towers
New York, NY 10047
(202) 488-4124

North Carolina
DEPARTMENT OF INSURANCE
Dobbs Bldg.

430 N. Salisbury St.
Raleigh, NC 27611
(919) 733-7343

North Dakota
INSURANCE DEPARTMENT
State Capitol, 5th Flr.
Bismarck, ND 58505
(701) 224-2440

Ohio
DEPARTMENT OF INSURANCE
2100 Stella Ct.
Columbus, OH 43215
(614) 466-2691

Oklahoma
INSURANCE DEPARTMENT
408 Will Rogers Memorial Bldg.
2401 N. Lincoln Blvd.
Oklahoma City, OK 73105
(405) 521-2828

Oregon
INSURANCE DIVISION
Department of Commerce
158 12th St., N.E.
Salem, OR 97310
(503) 378-4474

Pennsylvania
INSURANCE DEPARTMENT
1326 Strawberry Sq.
4th & Walnut Sts.
Harrisburg, PA 17120
(717) 787-5288

Rhode Island
INSURANCE COMMISSIONER
Department of Business
  Regulation
100 N. Main St.
Providence, RI 02903
(401) 277-2223

South Carolina
DEPARTMENT OF INSURANCE
Kittrell Center
2711 Middleburg Dr.
Columbia, SC 29240
(803) 758-3266

South Dakota
DIVISION OF INSURANCE
Insurance Bldg.
Broadway & Nicollet St.
Pierre, SD 57501
(605) 773-3563

Tennessee
DEPARTMENT OF INSURANCE
114 State Office Bldg.
5th & Charlotte Ave.
Nashville, TN 37219
(615) 741-2241

Texas
STATE BOARD OF INSURANCE
State Insurance Bldg.
1110 San Jacinto Blvd.
Austin, TX 78786
(512) 475-2273

Utah
INSURANCE DEPARTMENT
326 S. 5th East St.
Salt Lake City, UT 84102
(801) 533-5611

Vermont
DEPARTMENT OF BANKING
& INSURANCE
State Office Bldg.
120 State St.
Montpelier, VT 05602
(802) 828-3301

Virginia
BUREAU OF INSURANCE
Jefferson Bldg.
1220 Bank St.
Richmond, VA 23209
(804) 786-3741

Washington
INSURANCE COMMISSIONER
Insurance Bldg.
1306 Capitol Way
Mail Stop AQ-21
Olympia, WA 98504
(206) 753-7301

West Virginia
DEPARTMENT OF INSURANCE
2100 Washington St., E.
Charleston, WV 25305
(304) 348-3386

Wisconsin
INSURANCE COMMISSIONER
Loraine Bldg.
123 W. Washington Ave.
Madison, WI 53707
(608) 266-3585

Wyoming
INSURANCE DEPARTMENT
1 Pioneer Center
2424 Pioneer Ave.
Cheyenne, WY 82002
(307) 777-7401

Puerto Rico
INSURANCE COMMISSIONER
Intendente Alejandro Ramirez
    Bldg.
Covadonga Dr. Stop 1
San Juan, PR 00904
(809) 723-1122

Virgin Islands
INSURANCE COMMISSIONER
Lieutenant Governor's Office
18 Kongens Gade
Charlotte Amalie,
St. Thomas VI 00801
(809) 774-2991

40 HEALTH RISK APPRAISALS: A CONSUMER'S GUIDE

Jonathan E. Fielding, M.D., M.B.A., is professor in the UCLA Schools of Medicine and Public Health, where he concentrates on the organization and evaluation of employer-sponsored health programs. He is also founder and CEO of U.S. Corporate Health Management in Santa Monica, a producer of health risk appraisal instruments. He is the author of *Corporate Health Management* (Addison-Wesley, 1987).

Tracy Rodriguez is a specialist in the development and installation of health promotion products. She has written workbooks and audiotapes concerning stress management, weight control, nutrition, and women's health. She develops health risk appraisal programs for U.S. Corporate Health Management, and she is former director of marketing at the UCLA Center for Health Enhancement.

Health risk appraisals (HRAs) are tools used for assessing an individual's potential for developing certain diseases, particularly cancer and heart disease, and identifying the behaviors that increase that potential. Some HRAs also address dental health care, social support needs, self-care, and other important areas. In 1986, thousands of organizations used HRAs to increase awareness of health risks and to promote better habits. More companies offered HRAs to their employees than offered exercise classes, stress management seminars, or blood pressure control programs. In this chapter, public health researchers Jonathan Fielding and Tracy Rodriguez describe the increasing variety of evaluation tools and explain who will most benefit from their use.∎

Anyone who has heard footsteps in a dark alley or has felt a plane tremble in midair intuitively understands the notion of risk. Unfortunately, our notion of risk is more frequently based on media coverage and past experience than it is on cold, hard facts.

During the summer of 1986, for example, tens of thousands of Americans cancelled planned vacations in Europe after several terrorist attacks at European airports. Ironically, at that time the risk of being killed in a local driving vacation in the United States was much higher than being killed in a terrorist attack in Europe.

This example shows the importance of understanding personal risks in order to make meaningful choices to reduce those risks. An individual who perceives himself to be highly susceptible to attack and death by terrorism may avoid traveling abroad or walking near suspicious-looking individuals. This same individual may do little or nothing to make himself a safe driver, even though his chances of dying in a motor vehicle accident are greater and could be reduced by a far greater amount.

If our intuition often fails us, how do we assess our risk of developing disease and identify the behaviors that increase those risks? How do we know which behaviors have the greatest impact on our individual health and which deserve most of our attention? One of the newer and more popular tools for assessing individual risks is the health risk appraisal or HRA.

THE THREE STEPS TO ASSESSING RISKS

Although they come in a variety of shapes and sizes, most health risk appraisals assess risks using the following three steps:

1. **Collecting Information: The Questionnaire.** HRAs generally rely on questionnaires to collect personal information on health habits and practices. The questionnaires range from 10 to over 200 questions and can cover a variety of health areas. Table 40-1 shows the typical areas queried in a longer, more comprehensive questionnaire.

TABLE 40-1.

AREAS ADDRESSED IN MOST HEALTH RISK APPRAISAL QUESTIONNAIRES

Area	Question Examples
General information	Age, sex, and education
Personal history	History of diabetes
	History of hypertension
Family history	Family history of breast or colo-rectal cancer
Physiologic measurements	Weight
	Blood pressure
Personal health behaviors	Smoking
	Eating
	Exercise habits
Psychological health	Reaction to stressful situations
	General well-being
Safety practices	Seatbelt use
	Smoking in bed
Self-care practices	Breast self-exam
	Flossing and brushing teeth
Use of medical system	Pap smears for women

2. **Processing Information: Self- or Computer-Scored.** HRAs use responses from questions on current health status, health habits, and family history to estimate individual risk and to rate individual health practices. Processing can range from a simple rate-yourself paper-and-pencil test to a computer program based on hundreds of complicated algorithms or rules that tell the computer how to assess individual risk and assign personal statements.

To determine an individual's risk, HRAs consider the individual's risk factors. These are characteristics and practices such as age and smoking which affect a person's risk of developing specific diseases. To estimate a 10-year risk of dying from lung cancer for a 35-year-old male who smokes, for example, the health risk appraisal would estimate an average 10-year risk of dying for 35-year-old males. Drawing from population studies which show that smokers have a risk of developing lung cancer that averages 12 times higher than that of nonsmokers, the health risk appraisal would then multiply the nonsmoker's risk by 12 to obtain an estimate of the smoker's risk.

Of course, this is an oversimplification of many health risk appraisals; most computerized appraisals consider several variables at a time. In the example above, the HRA might also look at how much this person smokes and for how long. This picture grows even more complicated in conditions like heart disease where the HRA has to consider not only smoking but also exercise, past medical history, blood pressure, and other variables. As Table 40-2 shows, many of the common causes of death have more than one prominent risk factor.

TABLE 40-2.

PROMINENT CONTROLLABLE RISK FACTORS

Causes of Death	Risk Factors
Heart Disease	Smoking, high blood pressure, elevated blood cholesterol, diabetes, obesity, lack of exercise, Type A behavior
Cancer	Smoking, alcohol, sun exposure, radiation, worksite hazards, pollution, medications, infectious agents, diet, not obtaining pap smears
Stroke	High blood pressure, elevated cholesterol, smoking
Accidents other than motor vehicle	Alcohol, smoking (fires), product design, home hazards, handgun availability
Influenza/pneumonia	Vaccination status, smoking, alcohol
Motor vehicle accidents	Alcohol, no safety restraints, speed, automobile design, roadway design
Diabetes	Obesity (for adult onset), diet
Cirrhosis of liver	Alcohol
Suicide	Handgun availability, alcohol or drug misuse, depression, stress
Homicide	Handgun availability, alcohol, stress

3. **Providing Information: The Report.** An estimate of individual risk and an explanation of that risk is usually given to the individual in the form of a report. Some reports also rate health behaviors and provide suggestions for reducing risks and improving behaviors. Figure 40-1 shows one page of a computer-generated report which contains information about risks, a rating of health behaviors, and explanations and suggestions. This page of the report rates Jane's eating, exercising, and smoking habits and recommends that she give up smoking, lower her fat intake, increase her fiber intake, and consider adding stretching exercises.

Computerized and personalized reports enjoy considerable popularity in our high-tech, health-oriented and individual focused society. Anyone who has completed a personal and confidential questionnaire and received a report that appears to predict the future but indicates that one might be able to change it can attest to the appeal of this instrument! Self-scored instruments are also quite popular despite their lack of high-tech appeal. Popular wide-circulation magazines use these test-your-health type quizzes not only to increase their readers' awareness but also to interactively involve them with the magazine's content.

A growing number of community organizations and employers have also adopted the health risk appraisal. In 1986, thousands of organizations used health risk appraisals to increase awareness of health risks and stimulate changes in behavior.

WHO'S USING HEALTH RISK APPRAISALS?
Public and Private Worksites

A recent nationwide survey of worksites found that over 18% provided health risk appraisals to their employees. In fact, as Table 40-3 shows, health risk appraisals were the second most common health promotion program component, led only by smoking cessation. As this table in-

FIGURE 40-1.

Your major health risks

The four charts at the right show your risk of dying in a motor vehicle accident, dying from cancer, having a heart attack, or having a stroke, if you currenlty have a serious health problem your risk may be greater than reported here.

The percentage number for "Your Risk Now" compares your current risk to the average risk of a person of your age and sex.

The percentage rate for "Achievable Risk" shows what your risks would be if you follow the recommendations in this report.

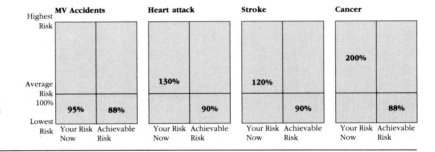

Your health habits

		Help!	Poor	Fair	Good	Tops!
Nutrition	Fat/Cholesterol	------- * * * ---------------------------------			+ + + + + + + + + + + + + + + + +	
	Salt	---			+ + + + + + * * * + + + + + + + + +	
	Fiber	---			* * * + + + + + + + + + + + + + + +	
	Sugar	---------------------------------------			* * * + + + + + + + + + + + + + + +	

Your fat intake is high, but your total blood cholesterol is satisfactory. Lowering your fat intake may not greatly reduce your heart attack or stroke risk, but may decrease your risk of colon and breast cancer. Increasing your fiber intake can improve your bowel functioning, reduce your risk of some bowel diseases, possibly including cancer.

	Help!	Poor	Fair	Good	Tops!
Exercise				* * *------------------------------	

You reported expending 2400 calories per week in regular exercise and other physical activities and engaging in aerobic exercise 1 to 3 times per week. Your exercise habits contribute to your good health by lowering your cardiovascular disease risk, helping you maintain your weight, manage stress, control blood pressure, and increasing your general sense of well-being. Consider doing some stretching exercises.

	Help!	Poor	Fair	Good	Tops!
Tobacco use	--------- * * * ------------------------------				

Your cigarette smoking habit increases your risk of heart attack by 1.5 times, stroke by 1.5 times, lung cancer by 5.0 times, oral cancer by 1.7 times, laryngeal cancer by 4.4 times, esophageal cancer by 4.0 times, bladder cancer by 2.3 times, and pancreatic cancer by 2.2 times. Your risk of chronic lung disease is also greatly increased. In addition, smoking decreases your exercise capacity, ages your skin faster and impairs your ability to taste and smell.

Jane Smith 10524388851

FIGURE 40-2.

... And what can be done about them

Nutrition

The choices you make each day about what you eat and drink affect every muscle, nerve, bone and other tissue in your body. Nutrition influences your risk of developing obesity and many major diseases, including heart disease, stroke and probably a number of cancers. In general, the best nutritional approach to maximize health is to limit the amount of fat, sugar and salt you eat and to increase the amount of complex carbohydrates and fiber. Eating a variety of foods from the basic food groups will assure that you receive the nutrients you need for good health. Balancing the calories you eat with the calories you burn through exercise will help you maintain normal weight.

Exercise

Aerobic exercise, the kind you get from repeated activity involving your largest muscles, improves your changes of avoiding a heart attack, gives you more energy, helps reduce stress and promotes emotional well being. You can achieve and maintain a good aerobic capacity by doing exercise that increases your heart rate to 70 percent of your estimated maximum for at least 20 minutes three or more times per week. Other important reasons to exercise are to maintain muscle strength and flexibility to reduce risk of accidents and to remain self-sufficient into old age.

Tobacco use

Tobacco use (cigarettes, cigars, pipes and smokeless tobacco) remains the single largest preventable cause of death in the United States. As many as 500,000 Americans die each year from using tobacco. It is not surprising that most smokers want to stop. They realize that smoking increases their risk of lung cancer and other forms of cancer, heart disease, chronic bronchitis, emphysema and pneumonia. Most smokers have experienced a decrease in their sense of smell and taste; many have experienced persistent coughs and decreased exercise ability. It may take several attempts, but persistent efforts to stop smoking lead to permanent quitting, even for heavy smokers. Quitting is usually easier if family and friends are supportive.

Personal safety

Personal safety is protecting yourself against accidental injury and death at home and on the road. You can protect yourself from death and injury in a motor vehicle by wearing your seat belts and obeying the speed limit. Simple changes in your safety practices can have a dramatic impact on your risk of injury.

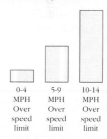

Risk of dying in a motor vehicle accident based on speed

| 0-4 MPH Over speed limit | 5-9 MPH Over speed limit | 10-14 MPH Over speed limit |

Simple changes in your health habits can dramatically reduce your risk.

Self care

Overexposing your skin to sun can cause cancer. Taking old prescriptions without consulting a physician can lead to serious illness. To have good health you have to take care of yourself. Self care, for example, brushing and flossing your teeth and breast self examination is important to preserving health. No matter how good your physician is, many health problems can only be avoided through the action you take yourself.

Alcohol use

Problem drinking and alcoholism are our number one drug abuse problem. Excessive drinking can damage the heart, blood vessels, liver, central nervous system, throat, stomach and intestines. It is also linked to cancer, heart attack and high blood pressure. High alcohol use often interferes with personal relationships and productivity at home and at work, and can result in serious legal and financial problems as well.

dicates, more companies offered health risk appraisals than offered exercise programs, stress management programs, and blood pressure control programs.

TABLE 40-3.

PERCENT OF WORKSITES OFFERING DIFFERENT TYPES OF HEALTH PROMOTION PROGRAMS

Type of Health Promotion Program	Percent of Worksites
Smoking cessation	19.4%
Health risk appraisal	18.9%
Exercise	16.1%
Stress management	14.8%
Healthy back	13.2%
Blood pressure control	11.7%
Weight management	11.2%

From: National Survey of Worksite Health Promotion Activities
The Office of Disease Prevention and Health Promotion
Department of Health and Human Services

Most companies use the health risk appraisal as a first step in a health promotion program. Objectives of using the health risk appraisal are to motivate employees and increase their awareness of the relationship between risk and disease. It can also direct them to the appropriate follow-up programs. Someone who discovers that smoking is increasing his risk of heart disease by 30% is probably more likely to join a smoking cessation program than someone without that information.

Some companies are using data from the health risk appraisal on a group of employees to plan and evaluate worksite health promotion programs. A sample of one page from such a report is shown in Table 40-4. In this company, 321 or 33% of the employees surveyed currently smoke. For most companies, this number would be large enough to justify a smoking cessation program. A year or two later this same company could determine if the percentage of smokers decreased after offering a smoking cessation program. In this way, a benefits manager or program director can use

summary data from the health risk appraisal to plan the components of a health promotion program, evaluate these components, and, in some cases, justify them to top-level managers.

Distributions of individual exercise, cigarette smoking, and alcohol habits are shown. Information from individual reports is placed in the categories listed under each area.

TABLE 40-4.

HEALTH HABITS
SPECIFIC HEALTH BEHAVIORS OF THE GROUP

	Number of Participants	Percent
Exercise		
2000 kcal/week or more in physical activity	344	35%
Exercise 20 minutes 3 times per week	251	26%
Cigarette Smoking		
Current cigarette smokers	321	33%
Former cigarette smokers	348	36%
Never smoked cigarettes	309	31%
Alcohol		
Drink 26 or more drinks/week	58	6%
Drink 15–25 drinks/week	141	14%
Drink fewer than 15 drinks/week	682	70%
Non-Drinker	97	10%
Drink as many as 8 drinks in a day	18	2%
Drink as many as 5–7 drinks in a day	39	4%

Health profile group report Notable Enterprises, Incorporated

Hospitals

Hospitals use health risk appraisals in programs for their own employees and in both community and worksite programs, often as a key component of a periodic health assessment or screening program. Because of the availability of nurses and other professional resources, hospitals frequently use health risk appraisals that place a greater emphasis on laboratory tests and physiologic measurements.

Health Maintenance Organizations

A growing number of HMOs (Health Maintenance Organizations) and PPOs (Preferred Provider Organizations) are mailing health risk appraisals to new and existing members to promote the organization and reinforce the interest of new members in personal health improvement. Because of their cost consciousness, HMOs and PPOs often use less expensive self-scored and simple one-page computerized appraisals.

Health Insurance Companies

Many insurance companies use HRAs as a promotional offering or premium to individuals and companies signing up for life insurance, health insurance, or disability insurance. In the future, insurance companies may also use HRAs to collect information that can help them project the costs of health insurance for a specific group.

Physicians and Other Health Care Professionals

The original health risk appraisal was developed to assist physicians in counseling their patients. Increasingly, physicians and other health care professionals are using the health risk appraisal as part of a physical or other initial assessment or as a starting point for more in-depth discussion concerning risk reduction and health improvement.

A wide variety of users with differing needs and growing demands have led to the growth of a new industry comprised of many small companies developing and offering HRAs. As a result of increasing competition within this industry, health risk appraisals have become more specialized and more diverse. Hundreds of variations on the original theme of collecting, processing, and providing risk information have been developed. Some of the major variations are described below.

1. **The Age-Group-Specific Health Risk Appraisal**. Most available health risk appraisals are of greatest value to the population aged 30 to 50. Many of these project the risk of dying from specific diseases in the next 10 years based on individual risk factors. Ten-year risk estimates based on bad health habits may be quite salient to a 45-year-old. For a 20-year-old, however, the same habits may lead to only a small increment in projected 10-year risk since cancer and acquired heart disease are rare in the 20s. Many HRAs are also less appropriate for the other end of the age spectrum. HRAs that mainly quantify risk will show a 70-year-old with excellent health habits that he still has a very high risk of dying in the next 10 years. This honest yet discouraging news is probably of less importance to him than his quality of life and ability to prevent disability.

   For these and other reasons, specific health risk appraisals have been and are being developed for the young and the old. In general, HRAs for the young place a greater emphasis on motor vehicle accidents and long-term prevention; HRAs for the older population tend to place less importance on risks and more importance on quality of living, safety, and other health issues most pertinent to this age group.

2. **The Disease-Specific Health Risk Appraisal**. Most health risk appraisals assess risks for the major causes of death: heart disease, cancer, motor vehicle accidents, stroke, and sometimes others. Some HRAs, however, focus on one disease. The appraisals developed by a few nonprofit voluntary agencies, for example, may focus exclusively or predominantly on cancer or heart disease.

3. **The Habit-Specific Health Risk Appraisal**. Just as there are HRAs that focus on one disease, there are also HRAs that focus on a particular health behavior, such as diet, stress, or fitness. These assessments generally do not include quantifiable risk information, since the risk of developing cancer, heart disease, or other conditions depends on many factors and cannot be assessed by looking at just one health habit. These instruments can have significant educational value in part due to their limited scope.

However, used alone, a particular instrument may give the false impression that its subject area is the most important to cover, and this will divert attention from other important opportunities for personal health improvement.

4. **The Interactive Health Risk Appraisal.** A few major companies and some software houses have developed interactive computerized HRAs using computer-based questionnaires. The questions asked of an individual depend upon the answers to his previous questions. For example, a man answering that he is male and 35-years-old will only receive those questions appropriate for his age and sex. Other computer programs simulate what effect changing certain habits would have on an individual's risk levels. For example, a person can see how increased exercise affects his risk of a heart attack or how driving with a safety belt affects his risk of serious motor vehicle injury.

The wide variety of health risk appraisals makes choosing among them difficult, especially when different types of HRAs fill different needs. A physician using an HRA as part of a comprehensive physical may choose, and appropriately so, a different appraisal than a company interested in increasing employee's knowledge of health risks.

Clearly defining how and why an appraisal will be used is the first step in selecting a health risk appraisal. Once the goals and uses have been determined, comparing several HRAs using the guidelines that follow may prove helpful in sorting through and selecting an instrument.

GUIDELINES FOR SELECTING A HEALTH RISK APPRAISAL: WHAT TO CONSIDER BEFORE YOU CHOOSE

1. **Your Goals.** Your goals and objectives will influence how you use and choose an HRA. Is the main purpose to increase personal awareness, to set a baseline, or to strongly encourage behavior change? Will the HRA stand alone or will it act as a gateway to other programs?

2. **Your Use.** How do you intend to use the health risk appraisal? Will the questionnaire accompany a health screening? Will lab results be included? Will a health educator or the post office deliver the results? Do you expect the results within minutes or within a month? Although you may have to make some compromises, the health risk appraisal you choose should fit your goals and uses.

3. **Your Target Group.** What is the age range and educational level of your target group? How varied is your group? Does the instrument need to be appropriate for a 25-year-old and a 60-year-old? Will most of your group be able to read and understand it?

4. **The HRA Design and Content.** As much as possible, the design and content of the instrument should help achieve your goals, fit your use, and reach your target group. Areas you may want to consider include the following:

   a. **The Length of the Questionnaire and Type of Report.** Questionnaires may require as little as 5 minutes and as much as an hour to complete. Some reports are designed to be explained by a health professional in a group session; others are designed so that they can be mailed directly to the individual, often with a number to call if there are any questions.

   b. **How the HRA Presents Risk.** Some HRAs don't quantify risk information at all, while others present results in terms of risk per 100,000 of dying over a 10-year period. Reporting that "You have a 800/100,000 risk of dying from lung cancer over the next 10 years" may be quite accurate but difficult for many users to interpret in a way that is personally meaningful.

   Some instruments convert total risk of dying into a health age or risk age—the sex-specific age for which the individual's risk would be average. For example, suppose a woman's overall risk of dying in the next 10 years is 2000/100,000. This may be much higher than the average for other women her age and similar to the average for women chronologically 15 years older. While this approach has intuitive appeal, it suggests to many that a person is aging biologically at a faster or slower rate than average. This is not correct and presents a misleading picture.

c. **The Health Areas Addressed.** Does the HRA address the health concerns of your group? The newer HRAs often incorporate more than risk information. They may also address safety, self-care, dental health, social support, and other important health areas. Many individuals report that this type of information is of greater personal importance than the quantification of their heart disease or cancer risks.

5. **The Credibility of the Vendor.** There is considerable variability in the validity of HRAs. Unfortunately, the relative validity of the models and programs are is difficult to assess. The following questions may help establish the credibility of the vendor:

- Who developed the instrument? Did the development include a team of recognized epidemiologists, statisticians, and behavioral experts?
- What are the major sources of data?
- How recently was the instrument revised?
- What types of internal edits exist to prevent an individual from receiving incorrect results?
- What procedures are followed to assure privacy and confidentiality?
- What types of model are used to assess risk?

Although having the absolute best estimate of risk may not be important to many users, it is critical to avoid providing incorrect or unreliable information. Incorrectly labeling an individual as anxious or falsely telling an individual that he

is at increased risk of cancer can have serious consequences.

Of course, health risk appraisals provide *probabilities, not predictions.* The most credible organization with the highest quality HRA can only provide estimates of risk. How accurate those estimates are depend not only on the program and the organization but also on current scientific knowledge. Understanding the limitations of this knowledge not only helps in choosing an instrument but will also help in using and explaining the appraisal.

Two of the more common limitations in the science of risk estimation are:

1. **Limited Information on Causes of Common Disease.** Although, as Table 40-2 shows, we know some risk factors for the major causes of death, we don't know the risk factors for other common and serious health problems, such as alcoholism, arthritis and stomach cancer. The indicators we know for heart disease, the major cause of death, can only predict about 50% of the deaths. In other cases, we may know that a risk factor contributes to a disease but we don't know how much. For example, we suspect that a lack of calcium contributes to high blood pressure and that depression increases the risk of suicide, but we're not sure by how much.

2. **Limited Ability to Account for Individual Differences.** At present, most HRAs are not sufficiently fine grained to account for individual differences. Consider the 50-year-old motorcyclist who has been riding for 30 years, drives defensively, never exceeds the speed limit, has a heavy motorcycle with fenders, and never drives at night. Does this motorcycle rider have the same risk of death from a crash per mile driven as an average motorcycle rider, which is about 9 times greater when compared to the average car driver? Probably not, since the average motorcyclist is in his early 20s, has limited driving experience, and is more likely to take chances. Although the HRA can provide

quite accurate information on large groups, its ability to provide accurate production information to an individual is more limited.

Some limitations of HRA won't change over time. Others, however, will greatly diminish with advances in biomedical and epidemiologi-cal research and improvements in computer hardware and software. Based on the rapid growth and increasing sophistication of HRAs in response to more discerning consumer demands, the future for HRAs as an integral part of personal health assessment is bright.

PART IX BIBLIOGRAPHY

Rochelle Perrine Schmalz, M.L.S., is director of the Planetree Health Resource Center, an innovative medical library for the layperson in San Francisco. She has extensive experience in the areas of patient education and consumer health information. Her book reviews have been published in *The San Francisco Chronicle, Medical Self-Care,* and *The Whole Earth Catalog.*

I. A FRAMEWORK FOR HEALTH

AMERICAN MEDICAL ASSOCIATION FAMILY MEDICAL GUIDE. New York: Random House, 1982.

Every home needs a basic medical reference book, and this is a good choice for those who want solid information and quick answers. A great 188-page section called "Symptoms and self-diagnosis" tells you when to apply home treatment and when to seek medical advice.

Ardell, Donald. 14 DAYS TO A WELLNESS LIFE-STYLE. Mill Valley, CA: Whatever Publ., 1982.

A game plan for achieving a higher state of well-being: improved physical health and emotional tranquility. Through self-diagnostic tests, charts, graphs, questionnaires, and a day-by-day program you should be able to improve your diet, physical fitness, stress response, and overall total health.

Arnot, Robert. THE COMPLETE MANUAL OF FITNESS AND WELL-BEING. New York: Viking Penguin, 1984.

This book, conceived and designed in England, has wonderful illustrations and pithy articles on how you can improve your overall quality of life. Covers everything from pregnancy to growing old gracefully. Motivating.

Berkeley Holistic Health Center. THE NEW HOLISTIC HEALTH HANDBOOK. Lexington, MA: The Stephen Greene Press, 1985.

An update of one of the first and best books on holistic health. A series of essays by experts covering everything from cancer prevention to nutrition to bodywork to the legal aspects of nontraditional medicine. A wonderful book for reference and inspiration.

Berkeley Holistic Health Center. THE HOLISTIC HEALTH LIFEBOOK: A GUIDE TO PERSONAL AND PLANETARY WELL-BEING. Berkeley: And/Or Press, 1981.

A companion volume to *The New Holistic Health Handbook*. How to apply holistic principles to your daily life.

Bricklin, Mark. THE PRACTICAL ENCYCLOPEDIA OF NATURAL HEALING. Rev. Ed. Emmaus, PA: Rodale Press, 1983.

From acne to yoga therapy, every common illness and natural healing modality is discussed. Good for quick reference and everyday use.

Brody, Jane. JANE BRODY'S THE NEW YORK TIMES GUIDE TO PERSONAL HEALTH. New York: Times Books, 1982; New York: Avon, 1983.

A comprehensive, authoritative guide to preventive health care and common illnesses. A traditional, scientific approach that provides solid information.

Dossey, Larry. BEYOND ILLNESS: DISCOVERING THE EXPERIENCE OF HEALTH. Boulder, CO: Shambala, 1984.

Dr. Dossey, physician and philosopher, uses both his commanding intellect and literary knowledge to write an insightful treatise on the nature of health and illness. These 14 essays challenge existing concepts of medicine and the doctor-patient relationship and offer a new way of defining health.

Dossey, Larry. SPACE, TIME AND MEDICINE. Boulder CO: Shambala, 1982.

The physics of health. Dossey advances the argument that the West's obsession with linear time profoundly affects our health and that changing our view of time can positively influence the course of disease. He also argues that there is a crisis in Western medicine which can only be resolved by radical change in attitude and practice. A compelling book.

Fries, James F., M.D. and Donald M. Vickery, M.D. TAKE CARE OF YOURSELF: A CONSUMER'S GUIDE TO MEDICAL CARE. 3rd ed. Reading, MA: Addison-Wesley, 1986.

One of the first and best books on self-care and self-diagnosis. Through the use of flow charts the book tells you when to use home treatment and when to seek medical care. A very useful book for home reference.

Griffith, H. Winter, M.D. COMPLETE GUIDE TO SPORTS INJURIES. Tucson, AZ: The Body Press, 1986.

A great book covering every conceivable athletic injury. Covers signs and symptoms, causes, risk assessment, appropriate health care, possible complications, treatment, and rehabilitation.

Inglis, Brian and Ruth West. THE ALTERNATIVE HEALTH GUIDE. New York: Knopf, 1983.

A delightful book from England that explores the variety of available alternative therapies. Divided into three sections—physical, psychological, and alternative therapies—this guide is well-written and well-illustrated. Particularly useful are the step-by-step illustrations showing you what to expect on a visit to an alternative practitioner.

Kaptchuk, Ted J. THE WEB THAT HAS NO WEAVER: UNDERSTANDING CHINESE MEDICINE. New York: Congdon & Weed, 1983.

The essentials of Chinese medicine explained with elegance and sensitivity. Understanding the Chinese philosophy of medicine requires new modes of thought and a dispelling of Western beliefs concerning how the body functions. Kaptchuk gently introduces his readers to new thought patterns and ways of conceptualizing health. Destined to become a classic.

Pelletier, Kenneth. HOLISTIC MEDICINE: FROM STRESS TO OPTIMUM HEALTH. New York: Delta, 1980.

A scholarly study of the essentials of holistic health with a particular focus on the importance of diet, exercise, and stress reduction. Citing current research in the field, Dr. Pelletier provides a cogent argument for the lifestyle changes that will result in optimum health and longevity.

Sobel, David, ed. WAYS OF HEALTH: HOLISTIC APPROACHES TO ANCIENT AND CONTEMPORARY MEDICINE. New York: Harcourt Brace Jovanovich, 1979.

An anthology of holistic views of health incorporating such healing systems as Navaho medicine, yogic theory, the laying on of hands, homeopathic medicine, and Chinese medicine. There is an intriguing chapter on the limits of modern medicine. An important collection for the reader who is interested in implementing changes in the medical system.

Weil, Andrew. HEALTH AND HEALING: UNDERSTANDING CONVENTIONAL & ALTERNATIVE MEDICINE. Boston: Houghton Mifflin, 1983.

A thought-provoking book on the concept of health, offering such ideas as: "illness is a necessary complement to wellness," "the body has innate healing abilities," "every body is different and every body has a weak point." Explores the various therapies from allopathic to homeopathy to faith healing. Helps you choose the best therapy for you. Good section on the placebo response.

II.   HEALTH EMPOWERMENT: YOURSELF

Adler, Robert. PSYCHONEUROIMMUNOLOGY. New York: Academic Press, 1981.

A thoroughly documented academic treatise on the interaction of mind, endocrines, and the immune system. Chapter titles include: "Immunologic abnormalities in mental illness," "Stress and immunologic competence," "Psychosocial factors in human cancer." This book is for those who seek scientific basis for the mind/body effect.

Benson, Herbert. THE MIND/BODY EFFECT. New York: Berkley, 1980, c1979.

A readable book on the relationship between illness and psychological factors. Dr. Benson combines an easy writing style with extensive research into the medical literature to produce a book that encourages the patient to take responsibility for his/her own health and develop a more productive doctor/patient relationship.

Cousins, Norman. ANATOMY OF AN ILLNESS AS PERCEIVED BY THE PATIENT. New York: Bantam, 1981, c1979.

If there is one single book that has revolutionized thinking on the ability of the patient to effect his own recovery from illness, this is it. A remarkable, inspirational book.

Dychtwald, Ken. BODY-MIND. New York: Jove, 1984, c1978.

A fascinating book that teaches you how your physical self reflects the shape of your mind. Taking the body from the head to the feet, Dychtwald describes body-mind interrelationships.

Gawain, Shakti. LIVING IN THE LIGHT. Mill Valley, CA: Whatever Publ., 1986.

Gawain, author of *Creative Visualization*, further develops her ideas and encourages readers to listen to their intuition while challenging the old behavior patterns and beliefs that may be holding them back.

Gawain, Shakti. CREATIVE VISUALIZATION. Mill Valley, CA: Whatever Publ., 1978. (Book and audiocassette)

A great introduction to the art of visualization. Gawain employs simple instructions that guide the reader/listener through the processes of mental imagery and relaxation. Good for beginners.

Goleman, Daniel. THE ESSENTIAL PSYCHOTHER-
APIES. New York: New American Library, 1982.

Hay, Louise L. SELF-HEALING. Los Angeles: Hay
House, 1984. (audio-cassette).

> A metaphysical approach to healing that teaches
> you how to recognize and change those negative
> thought patterns that may be creating poor health.

Hutschnecker, Arnold A. THE WILL TO LIVE. New
York: Simon and Schuster, 1983, c1951.

> A classic—one of the first, and still one of the
> best—in its field. Thirty-odd years after its initial
> publication, it still imparts a powerful message
> and shows you how to avoid illness by under-
> standing the emotional problems that may cause
> it.

LeShan, Lawrence L. HOW TO MEDITATE. New
York: Bantam, 1981, c1974.

> A simple, straightforward approach to the various
> types of meditation. Popular, good for beginners.

Locke, Steven E. MIND AND IMMUNITY: BEHAV-
IORAL IMMUNOLOGY: AN ANNOTATED BIBLI-
OGRAPHY 1976–1982. Praeger, 1983.

> Abstracts of over 1300 articles from 200 journals
> that discuss the interactions of the immune and
> nervous systems.

Peck, M. Scott. THE ROAD LESS TRAVELED. New
York: Simon and Schuster, 1978.

> An inspiring book that acknowledges that life is a
> painful process but that through confronting and
> resolving the pain, one can become more serene
> and fulfilled.

Samuels, Mike and Nancy Samuels. SEEING WITH
THE MIND'S EYE: THE HISTORY AND TECH-
NIQUES OF VISUALIZATION. New York: Random
House, 1975.

> A visually sumptuous in-depth look at visualiza-
> tion that opens the mind's eye to an inner world
> of exploration.

III. HEALTH EMPOWERMENT:
YOUR ENVIRONMENT

A. COMMUNITY/FAMILY/FRIENDS/SELF-HELP

Bezold, Clement. THE FUTURE OF PHARMACEU-
TICALS. New York: Wiley, 1981.

Cohen, Sheldon and S. Leonard Syme, ed. SOCIAL
SUPPORT AND HEALTH. Orlando, FL: Academic
Press, 1985.

> An academic treatise that addresses the impor-
> tance of social support networks in health and

well-being. It is "...a guide for doing further
> research on social support and health, and a
> source of information on the implications of exist-
> ing work for clinical practice and public policy."

Dass, Ram and Paul Gorman. HOW CAN I HELP?:
STORIES AND REFLECTIONS ON SERVICE. New
York: Knopf, 1985.

> A spiritual exploration on the nature of helping
> others either through work, volunteering, or in
> everyday life. People want to help others but are
> often confronted with such thoughts as "What can
> I do?" "Do I have anything worthwhile to con-
> tribute?" "What if I burn out?" Through vignettes
> and personal stories, the authors answer these
> questions and remind us that helping others is a
> basic tenet of society.

Duhl, Leonard, M.D. HEALTH PLANNING AND
SOCIAL CHANGE. Port Washington, N.Y.: Human
Science Press, 1986.

Fielding, Jonathan E. ANNUAL REVIEW OF PUBLIC
HEALTH. Palo Alto, CA: Annual Reviews Inc.

Gartner, Alan and Frank Riessman. THE SELF-HELP
REVOLUTION. New York: Human Sciences Press,
1984.

> This collection of essays is a scholarly treatise
> on the burgeoning self-help phenomenon. While
> focusing on specific self-help groups such as
> Recovery and Parent Anonymous, these evaluative
> essays are good guides to what does and doesn't
> work. This is an excellent resource for the layper-
> son who is interested in organizing a self-help
> group.

Lowell, Levin, Ph.D. SELF-CARE: LAY INITIATIVES.
Canton, MA: Watson, 1976.

> One of the first scholarly books written on the
> subject of self-care.

Rubin, Lillian. JUST FRIENDS: THE ROLE OF
FRIENDSHIP IN OUR LIVES. New York: Harper &
Row, 1985.

> Friendship, that fragile bond. What is it? What
> makes it work? Rubin, through interviews with
> over 300 people, focuses on the variety and
> importance of friendship. She explores friendship
> in marriage, friendship between men and wom-
> en, and the nature of best friends. A compassion-
> ate study of important relationships.

Simonton, Stephanie Matthews. THE HEALING
FAMILY: THE SIMONTON APPROACH FOR FAMI-
LIES FACING ILLNESS. New York: Bantam, 1984.

Serious illness not only profoundly affects the individual but can create disharmony within a family. Simonton draws on her extensive experience in cancer counseling and treatment to write a most valuable book on keeping families together during times of crisis while being supportive of the patient.

B.   YOUR WORK AND WORK PLACE

Jaffe, Dennis T. and Cynthia D. Scott. FROM BURNOUT TO BALANCE: A WORKBOOK FOR PEAK PERFORMANCE AND SELF-RENEWAL. New York: McGraw-Hall, 1984.

A guidebook for attaining mastery of those life situations which lead to people feeling overwhelmed by daily pressures and demands. Each chapter selects a problem area, presents a self-assessment questionnaire, and offers helpful techniques for coping with workplace stress.

Kriegel, Robert and Marilyn Harris Kriegal. THE C ZONE: PEAK PERFORMANCE UNDER PRESSURE. Garden City, NY: Anchor/Doubleday, 1984.

How to get from the D(rone) zone or the P(anic) zone to the C(onfidence) zone and turn stress and pressure into success. A real motivator for improving your work performance.

Lakein, Alan. HOW TO GET CONTROL OF YOUR TIME AND YOUR LIFE. New York: New American Library, 1973.

The best book on time management. Read it, apply the basic principles, and most of your time pressures will disappear.

Makower, Joel. OFFICE HAZARDS: HOW YOUR JOB CAN MAKE YOU SICK. Washington, D.C.: Tilden Press, 1981.

Documents hundreds of health and safety hazards that office workers face daily—photocopiers, video display terminals, boredom, and stress. The appendix includes office safety questionnaires, instructions for filing a complaint, and office exercises.

Pelletier, Kenneth R. HEALTHY PEOPLE IN UNHEALTHY PLACES. New York: Delacorte Press/Seymour Lawrence, 1984.

A scholarly study on the health problems inherent to the workplace—stress, burnout, toxic exposure, workaholic behavior—and how the individual and the corporation can work together to create a positive, healthy work environment. Reviews existent health promotion programs.

Polakoff, Phillip L. WORK & HEALTH: IT'S YOUR LIFE. Washington, D.C.: Press Assoc., 1984.

Dr. Polakoff is an expert in occupational health specializing in asbestos. He's written a highly readable book for the layperson explaining the physical, psychological, and emotional hazards of the workplace. Includes a glossary and resource lists of occupational health and safety organizations and agencies.

C.   HEALTH HAZARDS IN THE ENVIRONMENT

California Department of Consumer Affairs. CLEAN YOUR ROOM! A COMPENDIUM ON INDOOR AIR POLLUTANTS. Sacramento, CA: Department of Consumer Affairs, 1982.

How modern building design and the use of toxic building materials are endangering health and life. A very thorough report with excellent references.

HEALTH LETTER. 2000 P Street, N.W., Washington, D.C. 20036. $9.00/year for six issues.

This is a new activist newsletter conceived with the intention of warning the health care consumer about environmental and occupational hazards. An up-to-date informative publication.

Laws, Priscilla W. THE X-RAY INFORMATION BOOK: A CONSUMER'S GUIDE TO AVOIDING UNNECESSARY MEDICAL AND DENTAL X-RAYS. New York: Farrar, Straus, Giroux, 1983.

Researched with the help of Ralph Nader's Public Citizen Health Research Group, this book gives a clear perspective on the benefits and risks associated with medical x-rays, and how you can minimize your exposure. Discusses diagnostic x-rays only.

McCann, Michael. ARTIST BEWARE. New York: Watson-Guptill, 1979.

A comprehensive guide to the dangers of working with arts and crafts materials. Part one lists general hazards and warnings (materials, studio ventilation, protective equipment); part two lists the hazards of specific techniques (painting, printmaking, sculpture, etc.). A necessary book for the working artist.

Ott, John N. HEALTH AND LIGHT. New York: Pocket Books, 1983, c1973.

A fascinating book on the effect of artificial and natural light on man, how the right kind of light can cure certain illnesses, and how the wrong type of light can inflict harm. A real mind-opener.

Saifer, Phyllis and Merla Zellerback. DETOX. Los Angeles, Tarcher, distributed by Houghton Mifflin, 1984.

> A highly useful book for freeing yourself from the effects of nicotine, drugs, chemical pollutants, junk food addiction, and other environmental toxins. There is a general detox program plus nine programs for specific toxins. The excellent resource section lists toxins and detoxification centers.

Samuels, Mike and Hal Zina Bennett. WELL BODY, WELL EARTH: THE SIERRA CLUB ENVIRONMENTAL HEALTH SOURCEBOOK. San Francisco: Sierra Club Books, 1983.

> The authors write books which illuminate their subject in a wonderfully sensitive, informative manner. Through statistics, essays, and illustrations they, outline a program for dealing with environmental hazards in daily life. The best overall guide for the layperson.

Van Strum, Carol. A BITTER FOG: HERBICIDES AND HUMAN RIGHTS. San Francisco: Sierra Club Books, 1983.

> A well written expose on how herbicidal spraying in the United States affects human health. The book focuses on the spraying of Agent Orange in rural Oregon and the subsequent campaign by private citizens against herbicides. Provides a strong warning to the rest of the country.

IV.   STRESS AND STRESS MANAGEMENT

Benson, Herbert. BEYOND THE RELAXATION RESPONSE: HOW TO HARNESS THE HEALING POWER OF YOUR PERSONAL BELIEFS. New York: Berkley, 1985, c1984.

> Dr. Benson introduces the concept of the "Faith Factor," an individual's belief system which, when combined with meditation, can be used to reduce or alleviate many health problems such as backache, hypertension, and panic attacks. His theories are backed by extensive research into the medical literature and experiences taken from his own practice.

Benson, Herbert. THE RELAXATION RESPONSE. New York: Avon, 1975.

> The classic book on stress reduction. How to meditate and why.

Brod, Craig. TECHNOSTRESS: THE HUMAN COST OF THE COMPUTER REVOLUTION. Reading, MA: Addison-Wesley, 1984.

> Is "technostress" a new disease, stemming from the computer revolution? This book advances the theory that living in an increasingly computerized society has a profound effect on people's lives. A challenging book.

Davis, Martha and others. THE RELAXATION AND STRESS REDUCTION WORKBOOK. Oakland: New Harbinger, 1984, c1980.

> A step-by-step guide to learning the techniques of stress reduction and management.

Eliot, Robert S. IS IT WORTH DYING FOR? A SELF-ASSESSMENT PROGRAM TO MAKE STRESS WORK FOR YOU, NOT AGAINST YOU. New York: Bantam, 1984.

> A highly practical book on how you can take responsibility for reducing negative stress elements in your life through fitness, relaxation techniques, and changes in lifestyle. Has a great chapter on determining whether you are a "hot reactor."

Konicov, Barrie. POTENTIALS UNLIMITED, 9390 Whitneyville Road, Alto, MI 49302.

> This series of audio-cassettes offers two different approaches: voice/hypnosis on one side and music/subliminal (hidden messages) on the other side. The hypnosis side is straightforward. Dr. Konicov's voice is soothing and his text makes sense. The subliminal side combines music and ocean sounds and may be effective for those people who tend to overanalyze. The series covers unique topics, most of which are stress-related: stop nail-biting, agoraphobia, painless dentistry.

Miller, Emmett. SOURCE TAPES, 945 Evelyn Street, Menlo Park, CA 94025

> Dr. Miller has produced this wonderful series of hypnotically relaxing audio-cassettes which are immensely popular and effective. Topics range from stress reduction to preparing for surgery. Tapes combine music, voice, and mental imagery, and are excellent for people who have difficulty sticking with books. Some of his best-selling titles are *Rainbow, Butterfly, Healing Journey*, and *Letting Go of Stress*.

Pelletier, Kenneth R. MIND AS HEALER, MIND AS SLAYER. New York: Dell, 1984, c 1977.

One of the classic books on the role of stress in the etiology of disease. Describes the psychological and emotional factors that predispose one to illness. An academic approach that deserves time and attention.

Tubesing, Donald. KICKING YOUR STRESS HABIT. Duluth, MN: Whole Person Press, 1983, c1981.

A great introductory course on stress reduction that offers practical guidelines and exercises. The underlying theme is stop and reflect.

WINDHAM HILL RECORDS, P.O. Box 9388, Stanford, CA 94305.

The records produced by this company have nothing to do with health but everything to do with making you feel relaxed and easy. They're great for the evening commute home. The best artists are William Ackerman and George Winston.

V.   NUTRITION AND DIET

Freydberg, Nicholas and Willis A. Gortner. The Food Additives Book. New York: Bantam, 1982.

Explains the nature and function of additives and reviews 6000 brand-name foods.

Gussow, Joan Dye. THE FEEDING WEB: ISSUES IN NUTRITIONAL ECOLOGY. Palo Alto: Bull, 1978.

A most relevant book about food and the environment—both social and natural. It's distressing to see issues Gussow raised in 1978 still unsolved almost a decade later.

Haskell, William, James Scala, and James Whittam, eds. NUTRITION AND ATHLETIC PERFORMANCE: PROCEEDINGS OF THE CONFERENCE ON NUTRITIONAL DETERMINANTS IN ATHLETIC PERFORMANCE, SAN FRANCISCO, CALIFORNIA, SEPTEMBER 24–25, 1981. Palo Alto: Bull, 1982.

This compilation of scientific articles is a state-of-the-art review of the role of nutrition in vigorous competitive exercise.

Schell, Orville. MODERN MEAT. New York: Random House, 1984.

A truly important book that investigates the use of antibiotics and hormones in the livestock industry. Thoroughly researched, well-written, but you may never want to eat a hamburger again.

Winter, Ruth. A CONSUMER'S DICTIONARY OF FOOD ADDITIVES. Rev. ed. New York: Crown, 1984.

Food additives—what they are and where they're found. The dictionary approach makes this a handy reference tool.

B.   NUTRITION AND YOUR HEALTH

Ballentine, Rudolph. DIET AND NUTRITION: A HOLISTIC APPROACH. Honesdale, PA: Himalayan International Inst., 1982, c1978.

Compares and contrasts Eastern and Western attitudes about nutrition. Covers biochemistry, physiology, and pharmacology of nutrition for the lay reader. A well-researched book that also discusses the philosophy of nutrition.

Bricklin, Mark. THE NATURAL HEALING COOKBOOK. Emmaus, PA: Rodale, 1981.

A detailed, nicely illustrated book that gives sound advice on how to increase resistance, prevent illness, and speed recuperation when ill. Its particular value is in providing recommendations for specific illnesses.

Brody, Jane. JANE BRODY'S NUTRITION BOOK. New York: Norton, 1982.

A comprehensive book on nutrition and weight control by *The New York Times* health columnist. A well-documented, traditional view of the subject. Good for reference. Brody and Ballentine would be excellent selections for a core home nutrition library.

Brown, Gene. LOWER YOUR CHOLESTEROL. New York: Tribeca, 1984.

An inexpensive, useful book loaded with good information on how you can lower your cholesterol level. Detailed guide to the fat and cholesterol content of over 850 foods. A great bargain.

Faelton, Sharon and the Editors of Prevention Magazine. THE COMPLETE BOOK OF MINERALS FOR HEALTH. Emmaus, PA: Rodale Press, 1981.

How minerals can be incorporated into the diet to improve health and prevent disease. With recipes.

NUTRITION ACTION. (Center for Science in the Public Interest, 1775 S Street, N.W., Washington, D.C. 20009.) $20.00/year for 12 issues.

A consumer advocacy magazine for the layperson. Good content with an activist orientation.

Penington, Jean A.T. and Helen Nichols Church. FOOD VALUES OF PORTIONS COMMONLY USED. 14th ed. New York: Harper & Row, 1985.

The single most useful book on the nutritional content of foods. Covers calories, fat, cholesterol, fiber, protein, carbohydrates, saturated and polyunsaturated fatty acids, vitamins, minerals, salicylates, sugar, purine, and many more. Invaluable.

Prevention Magazine. THE COMPLETE BOOK OF VITAMINS. Emmaus, PA: Rodale Press, 1984.

Everything you could want to know about vitamins and vitamin therapy for disease. The book has a nontraditional slant, but is backed up by research in the medical literature. Encyclopedic format.

Robertson, Laurel and others. LAUREL'S KITCHEN: A HANDBOOK FOR VEGETARIAN COOKERY. Petaluma, CA: Nilgiri Press, 1984, c1976; New York: Random House.

In its 12th printing, it's the classic book on vegetarianism. Commonsense approach to buying and cooking food along with extensive and excellent nutritional tables.

Rohe, Fred. THE COMPLETE BOOK OF NATURAL FOODS. Boulder, CO: Shambala, 1983.

A nice book written from the heart, but backed by thorough knowledge of the subject. This handbook tells you how to buy, cook, process, and store natural foods. A guide for anyone who seriously wants to develop a healthier lifestyle.

Silverman, Harold and others. THE VITAMIN BOOK: A NO-NONSENSE CONSUMER GUIDE. New York: Bantam, 1985.

A much-needed reference book that helps clear up the confusion and contradictory information about vitamins and minerals. Written by pharmacists, this handy book profiles 35 different vitamins, therapeutic effectiveness, vitamin/-drug interactions, and the value of megadoses. Compares 10 popular weight-loss diets for nutritional content. The extensive bibliography makes this book invaluable.

TUFTS UNIVERSITY DIET & NUTRITION LETTER. (475 Park Avenue South, New York, NY 10016.) $18.00/year for 12 issues.

A newsletter with a traditional viewpoint on diet and nutrition. Emphasizes current research from the scientific literature combined with helpful eating hints and recipes.

C.   EATING DISORDERS

Chernin, Kim. THE HUNGRY SELF: WOMEN, EATING & IDENTITY. New York: Times Books, 1985.

Chernin explores the mother-daughter relationship as elemental in the evolution of eating disorders. At times her rhetoric becomes overblown; more often her words strike chords of immediate and profound recognition. For women struggling with anorexia, bulimia, or compulsive eating, reading Chernin and Orbach is essential.

Chernin, Kim. THE OBSESSION: REFLECTIONS ON THE TYRANNY OF SLENDERNESS. New York: Harper, 1981.

A landmark work on the cultural attitudes that influence women's preoccupation with weight and body size. It stands out for its intelligence, compassion, and insight into a disquieting subject.

Orbach, Susie. FAT IS A FEMINIST ISSUE II: A PROGRAM TO CONQUER COMPULSIVE EATING. Berkeley Books, 1982.

A psychotherapist's view of obesity with emphasis on compulsive eating and cultural responses. An excellent book for understanding what it means to be fat and how to change your habits if you really do wish to lose weight.

A practical guide to psychological exercises which address the persistent barriers that many women experience in dealing with their eating problems. The author points out the difference between emotional and physiological hunger and offers techniques to improve body image.

Pope, Harrison J. and James I. Hudson. NEW HOPE FOR BINGE EATERS: ADVANCES IN THE UNDERSTANDING AND TREATMENT OF BULIMIA. New York: Harper & Row, 1984.

A thorough explanation of bulimia written by two physicians. There is an excellent review of treatment options backed by research in the medical literature. Includes a comprehensive bibliography and list of treatment centers.

VI.   EXERCISE

Alter, Judy. SURVIVING EXERCISE. Boston: Houghton Mifflin, 1983.

How to work out without injuring yourself. An excellent book for beginners on how to devise a safe exercise program. Alter tells you which exercises may be destructive (forget deep knee bends and back arching) and which will help you develop strength and suppleness. Reassurance for the wary.

Anderson, Bob. STRETCHING. Bolinas, CA: Shelter Publ., 1984, 1980.

Whatever your age or physical condition this will be a most beneficial book. Clear diagrams for easy methods of stretching. Over 400,000 copies sold by an obscure publisher is a tribute to the excellence of this book.

Bailey, Covert. FIT OR FAT?: A NEW WAY TO HEALTH AND FITNESS THROUGH NUTRITION AND AEROBIC EXERCISE. Boston: Houghton Mifflin, 1977.

Everybody's favorite book on fitness. Explains why aerobic activity is the key to reducing body fat and body weight. The book presents a sensible balance of eating and activity that should increase metabolic rate and thus burn off fat. One of the most important books on exercise and nutrition.

Bailey, Covert. FIT-OR-FAT TARGET DIET. Boston: Houghton Mifflin, 1984.

A companion volume to *Fit or Fat?* that stresses the importance of removing fat from the American diet. Offers basic dietary principles and sound ideas for health improvement.

Cooper, Kenneth. THE AEROBICS PROGRAM FOR TOTAL WELL-BEING. New York: Bantam, 1982.

Dr. Cooper, the major writer on aerobics, tells how to improve your quality of life through fitness. Details on how to gauge, improve, and maintain individual fitness levels. Good sections on weight loss diets, food myths, and the principles of nutrition. There are fitness training charts for most sports and a list of sports medicine clinics.

Galloway, Jeff. GALLOWAY'S BOOK ON RUNNING. New York: Random House, 1984.

Galloway, a 1972 Olympian in the 10,000 meters, runs the gamut from training to injuries to nutrition to physiology in this book that is appropriate for both the beginner and the experienced marathoner. The writing style is easy and the advice practical.

Glover, Bob and Jack Shepherd. THE RUNNER'S HANDBOOK. New York: Penguin, 1985.

Smart running guidelines for all ages and abilities. Advice on pacing, diets, mental attitude, injury prevention and treatment. Very helpful sections on running for those with physical handicaps and health problems such as alcoholism and hearing loss. A good book for getting started.

Johnson, Don. BODY. Boston: Beacon Press, 1983.

A philosophy of the body. Johnson links body movement, body image, and body ideal with such social institutions as school, religion, and the military. He makes us aware of how we are pressured to mold ourselves to fit others' needs and we therefore lose the connection with our own body. A provocative author, Johnson urges us to reunite our feeling and thought, mind and body.

Lidell, Lucy. THE SIVANANDA COMPANION TO YOGA. New York: Simon and Schuster, 1983.

Of the many books written about yoga, this one is the most inspiring and beautifully done. Some of the postures are very advanced, but many are aimed at the beginner or intermediate practitioner. Very well photographed with good explanations of the philosophy behind yoga.

Morris, Alfred. SPORTS MEDICINE HANDBOOK. Dubuque, IA: Wm.C. Brown, 1985.

Gives useful advice on recognizing the difference between proper training and the overtraining that creates body stress. Strength training and flexibility exercises are emphasized to reduce the possibility of injury. Good sections on weather and environmental hazards.

Shangold, Mona and Gabe Mirkin. THE COMPLETE SPORTS MEDICINE BOOK FOR WOMEN. New York: Simon and Schuster, 1985.

A reference book for the active woman who doesn't have the time to read a long treatise on sports medicine. Answers questions on diet, proper clothing, prevention and treatment of injury, exercise throughout the life cycle (menopause, pregnancy). Discusses special medical problems such as asthma, earaches, and nosebleeds.

Ullyot, Joan. THE NEW WOMEN'S RUNNING. Brattleboro, VT: Stephen Greene Press, 1984.

Running for women at all levels of experience. Includes training tables, advice for getting started, equipment, safety, and specific advice on preventing injuries to the female body.

VIII.   SPECIFIC HEALTH ISSUES

A.   A HEALTHY HEART

Amsterdam, Ezra A. and A.M. Holmes. TAKE CARE OF YOUR HEART. New York: Facts on File, 1984.

The best general book for the layperson. Explains how the heart works, symptoms and prevention of heart disease, medical and surgical treatments, rehabilitation methods following a heart attack. Full of interesting facts and useful information.

American Medical Association. THE AMERICAN MEDICAL ASSOCIATION STRAIGHT-TALK, NO-NONSENSE GUIDE TO HEART-CARE. Rev. ed. New York: Random House, 1984.

A very helpful book for the heart patient and people who wish to prevent heart disease. Stresses the importance of diet, exercise, and stress reduction for maintaining a healthy heart.

Bennett, Cleaves M. CONTROL YOUR HIGH BLOOD PRESSURE WITHOUT DRUGS. New York: Doubleday, 1984.

This is a great book for anyone who wants to improve their health and lower their blood pressure. Offers a sensible 12-week program for learning positive nutrition, exercise, and stress reduction habits.

CORONARY CLUB BULLETIN. (3659 Green Road, #200, Cleveland, OH 44122.) Monthly. $12.00/year.

This valuable newsletter offers information on current trends in cardiovascular medicine and practical advice for the layperson. A recent issue had an article on what to eat while travelling in Great Britain. Up-to-date and reliable.

De Bakey, Michael E., M.D. THE LIVING HEART DIET. New York: Raven, 1984.

A sensible, medically-tested diet for people with, or at risk for, heart disease. Recipes, tables, discussion of risk factors.

Farquhar, John W., M.D. THE AMERICAN WAY OF LIFE NEED NOT BE HAZARDOUS TO YOUR HEALTH. Stanford, CA: Stanford Alumnni Association, 1978.

An important book that discusses the significance of exercise, smoking, body weight, diet, and stress in the role of heart disease. Guidelines for implementing a program to reduce the risk of heart disease.

Friedman, Meyer and Diane Ulmer. TREATING TYPE A BEHAVIOR. New York: Knopf, 1984.

Takes the original concept of Type A behavior one step further by telling you how to treat it. Based on an extensive 5-year study, this book shows you how to change your behavior and reduce your risk of heart attack.

Friedman, Meyer and Diane Ulmer. TYPE A BEHAVIOR AND YOUR HEART. New York: Fawcett, 1981, c1974.

Defines Type A behavior and gives guidelines on how to reduce the possibility of a heart attack. Discusses correlation between behavior and heart disease.

Ornish, Dean. STRESS, DIET, & YOUR HEART. New York: New American Library, 1982.

An informative book about preventing heart disease through stress reduction and changes in diet. Includes recipes.

Piscatella, Joseph C. DON'T EAT YOUR HEART OUT COOKBOOK. New York: Workman, 1982.

A heart patient's guide to healthy cooking. Interesting, inventive recipes that reduce cholesterol, salt, fat, and sugar. Helpful meal planning tips.

B.   CANCER PREVENTION

Alabaster, Oliver. WHAT YOU CAN DO TO PREVENT CANCER. New York: Simon and Schuster, 1985.

Given the theory that 50% of cancer in women and 40% of cancer in men may be caused by diet, this is a helpful book for putting the anticancer diet into practice. The author, the head of cancer research at Washington University Medical Center, establishes the link between diet and cancer and offers recommendations for reducing your cancer risk. The dietary advice given in this book is sound and helpful for anyone who is looking for a disease prevention diet.

MALIGNANT NEGLECT. New York: Knopf, 1979.

One of the first books written on known or suspected environmental carcinogens. A complete rundown on consumer products (food dyes, artificial sweeteners), radiation, air pollution, and airborne carcinogens (asbestos, vinyl chloride).

Lerner, Michael with Naomi Remen, M.D. "Varieties of Integral Cancer Therapies". Advances 2(3); Summer, 1985, pp. 14–33.

Lerner expounds upon his theory that "the course of an illness could be influenced by the way doctors behave toward patients and by the opportunities open to patients to become involved in combatting their illness." A stimulating article.

Rosenbaum, Ernest H. CAN YOU PREVENT CANCER?: REALISTIC GUIDELINES FOR DEVELOPING CANCER PREVENTIVE LIFE HABITS. St. Louis: Mosby, 1983.

Realistically explains what you can do to lessen your chances of getting cancer. Talks about cancer screening, environment and occupational risks, genetic susceptibility, lifestyle, and nutrition.

C.   HOW TO KEEP YOUR BODY
     HAPPY AND HEALTHY

Bay Area Consumers' Checkbook. Spring 1985. (Checkbook, 222 Agriculture Building, 101 The Embarcadero, San Francisco, CA 94105). $.95 per issue.

Most people really care about keeping their teeth and gums healthy. This issue of CHECKBOOK has the most up-to-date information about prevention of tooth and gum disease. Although the focus is on the San Francisco Bay Area, this guide is helpful for anyone interested in dental health.

Block, Barry H. FOOT TALK. New York: Kensington, 1985, c1984.

Whether you're an athlete or sit at a desk all day, you should read this book. It's a fascinating mixture of the history of shoes, foot erotica, solid medical information, and basic foot care. Includes a foot health test, glossary, and foot exercises.

The Boston Women's Health Book Collective. THE NEW OUR BODIES, OURSELVES. New York: Simon and Schuster, 1984.

The most comprehensive view of women's health—physical, mental, and emotional—in print. It covers every aspect of a woman's life with sensitivity and intelligence. The resources following each chapter are superb.

Cailliet, Rene. UNDERSTAND YOUR BACKACHE: A GUIDE TO PREVENTION. TREATMENT, AND RELIEF. Philadelphia: F.A. Davis, 1984.

Dr. Cailliet very simply writes the best books on the diagnosis and treatment of various body pains (back, shoulder, knee, etc.). This is his only book for the layperson and he applies his considerable expertise in clearly explaining the spine, its function, and the varieties of pain that can occur when it is misused or injured. He gives advice for distinguishing between physical and psychological pain and the necessity for home office therapy.

Danzi, J. Thomas, M.D. FREE YOURSELF FROM DIGESTIVE PAIN: A GUIDE TO PREVENTING AND CURING YOUR DIGESTIVE ILLNESS. Englewood Cliffs, NJ: Prentice-Hall, 1984.

A very popular book that helps you understand and live with ulcers, heartburn, intestinal gas, diverticulosis, irritable bowel syndrome, and gallbladder disease.

Erlich, David. THE BOWEL BOOK: A PRACTICAL GUIDE TO GOOD HEALTH. New York: Schocken Books, 1981.

This is a subject nobody talks about but everybody cares about. The book is written in an informal, friendly style and offers advice on the prevention and cure of many common bowel complaints— constipation, diarrhea, hemorrhoids. Diet and exercise are covered.

Greenberger, Monroe E. and Mary-Ellen Siegel. WHAT EVERY MAN SHOULD KNOW ABOUT HIS PROSTATE. New York: Walker, 1983.

The prostate causes more problems for more men than almost any other body part. Written by a urologist with many years of experience, the book discusses prostate disorders, their prevention and treatment. A valuable book for men of any age.

Madaras, Lynn and Jane Patterson. WOMANCARE: A GYNECOLOGICAL GUIDE TO YOUR BODY. New York: Avon, 1984. Rev. ed.

An excellent guide to women's health and disease. Answers your questions on any subject from breast self-exam to endometriosis. The good explanations of female anatomy combined with the excellent resource guide makes this a useful book.

Rezen, Susan V. and Carl Hausman. COPING WITH HEARING LOSS: A GUIDE FOR ADULTS AND THEIR FAMILIES. New York: Dembner Books, 1985.

A book on hearing loss: why it occurs, how to prevent it, and what to do about it. Good information on the selection of hearing aids, how to choose an audiologist, and how to cope with social situations where hearing loss may cause problems.

Schneider, Myles J., D.P.M. and Mark D. Sussman, D.P.S. HOW TO DOCTOR YOUR FEET WITHOUT A DOCTOR. Washington, D.C.: Acropolis Books, 1984.

Two podiatrists tell you how to recognize and treat many foot problems and offer practical advice for preventing and alleviating foot pain. The illustrations, exercises, and clear instructions cover everything from blisters and bunions to foot care for the athlete and the elderly.

D. ALCOHOL AND DRUG ABUSE

Black, Claudia. IT WILL NEVER HAPPEN TO ME. Boulder, CO: M.A.C., 1981.

Understanding the effect of alcoholism on the family. Black explains roles and coping mechanisms adopted by children of alcoholics and carried into adulthood. Case histories of children are interspersed with guidelines for developing family interaction. Self-help and professional resources are included.

Brecher, Edward M. and the Editors of Consumer Reports. LICIT AND ILLICIT DRUGS: THE CONSUMERS UNION REPORT ON NARCOTICS, STIMULANTS, DEPRESSANTS, INHALANTS, HALLUCINOGENS, AND MARIJUANA—INCLUDING CAFFEINE, NICOTINE AND ALCOHOL. Boston: Little, Brown and Co., 1972.

After 15 years this book is still in print and still valuable as a general reference book on the pharmacology, sociology, and history of drugs in American culture. The statistics may have changed, but the problems haven't.

Chilnick, Lawrence D., ed. THE COKE BOOK. New York: Berkley, 1984.

A reliable reference book on what cocaine is, its uses and abuses, its effects on mind and body, and how the drug can profoundly affect many respectable lives. The authors don't preach; they do provide straightforward facts that allow you to make your own decisions about cocaine. Includes a list of cocaine treatment centers.

Chilnick, Lawrence D., ed. THE LITTLE BLACK PILL BOOK. New York: Bantam, 1983.

The average American may be appalled at the thought of using street drugs yet may be unwittingly addicted to prescription drugs. This book makes readers aware that although they may be under the care of a physician, they still have a responsibility to decide whether they are abusing their medication. It approaches addiction, not as a moral issue but as a disease that can be helped. Includes self-assessment lists to determine whether a potential for addiction exists.

DuPont, Robert L., Jr., M.D. GETTING THOUGH ON GATEWAY DRUGS. Washington, D.C.: American Psychiatric Press, 1984.

A hard-hitting family guide to the use and abuse of alcohol, marijuana, and cocaine. Offers guidance to families whose children, both adult and adolescent, have a problem with drugs.

Ketcham, Katherine. EATING RIGHT TO LIVE SOBER. Seattle: Madrona Publ., 1983.

A much-needed book on the role of diet and nutrition in the treatment of alcoholism. How to avoid those foods that alter the body's chemistry and substitute foods that renew the body. Thoroughly researched with good explanations of vitamins and minerals. Includes recipes.

McConville, Brigid. WOMEN UNDER THE INFLUENCE. New York: Schocken Books, 1983.

The effect of alcohol consumption on women's lives, from society's attitudes toward women and drinking to the physiological effects of alcohol on women's bodies. Special attention is given to alcohol and pregnancy and the prevention of fetal alcohol syndrome. Includes lists of alcohol treatment programs and further resources.

Milam, James R. and Katherine Ketcham. UNDER THE INFLUENCE: A GUIDE TO THE MYTHS AND REALITIES OF ALCOHOLISM. Seattle, WA: Madrona, 1981; New York: Bantam, 1983.

This book treats alcoholism as a physiological disease rather than a psychological weakness, thus removing the stigma of guilt from alcoholics. Includes important discussions of how nutrition and hypoglycemia relate to the disease, why typically prescribed drugs are dangerous, guides to treatment, and how families can help. The best book on understanding the physical aspects of alcoholism.

Mumey, Jack. THE JOY OF BEING SOBER. Chicago: Contemporary Books, 1984.

Now that you've given up drinking, how do you remain sober and still live in a society where alcohol plays an important part in daily life? This is a frank, gutsy approach to coping with family holidays, business lunches, and flying if you can only get on a plane if you're drunk.

Seixas, Judith and Geraldine Youcha. CHILDREN OF ALCOHOLISM: A SURVIVOR'S MANUAL. New York: Crown, 1985.

A guide for coping with and changing evolved behavior patterns associated with alcoholic families. Addresses concerns the adult child may have regarding his/her own social drinking and family dynamics. Resource lists for support groups and further information.

Silverman, Milton, Philip R. Lee, and Mia Lydecker. PRESCRIPTIONS FOR DEATH: THE DRUGGING OF THE THIRD WORLD. Berkeley: University of California Press, 1982.

An expose of multinational pharmaceutical companies and their practices, including "drug dumping" and marketing in developing countries.

Wholey, Dennis. THE COURAGE TO CHANGE. Boston: Houghton Mifflin, 1985.

If you read only one book on alcoholism, this should be it. Wholey, a recovering alcoholic, had a series of personal conversations with many well-known alcoholics on just what it took to get them to quit drinking. A powerful book that offers much encouragement to anyone wishing to make a major change in their life.

Young, Lawrence A. and others. RECREATIONAL DRUGS. New York: Berkley Books, 1982.

Everything you need to know about mind-altering drugs from cocaine to heroin, including some drugs you may never know existed (Hawaiian baby wood rose, yage). This book doesn't preach; it talks about effects, dangers, and warning signs. Lists the common names of the 88 drugs referenced.

E. PRESCRIPTION AND NONPRESCRIPTION DRUGS

Bezold, Clement, Rick Carlson, and Jonathan Peck. THE FUTURE OF WORK AND HEALTH. Auburn House, 1986.

Bezold, Clement, Jerome Halperin, Richard Ashbaugh, and Harold Binkley, eds. PHARMACY IN THE 21ST CENTURY. Auburn House.

Long, James W. THE ESSENTIAL GUIDE TO PRESCRIPTION DRUGS. 4th ed. New York: Harper & Row, 1985.

The best, most comprehensive book written for the layperson on drugs and their side effects. Gives generic and brand names, explains how the drug works, who shouldn't take it, adverse effects, precautions, and interactions.

United States Pharmacopeial Convention. ABOUT YOUR MEDICINES. (12601 Twinbrook Parkway, Rockville, MD 20852.) $12.00/year for 6 issues.

Recent articles discussed breast-feeding and pregnancy, antibiotic use and abuse. A regular feature keeps the consumer abreast of new drug product information.

United States Pharmacopeial Convention (USP DI): Vol. I, DRUG INFORMATION FOR THE HEALTH CARE PROVIDER; Vol. II, ADVICE FOR THE PATIENT. USPC, 12601 Twinbrook Parkway, Rockville, MD 20852.

May be purchased separately. Published annually. A useful compendium of drug information written by the organization that sets the standards for drug quality in the United States. The volume for patients is written in easy-to-read type and terminology. Covers precautions, proper use of medications, side effects.

Zimmerman, David R. THE ESSENTIAL GUIDE TO NONPRESCRIPTION DRUGS. New York: Harper & Row, 1983.

If you ever have wondered about the effectiveness of an over-the-counter drug, this is the book you need. Over 100 brand names from acne medication to reducing aids are evaluated for their efficacy and safety. A money saving book.

F. SMOKING

Geisinger, David L. KICKING IT: THE NEW WAY TO STOP SMOKING PERMANENTLY. New York: Grove Press, 1977.

A tough but supportive book discussing physiological and emotional dependency on cigarettes. Through a series of habit-breaking techniques it teaches the reader to conquer smoking addiction. Geisinger also gives a thorough analysis of the sociology of smoking.

Rogers, Jacquelyn. YOU CAN STOP. New York: Pocket Books, 1977.

Rogers, a cofounder of Smokeenders, looks at the reasons people smoke, and offers insights into why smoking doesn't really fulfill these needs. A nonthreatening, empathetic discussion.

Ross, Walter S. HOW TO STOP SMOKING—PERMANENTLY WITH THE NEW NICOTINE GUM. Boston: Little, Brown, 1985.

Discusses the hazards of smoking and the benefits of quitting by using the new nicotine gum. Endorsed by the former U.S. Surgeon General, tells how the gum eases the physiological withdrawal from cigarettes.

G. HEALTHY ELDERS

Christensen, Alice and David Rankin. EASY DOES IT YOGA FOR OLDER PEOPLE. New York: Harper & Row, 1975.

A gentle introduction to the practice of yoga for older people. The spiral binding allows the book to lie flat, making exercise easier. A real motivator for the inactive.

Comfort, Alex. A GOOD AGE. New York: Crown, 1976.

A classic. An encyclopedia of topics related to aging, covering everything from depression to rejuvenation research. Profiles of people engaged in a productive and creative old age makes this an uplifting book.

Ellison, Jerome. LIFE'S SECOND HALF: THE PLEASURES OF AGING. Old Greenwich, CT: Devin-Adair Co., 1978.

It is Ellison's theory that after age 40 life takes on a different tone and nature for which most people are unprepared. His book is both an encouragement and preparation for addressing the trials of aging. Sensitively written. Particularly good for those of retirement age.

Fonda, Jane. WOMEN COMING OF AGE. New York: Simon and Schuster, 1984.

Somebody once asked me, "Doesn't Jane Fonda give you an inferiority complex? I mean she looks so great for her age." I replied, "No, I'm glad she's there as an example and an inspiration." Her book is a little self-centered, but mostly it encourages and motivates women toward a positive, dynamic middle age.

Greenwood, Sadja. MENOPAUSE NATURALLY: PREPARING FOR THE SECOND HALF OF LIFE. San Francisco: Volcano Press, 1984.

A wonderful, joyous book on the menopause. Dr. Greenwood presents the physical, emotional, and psychological aspects of this special time of life. Great suggestions for how to deal with hot flashes, depression, and osteoporosis through diet and exercise. Highly recommended.

Henig, Robin Marantz and the editors of ESQUIRE. HOW A WOMAN AGES. New York: Ballantine Books, 1985.

A useful book designed to help you understand the aging process so you can get better as you get older. Examines the female body and how to keep all systems working efficiently throughout your life.

Minkler, Meredith, Ph.D., and Carroll L. Estes, eds. READINGS IN THE POLITICAL ECONOMY OF AGING. Farmingdale, NY: Baywood; Policy, Politics, Health, and Medicine Series: Vol. 6.

Natow, Annette and Jo Ann Heslin. NUTRITION FOR THE PRIME OF YOUR LIFE. New York: McGraw-Hill, 1983.

As people age, their eating habits often become lax and indifferent. This book gives good advice on adapting nutrition needs to aging and includes special diet information for osteoporosis, high blood pressure, and heart problems. There are sections on food and drug interactions, food additives, and a nutritional analysis of fast foods.

Notelovitz, Morris and Marsha Ware. STAND TALL! THE INFORMED WOMAN'S GUIDE TO OSTEOPOROSIS. New York: Bantam, 1985, c1982.

Osteoporosis (excessive loss of bone mass) is a condition that affects many women in their later years. This preventive guide discusses the role of hormones, diet, and exercise in the etiology, prevention, and treatment of this disabling disorder. Every woman should read this book.

Pelletier, Kenneth. LONGEVITY: FULFILLING OUR BIOLOGICAL POTENTIAL. New York: Delacorte, 1981.

An academic analysis of the relationship of longevity to lifestyle, nutrition, and exercise that offers insight into the current research on aging. Pelletier is an authority on holistic and psychosomatic medicine and a thoroughly interesting writer.

Pesmen, Curtis. HOW A MAN AGES: GROWING OLDER: WHAT TO EXPECT AND WHAT YOU CAN DO ABOUT IT. New York: Ballantine, 1984.

Have you every wanted to know if you fit the norm? Are you losing your hair earlier than most men, are you having sex as often, is your memory failing? Then this is the book for you. Aside from the statistics and the time lines, there is good information on how to maintain your body at a healthy level.

Porcino, Jane. GROWING OLDER, GETTING BETTER: A HANDBOOK FOR WOMEN IN THE SECOND HALF OF LIFE. Reading, MA: Addison-Wesley, 1983.

A terrific book dealing with older women's lives as they continue to grow and change. Physical, social, and psychological needs and changing life situations are described. Lists of resources in each chapter (women in crisis, fitness after 40, economics of good health . . .).

H.   HEALTHY ADOLESCENTS

Bell, Ruth and others. CHANGING BODIES, CHANGING LIVES. New York: Random House, 1981.

> The best book for teens on all aspects of sexual and emotional life. Both physical and biological information is represented in a logical and caring way, including pregnancy and contraception. Also covered are potentially traumatic issues such as rape and homosexuality.

Gallagher, J. Roswell, Felix P. Heald, and Dale C. Garrell. MEDICAL CARE OF THE ADOLESCENT. 3rd ed. New York: Appleton-Century-Crofts, 1976.

McCoy, Kathleen. COPING WITH TEENAGE DEPRESSION. New York: New American Library, 1982.

> A parent's guide to recognizing teenage depression and how it manifests itself in school problems, pregnancy, eating disorders, or substance abuse. Good advice on coping with your own frustrations over your child's behavior and excellent suggestions for when, where, and how to choose professional help.

Madaras, Lynda with Dane Saavedra. THE WHAT'S HAPPENING TO MY BODY? BOOK FOR BOYS: A GROWING UP GUIDE FOR PARENTS AND SONS. New York: Newmarket, 1984.

> A guide for helping boys (and their parents) make the difficult transition into young manhood. A comfortable discussion of changing body size, growth, voice change, sexual development, and many other things boys want to know when they ask "Am I normal?"

Madaras, Lynda with Area Madaras. WHAT'S HAPPENING TO MY BODY? A GROWING UP GUIDE FOR MOTHERS AND DAUGHTERS. New York: Newmarket, 1983.

> Lynda Madaras writes wonderful, honest, informative books. Female puberty is discussed in a direct manner using language a young girl can understand. Provides a good basis for discussion between mother and daughter.

York, Phyllis, David Wachtel, and Ted Wachtel. TOUGHLOVE. New York: Bantam, 1982.

> Raising teenagers can be a most difficult experience, incurring problems with which many parents are unable to cope. *Toughlove* is a supportive self-help program which attempts to restore sanity and serenity in troubled relationships.

VIII.   THE HOW-TO OF HEALTH CARE

A.   HEALTH RISKS, ASSESSMENTS AND TESTS

Andrews, Lori. NEW CONCEPTIONS. New York: St. Martin's Press, 1984.

> A comprehensive guide to the medical, legal, and ethical aspects of the new, controversial treatments for infertility, sex preselection, surrogate mothering, and the future of reproductive technology.

Moskowitz, Mark A. and Michael E. Osband. THE COMPLETE BOOK OF MEDICAL TESTS. New York: Norton, 1984.

> A detailed layperson's guide to medical tests. Includes current information on medications that may interfere with test results.

Newman, Ruth G., Ph.D., and Nicholas J. Long, et al. 4th ed. CONFLICT IN THE CLASSROOM. Belmont, CA: Wadsworth, 1980.

Pinckney, Cathey and Edward R. Pinckney. DO-IT-YOURSELF MEDICAL TESTING: MORE THAN 160 TESTS YOU CAN DO AT HOME. New York: Facts on File.

> How to save money, protect your privacy, and become a more active participant in your own health care. Not a substitute for a doctor's visit, but a thorough preliminary screening.

Sobel, David, M.D. and Tom Ferguson, M.D. THE PEOPLE'S BOOK OF MEDICAL TESTS. New York: Summitt, 1985.

> The most comprehensive book on medical tests currently available for the layperson. For each of the 200 tests there is a brief overview and sections on preparation, why performed, normal values, interfering factors, costs, and special considerations.

Urquhart, John. RISK WATCH: THE ODDS OF LIFE. New York: Facts on File, 1984.

> How to put risk into perspective whether it be flying on a jumbo jet or eating processed foods. When does risk outweigh benefit and vice versa in surgery, the taking of prescription drugs, or just doing nothing? What are voluntary and involuntary risks? The self-assessment tests allow you to measure your health risk. A scientific, epidemiological approach.

Wurman, Richard Saul. MEDICAL ACCESS. Los Angeles: Access Press, 1985.

A true innovation in health care books. The flashy design and graphics present medical information in a whole new light. The information is solid and covers medical tests, surgical procedures, and patient's rights.

B. HOW TO BE AN INFORMED HEALTH CARE CONSUMER

Berman, Henry and others. THE COMPLETE HEALTH CARE ADVISOR. New York: St. Martin's, 1983.

Covers doctor-patient relationships, how to evaluate whether or not you need surgery, options for childbirth, what's the best insurance plan for you. Helpful information includes resources.

FDA CONSUMER. (Superintendent of Documents, Government Printing Office, Washington, DC 20402) $19.00/year for 10 issues.

Published by the Food and Drug Administration, this is an invaluable magazine for topical public health and safety issues (food additives, inoculations, nutrition, drugs). Reports court actions involving foods, drugs, devices, cosmetics.

Huttman, Barbara. THE PATIENT'S ADVOCATE: A COMPLETE HANDBOOK OF PATIENT'S RIGHTS. New York: Viking Press, 1981.

How to cope with hospitalization. The book is now out of print, but worth seeking out at a public library.

Inlander, Charles and Ed Weiner. TAKE THIS BOOK TO THE HOSPITAL WITH YOU. Emmaus, PA: Rodale Press, 1985.

The subtitle of this book—A CONSUMER GUIDE TO SURVIVING YOUR HOSPITAL STAY—encapsulates the essence of this book. A handy travel guide to the land of hospital.

Katz, Jay. THE SILENT WORLD. New York: MacMillan, 1984.

If you've ever been frustrated by a lack of communication with your physician, you should read this book. Examines the legal, psychological, moral, and medical issues in the doctor-patient relationship. A scholarly, provocative book.

People's Medical Society. HEALTH INSURANCE. Emmaus, PA: People's Medical Society, 1985.

A concise 34-page booklet on how to evaluate and select medical insurance. Includes an insurance comparison worksheet and an excellent glossary.

Planetree Health Resource Center. CHOOSING A GOOD DOCTOR. San Francisco: Planetree, 1983.

A basic booklet on how to interview a doctor, what to do on your first visit, and important questions to ask.

Rosenfeld, Isadore. SECOND OPINION: YOUR MEDICAL ALTERNATIVES. New York: Bantam, 1981.

A carefully written book about how, when, and where to ask for a second opinion before surgery. Discusses operations for heart disease, stroke, and gallbladder problems. Helpful for evaluating options.

INDEX

A

Abandonment by physician, patient rights on, 321

"Abnormal" test results, 324

Abortions, study of women with, 33

Absenteeism, employee, 314

Acetylcholine, 23, 24

Acne, adolescent and, 281

Action as phase in achieving food safety, 162

Activated Patient Program, 78

Active exercise, 244

Activities; *see also* Exercise
  high impact versus low impact, 182
  sports rating chart and, 195–196

Acupressure, adolescent and, 281

Acupuncture, court case on, 317

Acute disease, exchange of chronic disease for, 237

Addiction
  to caffeine, 203–204
  definition of, 203
  to opiates, 214, 215
  to smoking, 301–302

Ader, Robert, psychoneuroimmunology research of, 31–32, 35

Adolescence; *see also* Adolescent(s)
  changes in, over last 40 years, 277
  crisis in 276–282
  early, middle, and late, 268

Adolescent(s)
  activities for, in KidsPlace Project, 69
  alcohol and, 271
  compliance of, with treatment, 271–272
  counseling, advice on, 274
  crisis and, 276–282
  development of, 267–268, 277
  health behavior of, 268–269
  health problems of, approaches to, 269–272
    decision making and support in, 273–274
    future directions in, 274–275

Adolescent(s)—cont'd.
  health problems of, approaches to—cont'd.
    understanding and acknowledgment in, 272–273
  mortality rate of, 267
  motivation of, knowledge regarding, 267–268
  obesity and, 269–270
    approach to, 281–282
  physical illness and, 279–282
  RDAs for, 141, 142
  resiliency of, 277–278
  runaway, 278–279
  sexual activity of, 267–268
  smoking and, 270
  special needs and approaches to, 266–275
  working with individual, 272

Adolescent adults, suspicions about, 274

Advertisements and food chemicals, 162

Advocate groups on food safety, 163–164

Aerobic capacity, maximum, 181–182

Aerobic dancing, 197

Aerobic exercise, 193–194, 197, 244

Aerobics
  "big three," 194, 197
  caution about, 197
  origin of term, 193
  sports and, 194

The Aerobics Way, 194

Age, physiological versus chronological, 243

Age-group-specific health risk appraisal, 353

Ageism, 262

Aggressive behavior, violent images and, 30

Aging; *see also* Aging process; Elderly
  losses associated with, 260
  myths and realities about, 254–258
  personality and, 258

Aging process; *see also* Aging; Elderly
  exercise and, 242–253
    body systems and, 245–249
    chronic disease and, 249–250
    discussion on, 251
    need for further research on, 253
    summary of, 252
    utilization of findings on, 253
  stages in, 243
  versus disease, 249

AIDS
  adolescents and, 277
  heroin and, 216
  project on, 35
  stresses in patients with, 30

Air traffic controllers and stress, 99

Air, Water, and Places, 59

Alarm as phase of stress, 89

Alcohol, 201, 210–212
  abuse versus amphetamine abuse, 208
  adolescents and, 271
  balanced view of, 211–212
  barbiturates and, 212, 213
  dietary guidelines and, 137
  effects of, 210
  health consciousness and, 11
  health risk appraisal and, 351, 352
  marijuana and, 217–218
  morphine, heroin, and, 214

Alcoholic binge, 210

Alcoholics Anonymous, 271

Alcoholism, 210–211

Alcohol-like drugs, 212–213

Alice in Wonderland, 19th century factories and, 71

Altered States of Consciousness, 39

Alternative practitioner, 16, 317

Alternative therapies for cancer, 284, 288–290

Alternatives
  to drug experience, 218–220
  for primary care, 317

Athletic performance, supplements and, 140

Alzheimer's disease, 263
Ambulatory surgery, 311
American Academy of Pediatrics advice
  on supplements, 139
American Cancer Society
  advertisement of, 4
  dietary supplement statement by,
    138
  program of, for new patient, 293
  vitamin A recommendation by, 302
American dinner plate: today and
  tomorrow, 131
American Health, 3, 4
American Institute for Cancer Research
  mineral guide of, 145
  vitamin guide of, 144
American Journal of Cardiology, 94
American Medical Association and
  barbiturates, 213
American Medicine editorial on
  addicts, 215
American Psychiatric Association
  definition of runaway, 278, 279
Amphetamines, 96, 205
  balanced view of, 209
  effects of, 207
  Swedish study on, 207–208
  switch from cocaine to, 207, 209
Anaerobic exercise, 244–245
Analgesia, natural, 213
Anatomy of healing system, 28
Anatomy of an Illness, 291
Andrus Gerontology Center study
  findings, 257
Angina, 95
Angina pectoris and placebos, 17–18
Anticaffeine campaign, 204–205
Antismoking messages, 301
Appetite as guide to eating, 133
Appetite suppressants, 171
Aristotle, city theory of, 60–61
Arthritis
  exercise and, 182
  personality factors in rheumatoid,
    30–31
Ascorbic acid, 144
Assertiveness training, 108
Assignment in insurance, 331
Asthma
  biofeedback and, 47
  marijuana and, 217
  relaxation for, 40
Astronauts and stress, 99
Atherosclerosis
  chronic nature of, 237–238
  decline in, 239–240
  exercise and, 180–181

Atherosclerosis—cont'd.
  in monkeys, 97
Athletes and coronary disease, 184
At-home diagnostic tests, 11
Atkins diet, 171
Attitudes toward health, changing, 4
Atwater, Wilbur O., nutrition statement
  by, 132
Authority and power in adolescent
  counseling, 274
Autonomy of patient, 284–285

B

Baby boomers and morbidity, 240
Baby-sitting services and reduced job
  stress, 109
Bacardi rum advertisement, 11
Back injuries at workplace, 75
Balance in achieving food safety, 161
Balanced performance, 116
Barbital, 212
Barbiturates, 201, 212–213
  alcohol and, 212, 213
  balanced view of, 213
  warnings against, 213
Basal metabolic rate (BMR)
  calories and, 172
  exercise and, 174
Basic Four Food Groups, 136
"Baskin-Robbins society," 13
Behavior(s)
  of adolescents, 268–269
  changes in
    disease risk factors and, 51–52
    information and, 57
    social environment and, 52–53
    three ways to bring about, 55
  overeating, 168
  type A, 56, 99, 100–101, 106, 107,
    118
Behavioral modification
  adolescent health problems and,
    272–275
  changing food habits and, 173–174
  to manage job stress, 108–109
Belief system in health and healing, 27
Benefit in insurance, 331
Benefits of exercise, 189
Bennett and Eckman poll on elderly,
  256
Benson, Herbert
  psychoactive drug studies of,
    218–219
  relaxation studies of, 34, 39, 44
Bereavement
  elderly and, 261–262, 264

Bereavement—cont'd.
  immune system and, 33
Beta carotene and smoking, 302
Beta-endorphin, 213
Beverly Hills Diet, 171
Beyond Biofeedback, 45
Bias, Len, 96–97
Bicycle ergometer tests for fitness, 190
Bicycling as aerobic sport, 194, 197
Biochemical individuality, 160, 285
Biochemically unique profile, 232, 233
Biofeedback, 41–48
  apparatus of, 43, 47–48
  brain waves and, 45
  case example of, 42–44, 46
  frontiers of, 47–48
  healing and, 45–47
  for job stress, 108
  learning and, 42
  limitations of, 46
  self-control and, 44–45
  technology of, 43
Biofeedback machines, 43, 47–48
Biofeedback Society of America, 47
Biologically closed electric circuits,
  26–27
Biomagnetism, 26
Biomechanics, 74
Biopsychosocial AIDS Project, 35
Biotin, 144
Black market and cocaine, 208–209
Black, Stephen, hypnosis studies of, 35
Blood glucose test recommendation,
  327
Blood pressure; *see also* Hypertension
  biofeedback and, 42, 46
  exercise and, 180
  measurement, recommendation for,
    327
  relaxation and, 40
Blue Cross/Blue Shield
  service benefits of, 336–337
  supplemental insurance and, 341
Blue Shield, psychotherapy
  suit against, 317–318
Body
  exercise and systems of, 245–248
  metabolic efficiency of, 128
  nutritional wisdom of, 133
  relationship between mind and, 16
The Body Electric, 26
Boredom
  diet and, 170
  exercise and, 197
Borysenko, Joan, Mind/Body Group
  program of, 34
Brain damage and marijuana, 217

"Breakthroughs" in weight control plans, 170
Breast self-exam recommendation, 328
Breathing as stress management technique, 97
Bribery and adolescent counseling, 274
Bristol Cancer Help Center in England, 298
British physicians and opiates, 215
British Sports Council, 243
Broken Heart study, 33, 261
Bronchitis and marijuana, 217
Brown fat theory on weight gain, 169
Buber, Martin, 101
Bulk producers, 171
Bureau of Business Management study on elderly workers, 257
Burnout, 91, 112–119
    coping styles for, 116–119
    definition of, 113
    feedback and, 114–115
    performance and, 116
    persons at risk for, 114–115
    research on, 113–114
    self-renewal and major life changes for, 115–116
    signs of, 113
    stress resistant personality and, 116–119
    versus optimal zone, 117
    ways to overcome, 118–119
Burnout Inventory catalogues, 113
Bus drivers and hypertension, study of, 55–56

C

Caffeine, 96, 201–205
    addiction to, 203–204
    balanced view of, 205, 209
    campaign against, 204–205
    Coca-Cola and, 206
    cocaine and, 206, 209
    death from, 204
    effects of, 201
    as "evil" drug, 202, 203
    as psychoactive drug, 201
    reclassification of, 203
Calcium, 145
    supplement, 140, 147–149, 181
Caloric intake and longer life, 255
Calories
    in sound weight management program, 173
    weight control and, 172

Cancer
    alternative therapies for, 284, 288–290
    breast
        diet and, 290–291
        informed consent and, 319
        in mice, 32
        study of women coping with, 33–34
    colon, 150
    diagnosis of, 292–294
        Japanese versus Americans in, 293
    dietary guidelines and, 137–138
    fiber and, 150
    initial visit and diagnostic procedures for, 292
    integral therapies for, 283–289
        American medical history and, 288–290
        choice in, 294–295
        conclusion on, 298–299
        decision to terminate, 295–296
        historical and cultural context of, 287–290
        influence of established therapies on, 291–292
        nutritional research and, 290–291
        philosophy of, 298
        pivot points in, 292–296
        possible network for, 296–298
        principles of, 284–287
    lung, 240
        screening for, 324, 325
    nutrition and, 290–291
    occupational, 74, 75
    recurrence of, 295–296
    saccharin and, 159
    type C patient with, 35
Cancer and Common Sense, 287
Cancer therapy; *see* Cancer, integral therapies for
Capra, Fritjof, 61
Carbohydrates
    calories and, 172
    diet plans and, 171
    in sound weight management program, 173
"Carbos," 171, 172
Cardiorespiratory system and exercise, 189
Cardiovascular disease report in 1930s, 184; *see also* Heart disease
Cardiovascular system and exercise, 245–246
Carotene, 144
Cassileth, Barrie, cancer study of, 288, 290

CAT scanners, expense of, 310
Catastrophic insurance, 331, 335
Catecholamines and stress, 34, 96
Catholic Church and miraculous healings, 21–22
Celsus on cancer, 287
Cerebral cortex and alcohol, 210
Chemotherapy, 287, 291, 298
Chest x-rays, subjective interpretation of, 324
Chewing tobacco, 52
"The Child and the City" symposium, 66
Child ecology, 64
"The Child in the World of Tomorrow" symposium, 64–65
Childbirth education programs, 313
Children
    action agenda for, in Seattle, 66–69
    in cities, KidsPlace Project and, 63–69
    decline of, in Seattle, 65
    diets of, study on, 133
    mean heights and weights of, 143
    nutrition adaptation of, 129
    RDAs for, 141, 142
    recommended energy intake of, 143
    in 21st century, 69
    vitamin supplements and, 139
Children's hospitals, parental teaching at, 313
Cholesterol
    in blood, fiber and, 150
    in diet, 130, 171
    dietary guidelines and, 137
    heart disease and, 180–181
    LDL and HDL, 180, 181, 247
    level
        recommendation for test of, 327
        stress and, 97
Choline, 144
Chromium, dietary, 145
Chromosomes and remission theory, 25–26
Chronic alcoholism, 210–211
    phases of, 212
Chronic brain disorders, 262–263
Chronic disease; *see also* Disease(s)
    exchange of, for acute disease, 237
    exercise and, 249–250
    hospital patient and, 312
    incremental model of, 238
    nature of, 237–238
Cigarettes in heart disease study, 187, 188; *see also* Smoking
Cirrhosis of liver and alcohol, 210

City(ies); *see also* Community
  characteristics of healthy, 61–62
  children and youth in, 63–69
  dealing with unhealthy, 61–62
  definition of, 59
  focal point and success of, 61–62
  growth of, 64
  health of, 58–62
  health definition applied to, 62
  heterogeneity of, 60
  as patient, 61
  in 21st century, children and, 69
The City in History, 59
City-world of Lewis Mumford, 62
Civil War
  general, coffee and, 202
  morphine during, 214
Claim in insurance, 331
Climate of acceptability, 52, 55
Clinical pharmacist, role of
  in drug selection and cost
    containment, 227
  in patient care, 226
Clinics and self-care sponsorship, 83
A Closer Look publication on children
    studies, 66
Cobalamin, 144
Coca-Cola, cocaine and caffeine in, 206
Cocaine, 201
  addiction to, 206
  balanced view of, 209
  cardiac death from, 96–97
  "crack" and, 209
  derivation of, 205
  effects of, 205
  smuggling of, 208–209
  switch to amphetamines from, 207,
    208–209
Cod liver oil, 150–151
Coffee, 201, 202; *see also* Caffeine
Cognitive training in stress
    management, 108–109
Co-insurance/co-payment, 331, 333
Cola drinks and caffeine, 201
Color Additive Law, 158
Commitment and cancer patients, 295
Committee on Health Care Monitoring
    in Future, 232
Communicator molecules, 23
Community; *see also* City(ies)
  drug education and, 227–229
  elderly in, 255
    program for, 264
  health empowerment and, 81, 82, 84
  health and social services in, 264
  self-care and, 77–84
  as service area, 83

Community-controlled self-care
    program
  development of, 78–79
  evaluation of, 83–84
  example of, 79–84
Compliance of adolescents, 271–272
Computer report of health risk
    appraisal, 348, 349, 354
  sample page of, 350–351
Confidentiality of patient information,
    321
Constipation and fiber, 149
Consumer(s)
  changing health habits of, 3
  food safety and, 159–160
  in future, 233–235
  increased rights of health, 317
  risk and, 160
  role of, in assuring safe and effective
    drug use, 221–229
  state insurance departments
    protecting, 340, 343
  list of, by state, 343–346
Consumer Reports and natural foods,
    154
Consumer's guide to health risk
    appraisal, 347–356
Converse Rubber Company stress
    study, 110
Conversion clause in insurance, 333
Convoy metaphor of social networks,
    260
Cooper, Kenneth, aerobics and, 193,
    194
Coordination of benefits in insurance,
    333, 339
Coping styles
  with burnout, 116–119
  with stress
    immune response and, 33–34
    on job, 107–111
Copper, dietary, 145
Coronary angioplasty, 102
Coronary arteries, 95
Coronary artery spasm, 95
Coronary Artery Surgery Study, 102
Coronary bypass surgery, 101–102
Coronary heart disease
  as catalyst to transform individual,
    99
  exercise and reduced, 183–191
    benefits versus hazards of, 187
    early studies on, 184–185
    Harvard alumni study on,
      186–188
    longshoremen and, 185–186, 187
    Morris study on, 184–185, 186

Coronary heart disease—cont'd.
  exercise and reduced—cont'd.
    recent support studies on,
      188–190
    summary of considerations on,
      191
  parental history and, 187, 188
  relative risks of, tables on, 187, 188
  stress and, 93–103
    health policy implications of,
      101–103
    lifestyle factors in, 95–98
    new technology investigating, 94
    research studies into, 98, 99–100
Corporate management
  cities and, 61
  food safety and, 158
Cost containment and drug selection,
    227
Cost-sharing in health care, 311
Council of Better Business Bureaus'
    motto, 171
Council for Responsible Nutrition,
    138–139
Court cases
  on acupuncture, 317
  on breast cancer treatment, 319
  on cancer detection, 318
  on emergency care, 320
  on gynecologic exam, 320
  on negligence, 322
  on nerve operation, 320
  on patient-physician relationship,
    321
  on psychotherapy, 317–318
Cousins, Norman, on cancer, 291,
    292–293
"Crack," 205, 209
Crisis
  in adolescence, 276–278
    physical illness as, 279–282
    runaway as, 278–279
  Chinese character for, 91–92, 278
Cross-country skiing as aerobic
    exercise, 194, 195
Curare, meaning of, 285
Cyclophosphamide, 31

D

Dancing, aerobic, 197
Davis, Clara, nutrition study by, 133
Day care, KidsPlace Project and, 66
Death with dignity, 321
Death rate and weight, 167
Decaffeinated coffee and cola, 201–202
Deductible, 333

Delirium tremens and barbiturates, 213
Delta-9-tetrahydrocannabinol, 217
Department of Labor studies on elderly workers, 257
Dependence in addiction, 203, 204
Depersonalization and burnout, 113
Dermatologic disorders, work-related, 73
"Designer gene machines," 234
Diabetes
  in adolescents, 280
  exercise and, 180
  relaxation and, 40
Diacetylmorphine, 214
Diagnosis-related groups, 310
Diet; *see also* Nutrition
  adaptation and, 129–130
  avoid and abstain advice on, 137–138
  balanced, 122–134
    factors in, 123
    guidelines for, 130–132
    intuitive balance in, 132–133
    RDAs and, 124–126
    today and tomorrow, 131
    traditional wisdom of, 136–137
  breast cancer and, 290–291
  epidemiological approach to, 130, 132
  exercise, utilization, and, 247–248
  nutrition, weight control, and, 165–175
  plans
    adequacy of, 171–172
    calories in, 172
    high protein, low carbohydrate, 171
    ineffective, 170–171
    low protein, 171
    sound, 173
  throughout world, 123–124
Diet, Nutrition and Cancer, 290
Dietary goals, 137–138
The Dietary Guidelines for Americans, 130–132
Dietary supplements, 135–151
  balanced diet and, 136–137
  cancer and, 137–138
  changing professional attitudes about, 138–140, 147–151
  athletic performance and, 140
  calcium and, 140, 147–149
  fiber and, 149–150
  fish oils and, 150–151
  iron and, 149
  multiple vitamins and, 139–140

Dietary supplements—cont'd.
  dietary guidelines and, 137–138
  history of, 136
  product promotion of, 138
  summary of, 151
Disease(s)
  bereavement and, 261–262
  chronic and acute, 237
  dietary supplements and, 136, 137–138
  environment and, 53–54
  nature of chronic, 237–238
  occupational; *see* Occupational disease(s)
  prevention of
    friendship and, 54–55
    physical fitness and, 178–182
  screening tests for, 324–329
Disease-specific health risk appraisal, 353
Distress, 88
"Doctor within," 18
Dopamine, 213–214
Dopamine-norepinephrine system, 213–214
Doxiadas, Spyros A. and Constantinos, 64
Drug(s); *see also* Drug use; Prescription drugs
  alternatives to, 218–220
  education programs, community-based, 227–229
  future and, 233–234
  great American love affair with, 222, 229
  mind-affecting, 200–220: *see also* specific drugs
  psychoactive, 201
  questioning physicians about specific, 224–225
  selection, pharmacist's role in, 227
  written information about, 225–226
Drug abuse, amphetamines and, 207–208
Drug Price Competition and Patent Restoration Act, 227
Drug therapy
  benefits of, 222
  future of, 233
Drug use; *see also* Prescription drugs
  cost containment and, 227
  influence of mass media on, 224
  problems associated with, 222–223
Drugs and the Elderly, 229
Drunkenness, barbiturate and alcohol, 212
Dryden, John, 184

Duration in achieving food safety, 161
Durkheim, Emile, social environment study of, 53
Dynamic exercise, 244
Dysphoria, 213

E

"Eat all you want" foods, 170
Eating disorders, 168
Economic costs and food safety, 158
Ecos, 64
Education
  drug, 227–229
  nutrition, 130
  self-care, 78–79
Effective date in insurance, 333
Egypt, coffee in, 202
Egyptian mummies and cancer, 287
Eicosapentaenoic acid, 150
Ekistics, 64
Elbow breadth and frame size, 167
Elderly; *see also* Aging process
  bereavement and, 261–262
  capacities of, 257–258
  chronic brain disorders of, 262–263
  community-based services for, 264
  demographics on, 256
  dietary guidelines for, 137
  drug education programs for, 228–229
  exercise for, 181
    body systems and, 245–249
    chronic disease and, 249–250
    limitations and options in, 250–251
    need for further research on, 253
    programs and prescriptions for, 252–253
    types of, 244–245
    utilization of findings and, 253
  four-question poll about, 256
  friendship of, 260–261
  hospitals and, 312
  immune system of, 36, 40
  insurance and, 341
  loneliness of, 255
  mobility limitations of, 262
  motivation of, 248
  myths and realities about, 254–258
  national support systems for, 264–265
  poor, 262
  retirement and, 262
  "safehouses" for, 264
  sexual activity of, 258, 261
  social isolation of, 255, 259–265

Elderly—cont'd.
    social isolation of—cont'd.
        interventions for, 263–265
    social networks for, 259–265
    support groups for, 263–264
    true and false questions about,
        256–257
    work status of, 257
    versus younger people, 256
Electric current in body, 26–27
Electrolytes, RDAs for, 142
Electromagnetic biology, 26
Electromagnetic factor in healing,
    26–27
Electronic Biology and Cancer, 26
Emergency care, patient rights and,
    319–320
Emotional exhaustion and burnout,
    113
Emotional inoculation, 318
Emotional situations and overeating,
    168–169
Emotional stress and heart 95–98; *see
    also* Stress
Employee(s)
    absenteeism of, 34
    health promotion programs for,
        313–314, 315
    health risk appraisals and, 349, 352
    human service, burnout and, 114
    life insurance for at-risk, 71
    occupational disease and, 70–76
    questions for, 75
Employee assistance programs, 314
Employee health policies, 310–311
Empty calories, 172
The End of Medicine, 3–4
Endocrine/metabolic system and
    exercise, 189
Endorphin-like drugs, 214
Endorphins, 213–214, 216
Energy; *see* Food energy
Engineering controls for safe work-
    place, 73–74
Enkephalins, 213
Environment, growth of food in, 156
Environmental factors; *See also* Social
    environment
    in adolescent motivation, 269
    effect of, on health and disease,
        53–54
    longer life and, 255
    in smoking, 302, 303
Environmental intervention, ethics of,
    55
Environmental Protection Agency
    (EPA), 72

Ergonomics, 74
Erythoxlon coca, 206
Eskimos and heart disease, 150
Ethics
    of environmental intervention, 55
    medical
        patient autonomy and, 284–285
        president's commission on, 318,
            320
Ethiopia, coffee origins in, 202
Euphoria and drugs, 213, 218
European Cooperative Study of heart
    patients, 102
Eustress, 88, 91
Exclusions in insurance, 333, 339
"Executive's disease," 184
Exercise; *see also* Sports
    aerobics and, 193, 194, 244
    aging process and, 242–253
    as alternative to psychoactive drugs,
        219
    cholesterol and, 180–181
    degree of, 181–182
    diabetes and, 180
    for elderly, 244–249; *see also*
        Elderly, exercise for
    health risk appraisal and, 350, 351,
        352
    hypertension and, 180
    longevity and, 250
    as maintenance, 246–247
    mind and, 248
    obesity and, 180
    psychological benefits of, 181,
        193–194
    reduced coronary heart disease and,
        183–191
        benefits versus hazards of, 185,
            188, 189
        history of, 14
        representative studies on,
            185–190
        summary of considerations on,
            191
    relationship of, to disease
        prevention and health
        promotion, 178–182
    smoking and, 180, 302–303
    systems of body and, 245
        assimilative, 247–248
        cardiovascular/respiratory, 245–
            246
        musculoskeletal, 246–247
        neurosensory and cerebral, 248
    types of, 244–245
    weight control and, 174, 193
Exercise revolution, 185

Exhaustion as phase of stress, 89
Expectancy and placebo, 20
Extraordinary treatment, 321
Extreme old age, definition of, 243

F

Factory towns and occupational
    disease, 72
False despair, 17, 18
False negative test results, 324–325,
    326
False positive test results, 324, 326
Families in city, 60
Farmers and heart disease, study of,
    190
Fat
    body
        burning off, foods for, 170–171
        calories and, 172
        obesity and, 169
    in diet, 130, 131
        breast cancer and, 290–291
        dietary guidelines and, 137
        high, 171
Fat cell hypothesis on weight gain, 169
FD&C (Food, Drug, and Cosmetic)
    colors, 161
Federal Trade Commission, natural
    foods terms and, 153, 154
Fee-for-service arrangement, 310
Feedback
    biofeedback and, 44
    burnout and, 114–115
Females
    calcium supplement and, 140,
        147–148, 181
    mean heights and weights for, 143
    RDAs for, 141, 142
    recommended energy intake of, 143
Fertilizers and organic foods, 154, 156
Fiber
    cancer and, 138
    in diet, 124, 131, 149
        dietary guidelines and, 137
        supplement, 149–150
    "Fiber war," 138
Fight-or-flight response, 87–89, 96, 108
Fighter pilots and burnout, 115–116
Fine arts as alternative to psychoactive
    drugs, 218–220
Finland heart disease study, 190
Fish oil supplements, 150–151
Fitness center, hospital-affiliated,
    314–315
Fixx, Jim, 197
Flextime and job stress, 109

Fluctuations in nutrition requirements, 126–129
Folic acid, 144
Folklore on nutrition, 123–124
Food(s); see also Diet; Nutrition
  growth of, and environment, 156
  health, 152–156
  overeating and, 168
  safety; see Food safety
Food chemicals
  advocate-groups investigating, 163–164
  apologists for, arguments of, 162–163
  assimilation of information on, 162–163
  data on, 159
  debate surrounding, 158, 163; 164
  disorders associated with, 159
  guidelines to avoid risks of, 160–161
  individual response to, 160
  safety and, 158–159
  shopping plan for indentifying, 161–162
Food commercials, 133
Food and Drug Administration (FDA)
  barbiturates and, 213
  food safety and, 158
  NutraSweet and, 158, 159
  prescriptions and, 221, 223, 224, 227
  supplement use and, 137, 139, 140
Food energy
  intake
    distribution of, in hypothetical population, 125
    and output, 127–128
    recommended, table of, 143
    protein balance and, 128–129
  regulation
    homeostatic model of, 128
    mechanistic model of, 127
Food habits and behavior modification, 173–174
Food industry and market demands, 139
Food Safety, 157–164
  conceptual framework for, 158–160
  information on, 162–164
  publications on, 164
  rules behind, 158–160
  self-knowledge and, 160–161
  time allocation plan to achieve, 161–162
Food "sensitivities" and weight gain, 170
Football players and coronary disease, 184

Fortune 500 survey on cutting health costs, 311
Frame size and weight, 166–167
Framingham Heart Study, 188–189, 247
Franchise insurance, 334
Free fatty acids, 97
Free look provision in insurance, 340
Freud, 179
Freudenberger, Herbert, burnout of, 113–114
Friendship and disease prevention, 54–55
Friendship factor in smoking, 320
FUD factor and job stress, 107
Future of health care, 230–235

G

Galapagos tortoises, lifespan of, 238
Galileo, 94
Gallup Poll
  on physical fitness, 179
  on vitamin supplements, 139
Gastrointestinal system and exercise, 189
General Adaptation Sndrome, 89
Generic drugs, 227
Genetic defects
  chromosomal analysis and, 25–26
  marijuana and, 217
  thalidomide and, 159
Genetic explanations for obesity, 170
Genotoxin concept, 159
Germ theory, 237
Gerontophobia, 262
Glaucoma test recommendation, 327
God's Own Medicine, opiates as, 214
Goldstein and Kaizer study on coffee, 203-204
Grapefruit extracts for weight loss, 171
Gray Panthers, 265
Great Tranquilizer, opium as, 214
Green, Elmer and Alyce, yoga studies of, 44–45
Grief and immune system, 33
Grievances, ways to redress legal, 321–322
Group Health Cooperative of Puget Sound, 4
Group insurance, 334
Group support for social isolation, 99–100
"Guarantees" for weight loss, 170

H

Habit-specific health risk appraisal, 353–354
Haelen, meaning of, 285
Hall, Howard
  hypnosis studies of, 35–36
  psychology of healing and, 36, 37
HALT smoking acronym, 304
Hangover, 210
Harrison Narcotics Act, 214–215
Harvard alumni study on exercise and coronary disease, 186–188, 250, 251
The Harvard Medical School Health Letter and drug information, 225–226
Hazards of exercise, potential, 189
Headaches and biofeedback, 42, 47
Healing
  belief system and, 27
  biofeedback and, 45–47
  cancer therapy and, 285
  Eastern practices of, 19–20
  electromagnetic factor and, 26–27
  informational systems view of, 24
  inner mechanisms of, 27–28
  neurotransmitter plasticity and, 23–24
  prayer and, 22
  psychology of, 36, 37
  relaxation and, 40
  spiritual, 21–22
  as synergies of mind, body, and spirit, 15–28
Healing factor, 29–37
  AIDS and, 30, 35
  cancer and, 32, 33–34, 35
  hypnosis and imagery and, 35–37
  psychoneuroimmunology and, 29–33
  relaxation and, 34
  stress and, 32–34, 36
Healing system, proposed properties of, 27–28
Health
  of cities, 58–62
  definition, by World Health Organization, 62
  diet and, 136–137
  framework for, 2–8
  future of, self-care and, 14
  importance of social environment for, 50–57
  natural foods and, 154
  revolution in, 2–5, 11
  self-responsibility in, 10–14

Health Belief Model, 268
Health care
  expenditures in 1986, 105
  four legs of, 12, 14
  GNP and, 310
  as information flow, 13–14
  multiple options in, 13
  outcome measures in, of future, 232–233
  physician monopoly and, 317–318
  rising costs of, 310–311
Health Care Financing Administration (HCFA)
  health care cost estimates of, 105
  Medicare and, 342
Health care industry growth, 3
Health care system
  changes in, of future, 233
  expansion of, 309–310
  old and new, 11–12
  physician-centered, 12
Health education, 14; see also Education
  hospitals and, 312–313
Health field, changes in, 2–5
Health food stores, 153
Health foods, 152–156
  definition of, 153, 154,
Health information, 11, 13–14; see also Information
  confidentiality of, 321
Health insurance, 330–346
  for accidents, 335
  application for, 339
  benefit payments in, 336–340
  consumer protection and, 340, 343
  dental, 335
  disability income and, 335
  disease-specific, 336
  filing a complaint about, 343
  franchise, 334
  group, 334
  individual, 334
  long-term care, 336
  Medicare and, 332
  policies for, 334–336
  for psychotherapy, 317–318
  recommendations and advice in selecting, 340
  state departments regulating, 340, 343
    list of, by state, 343–346
  for travel, 336
  vocabulary of, 331, 333
  warnings about, 339–340
Health literacy, 14

Health Maintenance Organizations (HMOs), 3, 4, 319
  definition of, 311, 342
  health risk appraisal and, 353
  Medicare and, 341–342
Health profile group report, example of, 352
Health promotion
  health risk appraisal and, 352
  healthier lives in later life and, 236–241
  hospital and, 308–315
  law and, 317
  lifestyle programs in, 314–315
  movement in, 3
  physical fitness and, 178–182
  view of, 6–8
  at worksite, 313–314, 349, 352
Health revolution, 2–5, 11
Health risk appraisals (HRAs), 347–356
  age-group-specific, 353
  areas addressed in, 348
  computer report of, 348, 349
    sample page of, 350–351
  disese-specific, 353
  group report of, 352
  guidelines of selecting, 354–356
  habit-specific, 353–354
  HMOs and, 353
  at hospitals, 352–353
  information processing and, 348–349
  interactive, 354
  limitations of, 355–356
  questionnaire on, 355–356
Health risks, three steps to assessing, 348–349; see also Health risk appraisals (HRAs)
Healthy people, medical tests for, 323–329
  chart listing, 327–328
Hearing test recommendation, 328
Heart
  coronary disease and, 95
  emotional stress and, 95–98
Heart disease; see also Coronary heart disease
  biofeedback and, 47, 106
  cholesterol and, 180–181
  diet and, 130
  exercise and, 180, 193, 245–246
  fish oil and, 150–151
  Multiple Risk Factor Intervention Trial, study on, 51–52
  relaxation and, 40
  work-related, 73, 106

Hedley, O.F., cardiovascular disease report of, 184
Height
  mean, table of, 143
  Metropolitan Life Insurance tables on, 166
  weight and, 166–167
Hematocrit recommendaiton, 327
Hemiocorporectomy, 287
Heroin, 201, 204, 213
  addicts to, 215–216
  AIDS and, 216
  balanced view of, 216
  derivation of, 214
  smuggling of, 215
Herrick, J.B., on coronary disease, 184
High school survey, adolescent behavior and, 269
Hill-Burton Act, 309
Hippocrates
  benevolence principle of, 284
  on cancer, 287
  on diet and body, 123
  on exercise, 184
Hippocratic school, 59
HMOs; see Health Maintenance Organizations (HMOs)
Holistic Health Boards, 318
Holistic health revoluton, 3
Holland heart disease study, 189–190
Homans, Hilary, on nutrition, 124
Home health care, 309
  increase in, factors behind, 312
  monitoring system of future for, 231
  teaching programs on, 313
  trend toward, 13
Homeostasis, 133
  adaptation and, 129–130
  definition of, 126–127
  nutrition requirements and, 126–129
Homeostatic model of energy regulation, 128
Hope and cancer therapy, 286, 294
Hospital(s), 308–315
  admissions and stays at, 311–312
  changing role of, 309–310
  employee programs of, 313–314, 315
  health promotion programs of, 313–315
  health risk appraisal and, 352–353
  home care and, 312–313
  patient choice of, 319
  patient rights at
    emergency care and, 319–320
    in-patient care and, 320–321

Hospital(s)—cont'd.
  patient rights at—cont'd.
    negligence, malpractice, and, 321–322
Hospital insurance
  coverage by, 334
  Medicare and, 332
  questions concerning, 337–338
"Hospital on wrist" of future, 233
Human Options, 23
Human service workers and burnout, 114
Human Synergistics and job stress, 110
Hunger
  as guide to eating, 133
  overeating and, 168
Hydrolyzed vegetable protein (HVP), 159, 161
Hypertension; *see also* Blood pressure
  bus drivers and, 55–56
  calcium supplement and, 140, 148–149
  drug noncompliance and, 222
  exercise and, 180
  in heart disease study, 187, 188
  job stress and, 106
  meditation and, 39
Hypnosis and immune system, 35–36

I

"Ideal" body weight, 166–167
Identity and coronary heart disease, 99
"I-it relationship," 101
Illness; *see also* Disease(s)
  adolescent, 279–282
  drug-induced, 223
  stress-related, 90–91
Imagery and immune system, 35, 36–37
Immigration, 60
Immune system
  of elderly, studies on, 36, 40
  hypnosis and, 35–36
  imagery and, 35, 36–37
  of mice, 32
  mind and, 30–31, 32
  nervous system and, 32
  of rats, 31
  social relationships and, 54
  stress and, 32, 33–34, 36, 40, 106
  of widowers, 33
Inactivity and age, obesity and, 170
Indemnity benefits, 333, 336
India, marijuana in, 217
Individual(s)
  chemical differences among, 160

Individual(s)—cont'd.
  diet and, 133–134
  health and, 2
Individual insurance, 334
Individual Protection Association, 342
Industrial Revolution, 71
Infant(s)
  mean heights and weights for, 143
  RDAs for, 141, 142
  recommended energy intake of, 143
Information
  behavior change and, 57
  on dietary supplements, 136
  on food safety, 162–164
  in health risk appraisals, 348–349
  as leg of health care, 12, 14
  obtaining, from hospitals, 319, 320
  written, about drugs, 225–226
Information flow, health care as, 13–14
Informed consent, 318–319, 320
Inner contentment and stress management, 100
Inner Mechanisms of the Healing Response Program, 27
Inner self and burnout, 118
In-patient care, patient rights and, 320–321
Insominia and barbiturates, 212
Inspired performance, 116, 117–118
Instincts, stress, and primitive, 87, 88, 96
Institute for the Advancement of Health, 3
Institute for Labor and Mental Health stress groups, 110
Institute of Noetic Sciences healing and remission studies, 27
Insurance; *see* Health insurance
Insurance companies
  coronary surgery payment by, 102
  health risk appraisals and, 353
  job stress and, 105
  state insurance departments and, 343
Intelligence of elderly, 257
Interactive health rish appraisal, 354
International Medical Commission at Lourdes, 21–22
International Year of the Child, 65
Intuitive balance in diet, 132–133
Iodine, dietary, 145
Iron
  dietary, 145
  intake of, during pregnancy, 129–130
  supplement, 149
Iron deficiency anemia, 149

Isolated Elders, 261
Isolation; *see also* Social isolation
  coronary heart disese and, 99–100
  safe workplace and, 74
Isolators, 261
Isometric exercise, 244, 246–247
Isotonic exercise, 244

J

Japan, cancer diagnosis in, 293
Job stress; *see also* Stress
  burnout and: *see* Burnout
  cognitive trainint to manage, 107
  cost of, 104, 105
  future directions in management of, 111
  identifying causes of, 106–107
  illness and, 105–106
  illustrative programs for, 109–111
  physical fitness and, 109
  psychologic techniques to manage, 107–108
  results of, 110–111
  studies on, 105, 106
  training programs to manage, 107
Jogging, 109
  as aerobic sport, 194, 197
Journal of the American Dietetic Association on inadequate diet, 171

K

Kamiya, Joseph, biofeedback studies of, 45
Karolinska Institute stress tests, 32
Kids at Risk day camp, 67–68
KidsBoard program, 66
KidsDay in Seattle, 66
KidsPlace Action Agenda, 66–69
KidsPlace Project of Seattle, 63
  beginnings of, 64
  expansion of, 66
  goals of, 65
  origins of, 65
  program initiatives by, 65–66
  stepping stones to, 64–65
  30-point action agenda of, 66–69
Kiecolt-Glaser, Janice, elderly study by, 36, 40
Kilocalories/week in physical activity index, 187
Knorr, Dietrich, organic food study by, 155
Koran and coffee, 202
Korsakoff's syndrome and alcohol, 210

L

La Leche League, 313
Labels, food safety and, 161
Lactation
  Means heights and weights and
      recommended energy intake
      during, 143
  RDAs during, 141
The Lancet on mind/body skepticism,
    17
Law enforcement
  for amphetamines, 208
  for barbiturates, 213
  for cocaine, 206–207
  for heroin, 215–216
  for marijuana, 218
  for opiates, 214–215
Laws affecting patients, 317
  choice of hospital and, 319
  emergency care and, 319–320
  informed consent and, 318–319, 320
  in-patient care and, 320–321
  medical records and, 321
  and physician
      abandonment, 321
      monopoly, 317–318
  redress of grievances and, 321–322
  statute of limitations and, 322
  treatment refusal and, 320–321
Lay medical populism, 78
Laypeople
  professional services and, 12–13
  self-care by, 78
Leaf-chewing custom, cocaine and,
    205–206
Learning, biofeedback as, 42
"Letdown," amphetamines and, 207
Levy, sandra, breast cancer study by,
    33–34
Life
  biologic limits to, 238–239
  burnout and changes in, 115–116
  commitment to, cancer patients and,
    295
Life expectancy
  health promotion and, 236–241
  morbidity and, 239, 240
  two scenarios for, 236, 241
Life insurance for at-risk workers, 7
Life Skills Training Program for
    adolescent smokers, 270
Lifestyle factors
  in coronary heart disease, 95–98
    major influence of, 101, 102–103
    study of, 98, 99–100
  morbidity and, 239–240

Lifestyle programs, hospital-sponsored,
    314–315
Literature as alternative to
    psychoactive drugs, 219
"Live for Life" stress management
    program, 109, 111
Lives of a Cell, 60
Living will statutes, 321
Loneliness of elderly, 36, 255; *see also*
    Social isolation
Longshoremen and physical activity,
    study of, 185–186, 187, 246, 251
Love and cancer therapy, 286–287
Lung disease, occupational, 73

M

Magnesium, dietary, 145
Major Medical insurance, 331
  description of, 335
  questions concerning, 338–339
Males
  mean heights and weights for, 143
  RDAs for, 141, 142
  recommended energy intake of, 143
Malnutrition and adaptation, 129
Malpractice, 322
Mammography recommendation, 328
"Man as machine" nutrition concept,
    123, 127
Managers and burnout, 114, 117–118
Mandated benefits in insurance, 339
Manganese, dietary, 145
Manipulation and social environment,
    55
Mariani's wine, cocaine and, 206
Marijuana, 201, 217–218
  balanced view of, 218
  effects of, 217
  transcendental meditation and, 219
Marriage and health, 179
Mass media
  elderly and, 262
  influence of, on drug use, 224
Massage for adolescent stress, 281
The Mayo Clinic Health Letter, drug
    information and, 226
"Mayor for a Day" competition for
    children, 65
Meaning as link between mind and
    matter, 21
Mechanistic model of energy
    regulation, 127
Medicaid, 309, 310, 319
Medical model of disease, 237
Medical paternalism and patient
    autonomy, 284

Medical profession, amphetamine
    prescriptions and, 207, 208
Medical records and patient rights,
    321
Medical students and patient
    relationships, 7–8, 14
Medical-surgical insurance, 331
  description of, 335
  questions concerning, 338–339
Medicare, 309, 310, 319
  description of, 341
  payment by, 331, 332
  recipients, additional coverage
      options for, 341, 342,
Medicare Assignment, 341
Medicare Supplemental Insurance, 341
Medicine as a Human Experience, 285
Medi-gap insurance, 341
Meditation
  biofeedback and, 41, 45
  for job stress, 108
  overview of, 38–40
  stress and, 39
  as stress management technique,
    97–98
  versus relaxation, 39
Medjugorje, Yugoslavia, religious
    visions and healing at, 22
Megatrends, 12
Men; *see* Males
Metabolism
  adaptation and, 129–130
  nutrition and, 128–129
  weight loss and, 129
Meta-structure of healing system, 28
Methadone, 213, 216
Metropolitan Life Insurance height-
    weight tables, 166, 167
Mice, immune system of, 32
Middle age, definition of, 243
Middle-class migration, 60
Miller, Neal, biofeedback studies of,
    44, 46
Mind; *see also* Mind/body relationship
  exercise and, 248
  immune system and, 30–31
Mind-affecting drugs, 200–220; *see also*
    specific drugs
Mind/Body Group at Beth Israel
    Hospital, 34
Mind/body plasticity and placebos,
    19–21
Mind/body relationship, 16
  belief system and, 27
  electromagnetic factor and, 26–27
  hypnosis and, 36
  meaning in, 21

Mind/body relationship—cont'd.
  neurotransmitters and, 23–24
  placebos and, 17–19
  skepticism in, 16–17
Mindfulness meditation, 30
Mine Safety and Health Administration, 72
Mineral safety index, 148
Minerals
  guide to individual, 145
  RDAs for, 141
Minor tranquilizers, 212
Miraculous healings, 21–22
Mission and burnout, 118–119
Mohammedans and coffee, 202
Monitoring in future, 234–235
Monkeys, atherosclerosis in, 97
Monsodium glutamate, 159, 161
Mood factor in smoking, 302
Morbidity
  caveats on, 240
  compression of, 239–240, 241
  health promotion and, 237
  opportunity and, 241
  strategy for postponement of onset of, 239
Morphine, 213
  heroin and, 215
  opium and, 214
Morris, J.N., coronary disease study by, 184–185, 186
Mortality rate, 238–239
Mother Teresa, 286
Mothers Against Drunken Driving (MADD), 61, 275
Motivation
  of adolescents, 266–275
  behavior change and, 57
Mount Sinai School of Medicine study of widowers, 33
Multiple option, trend toward, 13
Multiple Risk Factor Intervention Trial, 51–52
Multiple vitamins, 139–140
Muscular relaxation to manage stress, 107–108
Musculoskeletal system
  exercise and, 189
  work-related injuries to, 73
Myocardial infarction, 95
Myths about elderly, 256–257

N

Narcomanias, 202
National Academy of Sciences cancer guidelines, 137–138

National Cancer Institute (NCI), 72
  on diet, 3, 138
  prevention estimate of, 239
  questionable statistics of, 292
  research and, 299
National Center for Cancer Research in Tokyo, 293, 302
National Council on aging study, 256
National Council on Patient Information and Education, 224–225
National Health Interview Study, vitamin supplements and, 139–140
National Institute on Heart, Lung, and Blood Disease, 3
National Institute for Occupational Safety and Health (NIOSH), 72
  list of work-related diseases by, 73
National Institutes of Health meditation report, 39
Natural death acts, 321
Natural food stores, 153
Natural foods
  definition of, 153, 154
  labels and, 154
  versus organic foods, 156
Negative thinking and weight gain, 174
Negligence in treatment, 321–322
Nervous system
  drugs and, 213–214
  immune system and, 32
  stress, and, 95–96
Nervousness and barbiturates, 212
Neurologic system and exercise, 189
Neurons and mind/body relationship, 23–24
Neuropeptides, 24
Neurotoxic disorders, work-related, 73
Neurotransmitter plasticity and self-repair, 23–24
Neurotransmitters, 23
New Aerobics, 194
New England Journal of Medicine, 6
  on genetics and weight, 170
  on mind/body skepticism, 16–17
New Health Revolution, 2–5
New populism, 61
New York Medical Journal and Harrison Act, 215
New York Telephone Company stress study, 109–110
Niacin, 144
Nicorette, 304–305
nicotine
  properties of, 302
  as psychoactive drug, 201

Nicotine gum, 304–305
NIH Consensus Conference calcium recommendation, 140
NIH Consensus Development Panel on the Health Implications of Obesity, 167–168
"No harm," food safety and, 158–159
Nomads of Sahara, diet of, 124
Noncaffeine stimulants, 205–209
Noncompliance, drug, 222–224
Nonsmokers, help for smokers from, 306
Nordenström, Björn, body electricity theory of, 26–27
Norepinephrine, 213
  relaxation and, 40
Normal range of values, test results and, 324
"Normal" test results, 324–325
Nuclear Regulatory Commission, 72
Nursing care, Medicare and, 332
Nursing home utilization, 240
NutraSweet, 158, 159, 161
Nutrient(s)
  allowances of, 125
  dietary supplements and, 136, 138–139, 140
  intakes, distribution of, for hypothetical population, 126
Nutrition; *see also* Diet: Dietary Supplements
  adaptation and, 129–130
  adequate, in diet, 171–172
  calories and, 172
  cancer therapy and, 290–291
  diet, weight control, and, 165–175
  dietary guidelines and, 130–132
  folklore to science of, 123–124
  health risk appraisal and, 350, 351
  homeostasis and, 126–129
  intuitive balance in, 132–133
  metabolism and, 128–129
  RDAs and, 124, 126
  requirements and time factors affecting, 126
  smoking and, 302
  sound weight management program and, 173
  tasks of science of, 156
  theories about, 4, 124, 127–129
Nutrition and Your Health: Dietary Guidelines for Americans, 137

O

Obesity
  of adolescents, 269–270

Obesity—cont'd.
exercise and, 180
in heart disease study, 187, 188
prejudice against, 168
risks associated with, 167–168
theories on, 169–170
Obesity Research Group, 169
Occupational disease(s), 70–76
in ancient times, 71
annual estimate of, 71
engineering controls for, 73–74
protective agencies against, 72
questions to determine, 75
stress and, 72–73
ten leading, 73
worker's compensation and, 75–76
Occupational health services, 314
Occupational health specialist, 71
Occupational physical activity, 185–186
Occupational Safety and Health Organization (OSHA), 72, 314
Old age, definition, 243
"Old old" population, 263
Old system of health care, 12
Older Women's League, 265
Opiates, 201, 214
addiction to, 214, 215
balanced view of, 216
effects of, 215
Opium, 214
Opportunity, crisis as, 91–92, 278, 282
Optimal performance, 116
versus burnout, 117
Oral contraceptives, 222
adolescents and, 272
Organic foods
definition of, 153, 154–155
farming versus conventional
farming, 155–156
versus natural foods, 156
Organic Gardening and Farming, 154
Oslo, Norway, heart disease study, 188
Osteoarthritis and exercise, 182
Osteoporosis
calcium supplement and, 140,
147–149
exercise and, 181
Outpatient testing, 311
Overeating; *see also* Obesity
causes of, 168–169
habits associated with, 173–174
"Overnight approach" to weight loss,
171
Overweight
behavior and, 51, 52
body area of, 168
definition of, 166, 167–168

P

Pacific Arts Center, 68
Pain and relaxation, 40
Pantothenic acid, 144
Pap smear recommendation, 328
Passive exercise, 244
"Passive volition", 43
Patience and adolescent counseling,
274
Patient(s)
autonomy of, 284–285
cancer
alternative therapies and, 288–289
assimilation period for, 294
diagnosis of, 292–294
integral therapy network for,
296–298
life-death choice of, 296
options of, 294–295
termination of therapy and,
295–296
three groups of, 289
city as, 61
clinical pharmacist and care of, 226
drug use by, 221–229
emotional needs of, 7
in hospital
admission and stay of, 311–312
changing role of, 309
home care teaching of, 312
programs for, 313
physician and, 6–8
rights of; *see* Patient's rights
Patient noncompliance with drug
treatment, 223–224
Patient-physician relationship, 6–8
abandonment and, 321
questionnaire on, 7–8
as "soft," 7, 8
Patient's rights, 316–322
on abandonment by physician, 321
on choice
of hospital, 319
of practitioner, 317–318
of procedure, 318–319
to death with dignity, 321
on emergency care, 319–320
informed consent and, 318–319, 320
on in-patient care, 319–320
on medical records, 321
in redressing grievances, 321–322
to refuse treatment, 320–321
Pedekistics, 64
Peninsula Wellness and Fitness Center,
314–315
People as social environment, 53–54

People's Medical Society, 234, 330
Perceived effort in aerobics, 194
Performance
inspired, 116, 117–118
levels and rhythms of, 116
stress and, 91, 92
Performance Zones, 116
Personal attention and cancer therapy,
286
Personal Environment/Biochemical
Matrix, 160–161
Personal enviromental context and
food safety, 160
Personal power and burnout, 118
Personal safety in health risk appraisal,
348, 351
Peru, cocaine use in, 206
Pesticides and organic foods, 155
Pets, stress and people with, 100
Pharmacy in 2010, 231–232
Pharmaceautical R&D of future,
233–234
Pharmaceauticals in future, 230–235
Pharmacist and drug information, 226,
227
Pharmacogenetics, 233
*The Pharmacological Basis of
Therapeutics*, 201
Phenylpropanolamine, 171
Philosophers of medicine, 7
Phosphorus, dietary, 145
Physical activity, 179; *see also* Exercise
aging and, 243, 257–258
occupational, 185–186
recreational, 186–188
sports rating chart and, 195–196
Physical activity index in studies, 187
Physicial exam recommendation,
327
Physical fitness; *see also* Exercise
disease prevention, health
promotion, and, 178–182
increase in, 179
job stress and, 109
Physician(s)
abandonment by, 321
alternative cancer therapy and,
288–290
burnout and, 115
cancer diagnosis by, 292–294
drug selection and, 227
health risk appraisal and, 353
negligence of, 321–322
noncompliance of patient, 223
patient and, 6–8
questioning, about specific drugs,
224–225

Physician(s)—cont'd.
  role of, in stress management and heart disease, 102–103
  surplus of, 8
Physician assistant laws, 318
Physician insurance, Medicare and, 332
Physician monopoly, 317–318
Physicians' Desk Reference (PDR), 225, 234
Placebo-prone personality, 19
Placebo—Theory, Research, and Mechanisms, 17
Placebos
  angina pectoris and, 17–18
  cognitive approach to, 20–21
  distrust of, 17
  as hidden paths between mind and body, 17–18
  mind/body plasticity and, 19–21
  neurotransmitter plasticity and, 24
  responder to, 18–19
  theory of, 20
Plasticity
  mind/body, 19–21
  neurotransmitter, 23–24
Platelet aggregation, 95
Platelets, 95
Playgrounds, Seattle programs for, 68
PNI; *see* Psychoneuroimmunology
Points in aerobics, 194
Pollution, 255
Populations and RDAs, 125–126
Positron emission tomography of heart, 94
Potassium, dietary, 145
Practitioner
  nonphysician, 318
  patient choice of, 317–318
Prayer and healing, 22
Pre-existing condition in insurance, 333, 339
Preferred Provider Organizations (PPO's), 311, 342
Pregnancy
  iron during, 129
  mean heights and weights and recommended energy intake during, 143
  nutrition adaptation during, 129
  RDAs during, 141
  vitamin B_6 and, 140
Prejudice against obesity, 168
Premium in insurance, 333
Prescription drugs; *see also* Drug(s); Drug use
  advertising of, 224

Prescription drugs—cont'd.
  expenditures on, 222
  information on, 225–226
  patient noncompliance and, 222–224
  questions concerning, 224–225
President's Commission for the Study of Ethical Problems in Medicine and Biomedical and Behavioral Research, 318, 320
"Prevention" centers, 3
Primary care, alternative approaches to, 317
Problem behavior proneness, 269
Procedure, patient choice of, 318–319
Professional care, shift from, to self-care, 12–13
Professional support for self-care, 12, 14, 82–83
Prospective epidemiology, 233
Prostress, 88
Protein
  diet plans and, 171–172
  in sound weight management program, 173
Protein-sparing diet, 173
Psyche, 21, 23
Psychoactive drugs, 201; *see also* specific drugs
  alternatives to, 218–220
  balanced view of, 220
Psychoimmunology, 31
Psychological benefits of exercise, 193–194
Psychological disorders, work-related, 73
Psychological techniques in stress management, 107–108
Psychological therapies for cancer, 288, 291
  examples of, 298
  patient commitment and, 295
The Psychology of Mind-Body Healing, 24
Psychoneuroimmunology
  definition of, 16, 29
  derivation of, 30, 31
  early research in, 30–32
  healing factor and, 29–37
  history of, 30–31
  immune system and, 106
  increased attention in, 8
  potential of, 35
  purpose of, 30
  recent focus of, 32–33
Psychosomatic, derivation of, 21

Psychotherapy, court case on, 317–318
Public health epidemiology, 130
Puerto Rican farmers, heart disease study of, 190
Pyridoxine, 144

Q

Quasim, Abdul, on cancer, 287
Questionnaire in health risk appraisal, 348, 354
Quieting response, 108

R

Rabbits, coronary disease study of, 100
Radiotherapy, 287, 291, 298
Ramazzini, Bernardo
  on exercise, 184
  on worker safety, 71
Rats
  biofeedback in, 44
  caffeine and, TV program on, 204–205
RDAs; *see* Recommended Daily Allowances; Recommended Daily Dietary Allowances; Recommended Dietary Allowances
"Reasonable certainty" and food safety, 158
Rebellion and marijuana, 217
Reciprocal maintenance in healthy city, 61
Recommended Daily Allowances
  average intakes and, 125
  iron and, for pregnant woman, 129–130
  useful application of, 124–126
  for Western versus African children, 129
Recommended Daily Dietary Allowances, table of, 141, 142
Recommended Dietary Allowances, 137
  diets lacking in, 171
  in sound weight management program, 173
  supplements and, 139, 140
Record keeping in future, 232–233
Recreational physical activity, 186–188
Reduced personal accomplishment and burnout, 113
Regional Outreach Educational Plan, 229
Rehabilitation of workers, 76

Relaxation
  for adolescent, 281
  for elderly, 36, 40
  heart disease and, 40
  immune system and, 36, 40
  versus meditation, 39
  overview of, 38–40
  problems with, 40
  stress and studies on, 34, 36, 39–40
Relaxation machines, 47–48
Relaxation response, 34, 39
  in stress studies, 109, 110
Remission, 25–26
Renewal clause in insurance, 333
Research
  on adolescent health behavior, 269
  consumer, on food safety, 162
  on integral cancer therapy network, 297
    pharmaceutical, in future, 233–234
Researchability of healing system, 28
Resistance as phase of stress, 89
Resources, self-care, 80–81
Respiratory system and exercise, 245–246
Retail health store, 4
Retirement, mandatory, 262
Reynolds Tobacco Company, 11
Riboflavin, 144
Rice Diet, 171
Rights for patients; *see* Patient's rights
Riley, Vernon, cancer research of, 32
Risk accepting consumers, 160
Risk averse consumers, 160
Risk factors; *see also* Health risk
    appraisals
  behavior changes and, 51–52
  controllable, causes of death and, 349
  of individual, 348–349
  sample report on, 350–351
Rogers, Don, 96–97
Routine in achieving food safety, 161
Rubella antibody titer
    recommendation 328
Runaway adolescents, 278–279

S

Saccharin, 159
"Safehouses" for elderly, 264
St. Vincent Wellness Centers, 313
Salk, Jonas, on mind-body issue, 23
Salt
  in diet, 124, 130
  dietary guidelines and, 137

"Saturday night special," cocaine as, 206
Schedule of benefits in insurance, 333
Schwartz, Jack, yoga feat of, 45
Screening tests, 324–329
  chart of, 327–328
  questions in choosing, 325–326
"Seattle in Transition" project, 65
Seleium, dietary, 145
Self-awareness, biofeedback and, 42
Self care
  biofeedback and, 40
  development of approach to
      community-controlled, 77–84
  education, 78–79
  health risk appraisal and, 351
  history of, 78
  information, 11, 78
  new health care system and, 12
  professional support for, 12, 14, 82–83
  project for, 79–84
  public policy issues in, 14
  shift from professional care to, 12–13, 78
  trend toward, 11, 78
Self-control, possibility of, 44–45
Self-esteem
  in adolescent behavior, 269
  coronary heart disease and, 99
Self-insurance, 343
Self-involvement and stress, 100–101
Self-renewal in burnout, 115–116
Self-repair; *see also* Healing
  neurotransmitter plasticity and, 23–24
  remission and, 25–26
Self-responsibility, 10-14; *see also*
    Self-care
Semi-starvation and diet plans, 172
Selye, Hans, stress theories of, 88, 91
Senate Select Committee on Nutrition, 137
Serax, 213
Service benefits in insurance, 336–337
Setpoint theory of weight gain, 169
Seven Countries Study on heart
    disease, 190
Sexual activity
  adolescents and, 267–268
  elderly and, 258, 261
Shapedown program for adolescent
    obesity, 269–270
Side effects
  alternate view of, 18
  of drugs, 225

Sigmoidoscopy recommendation, 328
Simmons, Richard, diet of, 171
Situations as focus of burnout, 113–114
Skills
  generic human and self-
      management, 117
  as leg of health care, 12, 14
Smokers; *see also* Smoking
  guilt and confusion of, 301
  social support for, 303
The Smoker's Book of Health, 301
Smoking, 300–306
  acceptability of, 55
  addiction to, 301–302
  adolescents and, 270
  chronic disease and, 237–238
  coronary heart disease and, 96
  decline in, 11, 52
  environmental factors in, 303
  exercise and, 180, 302–303
  health risk appraisal and, 350, 351, 352
  heart disease study and, 51, 52, 187, 188
  nutrition and, 302
  programs to stop, 53
  social stigma of, 301
  strategies for cutting down, 303–304
  tools for quitting, 304–305
  vegetables and, 302
  vitamin A and, 302
  weight gain and, 305–306
Snow, John, 59
Social ecology model of city, 60
Social environment
  behavior changes and, 52–53
  case example of importance of, 55–56
  disease prevention and, 54–55
  importance of, for well-being and
      health, 50–57
  people as, 53–54
  studies on, 53–54
  suicide and, 53
Social isolation
  definition of, 260
  of elderly, 255, 259–265
    factors in, 261–263
    intervention strategies for, 263–265
Social Learning Theory, 268–269
Social networks
  definition of, 260
  for elderly, 259–265
    community-based, 264

Social networks—cont'd.
  for elderly—cont'd.
    at individual level, 263–264
    at national level, 264–265
Social reality of dietary guidelines, 130–132
Social relationships
  disease and, 53–54
  stress and, 100
Society of victims, 61
"Soft technologies," future and, 235
Solomon, George, psychomimmunology research of, 30–31
Soma, 21, 23
Sound at workplace, 74
Speed freaks, 208
Spirit
  crisis of, in burnout, 113
  renewal of, 112–119
Spiritual healing, 21–22
Spiritual work of cancer patients, 295
Sports, 192–197; *see also* Exercise
  aerobic, 193–194, 197
  benefits from, 193
  history of, 193
  rating chart for, 195–196
  regularity and, 194
SRx: Senior Medication Program, 228–229
Starvation in Africa, 129
State insurance departments, 343
  list of, by state, 343–346
Static exercise, 244
Statute of limitations and negligence, 322
Steady state of body, 128
Stillman diet, 171
Stimulant(s)
  caffeine as, 203
  noncaffeine, 205–209
Stool blood test recommendation, 328
Strained performance, 116
Stress
  biofeedback and, 42, 47, 108
  body response to, 72
  build-up of, 90
  coronary heart disease and, 93–103
    effective management of, 98–101
    health policy implications of, 101–103
    lifestyle factors associated with, 95–98
  definition and effects of, 86–92
  exercise and, 181
  illness and, 90–91
  immune system and, 32, 40
  job; *see* Job stress

Stress—cont'd.
  management of; *see* Stress management
  meditation and, 39–40, 108
  occupational, 72–73; *see also* Job stress
  organizations and management of, 104–111
  performance and, 91, 92
  positive response to, 91–92
  problems related to, rise of, 87
  psychoneuroimmunology studies of, 32–34, 36, 40
  relaxation and, 39–40
  symptoms of, 87, 88
  warning signs of, 90
Stress and the Art of Biofeedback, 43
Stress-inducing cycles, 99
Stress management
  in burnout, 116–119
  cognitive training in, 108–109
  as corporate priority, 106
  future directions in, 111
  illustrative programs of, 109–1ll
  job stress and, 105–111
  physical fitness and, 109
  psychologic techniques in, 107–108
  results of, 110–111
  techniques, 97–98
    effectiveness of, 98–101
  training programs in, at worksite, 107
Stress resistant personality, 116–118
Stress response, 87
  in modern world, 88–89
StressMap, 116–117
Stressors, 88, 89
Stretching as stress management technique, 97
Structure of healing system, 28
Students Against Drunk Driving (SADD), 61, 275
Substitution technique for safe workplace, 73–74
Sugar
  calories and, 172
  in diet, 124, 130, 131
  dietary guidelines and, 137
Suicide, 53
Sulfite, partial ban on, 159
Supermarkets and food arrangement, 55
Support groups for elderly, 263–264
Support as leg of health care, 12, 14
Support nets for burnout, 118
Surgeon General's Report on Smoking, 11

Surgery for cancer, 287, 291, 297–298
Survival curves
  after elimination of disease, 240
  of 20th century, 239
Swami Rama, yoga feats of, 45
Swedish amphetamine study, 207–208
Swimming as aerobic sport, 194, 197
Synergies of mind, body, and spirit, 15–28

T

Take Care retail health store, 4
Tavistock Institute on Human Relations study of widowers, 33
Technology, hospital and new, 310, 312
Teenagers; *see* Adolescents
Telepathy and biofeedback, 44
Television program on rats and caffeine, 204–205
Temoshok, Linda, psychotherapeutic cancer studies of, 34–35
Tenderloin Senior Outreach Project, 264
Tennis, 194
Tension
  biofeedback and, 46–47
  exercise and, 181
Terrorist attacks and personal risk, 348
Test animals and food safety, 159, 163
Testicular self-exam recommendation, 328
Testimonials and weight loss gimmicks, 171
Tests
  at-home, sales of, 11
  medical, for healthy people, 323–329
    chart listing, 327–328
    false negatives and, 324–325
    false positives and, 324
    guidelines for, 326–329
    questions concerning, 325–326
Thalidomide and birth defects, 159
THC, 217
Theta waves and biofeedback, 45
Thiamin, 144
Thought restructuring and weight control, 174
"Thrill pills," 213
Thromboxane A_2, 96, 97
Thymosins and pituitary gland, 32
Tobacco industry, 11, 55
Tolerance in addiction, 203, 204
Tonometry recommendation, 327
Tools as leg of health care, 12, 14

Trace elements, RDAs for, 142
Tranquilizers, 212–213
Transcendental meditation, 39
  as alternative to psychoactive drugs, 218–219
Tranxene, 213
Tremolieres, Jean, on nutrition, 123
Triggers in healing system, 28
Truck drivers and amphetamines, 207
Tuberculin skin test recommendation, 327

U

UCLA School of Medicine survey on physician-patient relationship, 7–8
United States Department of Labor on occupational disease, 71
United States Supreme Court
  NutraSweet and, 158
  psychotherapy insurance and, 318
United States Pharmacopeia-Drug Information system, 226
University of Chicago study on self-care, 11
University of Maryland Elder-ED and Elder Health Programs, 228
Unprofessional physician conduct, 321
Urban clinicians, 69
Urbanization, 64, 65, 69
Uric acid levels and diet, 171
Urinalysis recommendation, 327
Usual, customary, and reasonable (UCR) fees, 337
Utilitarianism and patient autonomy, 284

V

Vaccines, 222
Valium, side effects of, 225
Values
  changing, toward health, 4
  coronary heart disease and, 99
Vendor credibility and health risk appraisal, 355
Ventiliation at workplace, 74
Very old age, definition of, 243

Veteran's Administration Collaborative Study of heart patients, 102
Victims, society of, 61
Vinyl chloride, 74
Virgin Mary, apparition of, 22
Vision test recommendation, 327
Visualization as stress management technique, 98
Vitamin(s)
  A, smoking and, 302
  B$_6$, pregnancy and, 140
  fat-soluble, 140, 141
  guide to individual, 144
  RDAs for, 141, 142
  water-soluble, 140, 141
Vitamin safety index, 147
Vitamin supplements, 139–140
  labels on, how to read, 146

W

Waiting period in insurance, 333
Walking
  aerobic exercise and, 194, 197
  for relief of tension, 181
Washington Consumer Checkbook, 234
Weight
  classifying body, 166–167
  how not to lose, 170–171
  mean, table of, 143
  Metropolitan Life Insurance tables on, 166
  problem, defining, 167–168
Weight control
  calories and, 172
  changing food habits for, 173–174
  diet, nutrition, and 165–175
  exercise and, 193
  sound program for, 173
  summary of, 175
  three guides to, 180
  unsuccessful approaches to, 170–171
Weight gain
  brown fat theory on, 169
  equation for, 169
  smoking and, 305–306
Weight loss; *see also* Weight control
  food intake and, 127–128
  metabolism and, 129

Weight obsessions, 168
Well-being
  importance of social environment for, 50–57
  physical fitness and, 179
Wellness programs, 3
Western Civilization and nutrition, 126, 129, 130, 132
White, Paul Dudley, exercise crusade of, 184
Whole foods, 154
Whole person, cancer therapy for, 284, 288
Widdowson, Elsi, diet study of, 126
Widowers, lifespan study of, 33
Women; *see* Females
Women's magazines and diets, 166
Work & Health, 75
Workers; *see* Employee(s)
Worker's compensation, 75–76, 335
Workplace(s)
  engineering controls for safe, 73–74
  health risk appraisals at, 349, 352
  identifying causes of stress at, 106–107
  major categories of, hazards and, 73
World Health Organization definition of health, 62
World Journal of Surgery on placebos, 18

Y

Yale-Kellogg Self-Care Education Demonstration Project, 79–84
  conclusions from 82–84
  empowerment approach of, 81, 82, 84
  resources of, 80–81
Yoga and relaxation, 34, 44–45
Your Medicine Handbook, 341
Youth in cities, 63–69
Yunis, Jorge, chromosomal analysis by, 25–26

Z

Zero-sum world view, 101
Zinc, dietary, 145